The Psychoses of Menstruation and Childbearing

The Psychoses of Menstruation and Childbearing

Ian Brockington
Professor Emeritus, University of Birmingham, Birmingham, UK

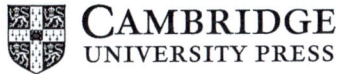
CAMBRIDGE
UNIVERSITY PRESS

CAMBRIDGE
UNIVERSITY PRESS

University Printing House, Cambridge CB2 8BS, United Kingdom

Cambridge University Press is part of the University of Cambridge.

It furthers the University's mission by disseminating knowledge in the pursuit of education, learning and research at the highest international levels of excellence.

www.cambridge.org
Information on this title: www.cambridge.org/9781107113602
DOI: 10.1017/9781316286517

© Ian Brockington 2017

First published 2017

Printed in the United Kingdom by Clays, St Ives plc

A catalogue record for this publication is available from the British Library

Library of Congress Cataloguing-in-Publication data
Names: Brockington, I. F., author.
Title: The psychoses of menstruation and childbearing / Ian Brockington.
Description: Cambridge, United Kingdom ; New York : Cambridge University Press, 2016. | Includes bibliographical references and index.
Identifiers: LCCN 2016016025 | ISBN 9781107113602 (Hardback : alk. paper)
Subjects: | MESH: Puerperal Disorders–psychology | Menstruation–psychology | Mother-Child Relations | Psychotic Disorders–etiology
Classification: LCC RG852 | NLM WQ 500 | DDC 618.7/6–dc23
LC record available at https://lccn.loc.gov/2016016025

ISBN 978-1-107-11360-2 Hardback

. . . .

Dedication

To my wife, Diana, who has given me so much happiness.

Si nos pères n'avaient pas la science que nous possédons aujourd'hui, ils avaient du moins une puissance d'observation et d'intuition supérieure à la nôtre: nous le reconnaissons tous les jours en découvrant dans leurs ouvrages les germes des plus beaux fleurons scientifiques de notre siècle [Icard 1890, reference 87, page XI].

[If our fore-fathers lacked the scientific tools we now have at our disposal, they had superior powers of observation and intuition. We find in their works, time and again, the seeds of our century's finest flowers of scientific achievement].

Contents

Foreword

I first met Ian Brockington in 1985 in Umeå, Sweden. I had to discuss my PhD thesis on schizoaffective and cycloid psychoses, and he was my 'opponent' (i.e., an internationally renowned expert on that topic who was supposed to challenge what I had written in the thesis). I immediately noticed on that occasion a peculiarity that clearly emerges from this book and makes Ian a very uncommon figure in the current international panorama of our discipline: he is at the same time a scholar whose knowledge of a specific area goes well beyond the usual limits for a prominent scientist and academician (extending to literally hundreds of papers that for the language in which they were written or the journals in which they appeared had been virtually inaccessible until he traced them), and an old-fashioned extraordinarily skilled and experienced clinician, one of those, to cite the quotation appearing at the beginning of this book, who have 'superior powers of observation and intuition.'

The area in which Ian has applied these nowadays so rare talents – that of psychoses of pregnancy and puerperium and more in general of perinatal mental health – is itself peculiar for being of exceptional clinical, scientific, public health, service and educational interest, while being remarkably neglected in clinical practice, research, curricula of students in medicine and residents in psychiatry, as well as – with some exceptions – national public health programs. Hence, the usefulness and timeliness of this volume.

As Ian observes, there are no surveys of puerperal psychoses in the general population in any country of the world. Although organic psychoses of pregnancy and puerperium are still not uncommon in some low-income countries, no recent documentation is available of this incidence, mostly because of lack of systematic attention to the issue. Narrative descriptions, which allow the interpretation of clinical records written many years earlier, have become increasingly rare in ordinary practice and in research projects, so that the transfer of knowledge and expertise about conditions that require that level of detailed description has become increasingly difficult. Long-term follow-up studies, which would be essential in this area, are made almost impossible by the fragmentation of services dealing with these conditions and the extremely limited number of interested research groups. Indeed, as Ian points out, the opportunity offered by psychoses that can be precisely located in time, and that are causally linked to events whose physical and psychological impact is relatively well understood, is being widely neglected. Ideally this volume can contribute significantly to getting the ball rolling.

Will clinicians and researchers be discouraged from reading a book of almost 400 pages with several thousand references? I do not think so. The structure of the volume, with its subdivision into several brief sections with clear descriptive titles, should allow the reader either to focus on specific topics of interests or to build up his or her own pathway starting from one of the topics listed in the initial contents and then extending attention to others. Furthermore, this book is obviously very suitable for consultation by the clinician confronted with any psychopathological condition arising in relation to pregnancy, puerperium, or menstruation.

I particularly recommend the final chapters 'What Is Known', 'Obstacles to the Growth of Knowledge', and 'Research Suggestions'. These could ideally be made open access on the Web, so that a vast audience of clinicians, researchers and policy makers can be sensitized to this neglected clinical and research area, with the hope that hundreds of them may be stimulated to read the full book.

Mario Maj, Past President, World Psychiatric Association

Preface

Childbearing, from the standpoint of psychological medicine, is the most complex event in human experience. Of the dozens of disorders that affect the generative process, or are unleashed as complications, many fall under the heading of 'psychoses' – profound disturbances of thought, perception, cognition and behaviour. These are heterogeneous, with a wide range of organic and non-organic forms. Some are relatively common and some are rare, indeed all but extinct in nations with advanced obstetric and medical services. The aim of this monograph, however, is not to describe the disorders now seen in high-income nations, but to explore all the psychoses that have complicated the reproductive process, throughout history and throughout the world. Rare disorders may be less rare in countries with high birth and high maternal mortality rates, and apparent rarity may result from the lack of recent reports. Circumstances may change and extinct disorders return.

These psychoses disrupt personal and family life, often at a critical time. Starting at the dawn of medicine, knowledge has accumulated through the contributions of many disciplines, many nations and in many languages. Armed with this knowledge, and wielding a range of interventions, many women can be restored to health and their vital roles in the family and community. There is much to discover, and there are untapped research opportunities, but we can be confident that, in the fullness of time, when the risk factors are known, multidisciplinary preventive strategies will transform the lives of vulnerable women.

In 1996[1], *Motherhood and Mental Health* reviewed 4,000 works on the whole span of mother–infant psychiatry; it included a chapter on puerperal psychosis (Chapter 4), with a discussion of the role of menstruation. During the last ten years I have taken a closer look at this literature and published a trilogy of monographs, dealing with the organic and non-organic psychoses of childbearing, and menstrual psychosis:

Eileithyia's Mischief: The Organic Psychoses of Pregnancy, Parturition and the Puerperium (2006)[2], 100,000 words with 1,300 references

What Is Worth Knowing about 'Puerperal Psychosis' (2014)[3], 90,000 words, reviewing 2,400 works with 800 selected references

Menstrual Psychosis and the Catamenial Process (2008)[4], 85,000 words with 1,250 references

These are scarce, handcrafted monographs, available in a few libraries[a]. In order to reach psychiatrists, obstetricians and gynaecologists, midwives, general practitioners, neuroscientists and other professionals worldwide, there is a need for an abridgement, at half the length, in a single volume. That is the purpose of the present work.

I thank my friend Professor Mario Maj for writing a Foreword. I admire his wise and inspired leadership of the World Psychiatric Association, and, indeed, of world psychiatry.

---

[a] The British copyright libraries, the Barnes Library at the University of Birmingham, the Markland Library at the Royal College of Obstetricians and Gynaecologists, the Institute of Psychiatry, the Becker Library at Washington University in St Louis, the Vanderbilt Library in Louisville, Kentucky, l'Académie de Medécine in Paris, and the University of Ulm have all three volumes.

Acknowledgements

The North Western Regional Health Authority (under its locally organized projects) funded two studies of puerperal psychosis conducted in Manchester in 1975–1980. The Endowment Fund of the Queen Elizabeth Hospital funded the search for recurrent puerperal psychosis, conducted by Anne Roper. Graham Pye contributed generously to a long-term study. The Welcome Trust gave £5,000 to obtain literature.

I thank the mothers for whom I had the privilege of care when they were suffering from 'puerperal psychosis', especially those who contributed to my catamnestic study. I also thank patients and parents from all over the world, who have corresponded with me about menstrual psychosis.

Abbreviations and Printing Conventions

I have used the following acronyms:

CAT   Computerized axial tomography
CSF   Cerebral spinal fluid
ECT   Electroconvulsive therapy
EEG   Electro-encephalogram
FSH   Follicle stimulating hormone
IQ   Intelligence quotient
LH   Luteinising hormone
MRI   Magnetic resonance imaging
RR   Relative risk

The term 'puerperal psychosis' is generally used by psychiatrists, but 'childbearing psychosis' is more precise because episodes erupt during all phases of the reproductive process and after abortion; I have used these terms interchangeably. The words *délire, folie* and *Tobsucht* are approximately equivalent to 'psychosis'. The word 'menses' here means menstrual bleeding. 'Day 1' is the first day of the puerperium.

Translations and comments are printed in MyriadPro-Regular font between square brackets. For statistical tests, Fisher's exact test has been used throughout.

The Data

The Literature

Over the course of 40 years I have accumulated literature on puerperal and menstrual psychoses. On puerperal psychoses, from a bibliography of more than 2,680 relevant publications, I obtained 2,451 (92 per cent of the literature known to me). On menstrual psychosis I collected 470 works (84 per cent of the literature known to me). These bibliographies are incomplete – there will be other unpublished theses, Russian articles and those in journals not listed in the indices. It was necessary to translate more than 70 per cent of these works. I am no linguist, so there will be errors, but this is better than not reading them at all.

This literature is surprisingly sparse, taking into account:

- Puerperal delirium was mentioned by Hippocrates[5], who lived in the fifth century BC; the first reports of menstrual psychosis appeared in the eighteenth century.
- PubMed lists about 1,000 publications on puerperal psychosis and 150 on menstrual psychosis; this is less than those on disorders only recently identified, for example post-traumatic stress disorder (more than 24,000).
- These psychoses are not trivial – they result in hospitalization, recur, disrupt young families, and sometimes lead to suicide and filicide.
- 'Puerperal psychosis' is not one, but a score of distinct disorders, and menstrual psychosis is also complex.
- The most common form – puerperal bipolar/cycloid disorder – occurs after 1/1,000 births, so that there are more than 100,000 cases per year worldwide.
- In the only polydiagnostic study that has compared its incidence with other psychoses (the Camberwell 1st admission study[6,7]), 5/119 cases were puerperal. This can be compared with 10 cases of schizophrenia (Feighner criteria[8]). Thus the ratio of schizophrenia (as now defined as a chronic disorder) to puerperal psychosis was 2:1; the respective numbers of publications, listed in PubMed at the time of writing, is 112,805 for schizophrenia and 1,012 for puerperal psychosis, a ratio of 111:1.

Puerperal Psychosis

Table 1.1 shows in each 25-year period the number of publications in different language groups:

This table shows that, before 1850, there were a little more than 250 case reports or brief annotations, half of which were in the German language and almost all the rest from France or Britain. Until 1975 the number of publications during each 25-year

Table 1.1 Publications on childbearing psychosis

Group	Before 1850	1851–1875	1876–1900	1901–1925	1926–1950	1951–1975	After 1975	Total
British Commonwealth	58	60	55	33	39	50	272	**567**
German-speaking nations	125	50	71	127	38	35	61	**507**
USA	6	36	87	48	60	85	152	**474**
French-speaking nations	54	53	69	75	63	61	87	**462**
All others	20	6	29	51	39	115	181	**441**
Total	**263**	**205**	**311**	**334**	**239**	**346**	**753**	**2,451**

period remained in the range 200–350. In the twentieth century more than 100 German articles appeared before the First World War; the number then fell sharply and the English language began to predominate. Since 1975 there have been few major contributions in other languages. A high proportion of all publications have been from Germany, the United States, France and the British Commonwealth, and it was not until 1950 that other nations made a substantial contribution. There has been a rise in the last 30 years, but this has been modest, when one takes into account

- The enormous increase in medical journals and publications
- An increase in the nations involved
- The foundation of the Marcé Society and the societies of Women's Mental Health
- The development of mother–infant psychiatry as an area of specialization

By now, 62 nations have contributed at least one case report or survey. Among the more populous nations, Indonesia, Bangladesh and the Philippines have not, to my knowledge, published on this subject.

Menstrual Psychosis

Table 1.2 shows the same data for menstrual psychosis. This distribution is curious:

- Since there were only 76 works published in 1976–2000 (and 24 since then), the peak was reached 100 years earlier.
- The pioneering observations were French, but their contribution came to an end in 1900, except for a cluster of papers on *hyperfolliculinaemia* (a concept with slight relevance) in 1938–1961.
- German-speaking nations followed, with their meticulous dating and have made the greatest contribution, although this suffered as a result of the world wars.
- The first Japanese paper appeared in 1934; since 1950, Japanese authors have contributed many valuable clinical and neuroendocrinological studies.
- Early American papers were about the treatment of mental illness by removal of the ovaries. Recently they have contributed some well-studied cases.

- The contribution of Britain (39 papers) and the Commonwealth (10 papers) has been relatively weak.
- Italy has contributed 21 papers, the Netherlands 7, Norway 5, Russia and Poland 4 each and 12 other nations the remaining 23 papers.

Table 1.2 Publications on menstrual psychosis

Group	Before 1850	1851–1875	1876–1900	1901–1925	1926–1950	1951–1975	After 1975	Total
German-speaking nations	9	11	39	49	17	7	11	**143**
French-speaking nations	18	20	26	13	24	7	1	**109**
USA			12	1	11	12	28	**64**
British Commonwealth	2	1	7	3	3	15	18	**49**
Japan				1		14	26	**41**
All others	2		8	11	15	11	16	**63**
Total	**31**	**32**	**92**	**77**	**71**	**66**	**100**	**469**

Citation Analysis

In order to track the spread of knowledge, I indexed the citations of 2,205 publications on puerperal psychosis and 357 on menstrual psychosis.

Case Lore

I summarized 4,029 cases of puerperal psychosis; this is also a small number, considering that the first 8 cases were published by Hippocrates[5], making up 20 per cent of all cases in the 1st and 3rd books of Epidemics, and nearly half his female cases, covering the whole of medicine. Most have been published in the last 200 years. There is no record of the number of children born in that time, but we can make a guess. Worldwide, Carl Haub[9] has estimated that 15–20 billion have been born since 1800. Some form of puerperal psychosis will have complicated 15–20 million; of this 4,000 cases is a minute proportion. In France, the largest contributor, about 200 million children were born in that time, which will have been complicated by 200,000 cases of puerperal psychoses. Those published in the French literature are about 1/200 of that number.

As for menstrual psychosis, the literature contains descriptions of 246 cases with at least three episodes linked to the menses. If the lifetime rate is 1/10,000 women (see Chapter 30) this is also a small proportion.

There are two sides to this coin:

- Published cases may grossly misrepresent what is happening in the population. This is a major limitation, but the only alternative is personal experience.
- Even a single case may illustrate a disorder that afflicts many women.

Personal Experience

Puerperal Psychosis

In 1970, while working as Senior House Officer to the late Professor RE Kendell, I encountered my first mother with this disorder:

> A 20-year old was admitted soon after childbirth: she 'went wild', broke things, hit her husband, threw powder in the baby's face, pulled off the wallpaper, and absconded with the infant: on admission to the Bethlem Royal Hospital, she was disinhibited, distractible and perplexed.

In 1972, we found five cases in a survey of Camberwell 1st admissions.

From 1975 to 1980, as Senior Lecturer in the University of Manchester, I had responsibility for the Withington Hospital mother & baby unit. Through the kindness of other consultants – Drs Hay, JJ Johnson, DAW Johnson, Atkinson, Hore, McGuire and Professor Goldberg, I was able to study more than 80 mothers with puerperal psychosis.

In 1982, on return from visiting professorships in the United States, this mother was admitted under my care:

> A 21-year-old developed puerperal mania. She made a rapid recovery but relapsed at her 1st menses. She was arrested by the police, trying to stuff an apple into the baby's mouth. It had begun to turn blue, its throat blocked by apple and banana; a policeman saved its life by mouth-to-mouth respiration.

As a result of this single episode, I began to suspect that menstruation might have a role.

In 1983 I was appointed to the Chair of Psychiatry at the University of Birmingham. Soon afterwards, my colleague Dr Peter Hall of Worcester drew my attention to a mother who suffered six menstrual relapses after an episode of puerperal psychosis. I began to collect literature on menstrual psychosis, and published various reviews[10–12] and a monograph. I had no service for menstrual disorders, but have received letters from many sufferers, or the mothers of teenagers, with this disorder.

It was nine years before the Queen Elizabeth Psychiatric Hospital, with its mother & baby unit, was built. During that time I had the valuable experience of working *without* this resource, treating mothers at home, or admitting them, with their babies, to acute psychiatric wards. From 1992 until my retirement in 2001, I worked as honorary consultant to the Queen Elizabeth mother & baby unit, except for three months as visiting consultant at the Princess Margaret mother & baby unit in Christchurch, New Zealand. Thus I spent 14 years working on three mother & baby units. After retirement I extended my experience through medico-legal work, and received letters and emails from many sufferers. In all I have records of 321 mothers with various forms of 'puerperal psychosis', consisting of three major series, plus some others that have reached me from various sources:

The Manchester series (1975–1982). While working on the Withington Hospital mother & baby unit, we conducted a controlled clinical study[13] of 56 mothers (58 episodes), who became ill within two weeks of the birth. After its completion I continued to collect information on mothers admitted to the unit, reaching a total of 86 cases. In September 2013, with the agreement of the National Research Ethics Service in Maple St London, and of the Caldicott Guardian, Dr Lennon, I visited the University Hospital of South Manchester to review the case records (six visits). I obtained data on 81 mothers, more than any series so far published in the literature. The data came from the psychiatric records. The median length of observation was 4 years, but four mothers were followed for more than 30 years.

The Birmingham Mother & Baby Unit series (1983–2001). During these 18 years more than 200 mothers suffering from puerperal psychosis came under my care. The 'Birmingham series' consists of 100 of these mothers not included in the Roper series. As with the Manchester series, the data came from the psychiatric records. The mean length of observation was 5 years.

The Roper series. In the late 1980s, I began a long-term study. With the agreement of ethics committees and the help of the late Anne Cox-Roper, I recruited mothers with recurrent puerperal psychosis. Later I included other mothers, especially *multiparae*, seeking to compare pregnancies affected, and not affected, by psychosis. All patients had the Anne Roper interview (see Appendix). In most, I reviewed the general practice records, and, in a few, psychiatric records as well. The Roper series consists of 84 mothers, the majority of whom were followed for at least 10 years.

Other patients. I encountered 56 other patients from various sources, including those seen in London in 1970–1975, legal reports, student case commentaries and correspondence.

This is by no means an unbiased population-based series, but is by far the largest opportunity series. Table 1.3 compares cases in the literature with my own. In 200 years of research more than half of those, described in detail and followed for more than 20 years, were from my series.

Table 1.3 Comparison of my series with puerperal psychosis with those in the literature

Category		Literature	My series
Organic		1,368	18
Non-organic		2,661	303
Total		4,029	321
Recurrent		453	135
Non-organic episodes		3,039	485
Prolonged observation	10–20 years	137	66
	21–30 years	43	45
	More than 30 years	14	28

Menstrual Psychosis

Although I had no dedicated clinical service, I have obtained details of some 60 sufferers with at least two episodes claimed to be related to the menses. These came from my mother & baby service (18), referrals by doctors and other professionals or student case commentaries (12) and correspondence with sufferers or their relatives (30). This can be compared with v. Kraff-Ebing's experience: his first publication was in 1878[14], and his last in 1902[15] (when he died), thus 24 years; he borrowed 9 from the literature and had 59 of his own, of which 27 were 'possible' (at least 3 dated episodes linked to the menses), 10 'probable' (at least 5) and 2 'confirmed' (at least 7). My interest began in 1982, with my first publication in 1988[16], and has lasted 33 years; of 60 cases, 19 were 'possible', 11 'probable' and 4 'confirmed'.

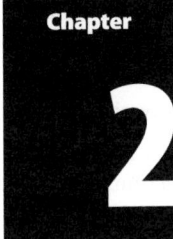

History

This chapter will focus on the main pioneering observations. After summarizing the relevant passages from Hippocrates[5], it will consider the contributions made in the sixteenth and seventeenth centuries, the eighteenth century (including a translation of Osiander's[17] description of puerperal mania), the two halves of the nineteenth century, the first half of the twentieth century and the last 65 years.

Hippocrates

Recognition of a link between psychosis and childbirth began with the dawn of medicine, at which time it had a prominence it has never regained. Hippocrates, who pioneered clinical description, briefly described eight cases of delirium associated with prepartum, postpartum or post-abortion sepsis: these comprised 8/42 cases in the 1st and 3rd books of Epidemics, and 8/17 of the women; all eight were complicated by delirium. These are the case histories:

In Thasos the wife of Philinus gave birth to a daughter. On day 14 she was seized with fever and a rigor. At first she suffered in the stomach and right hypochondrium, and from pains in the genitals, head, neck and loins. Six days later she had much delirium at night. On the 8th day of the illness she had another rigor and many painful convulsions with much delirium. She had no sleep. She had more convulsions on the 9th day and lucid intervals on the 10th day. On the 11th day she had a complete recovery of her memory, quickly followed by renewed delirium. Her urine contained much sediment. About the 14th day there were twitchings over all the body, and much wandering with lucid intervals followed by renewed delirium. On the 17th day she became speechless. On the 20th day she died, 34 days after delivery.

(1st book of Epidemics, case 4).

The wife of Epicrates was near her delivery when she was seized with a severe rigor. The same occurred the following day. On the next day she gave birth to a daughter. On day 2 she was seized with acute fever, stomach pain and pain in the genitals, head, neck and loins. She had no sleep. On the 6th and 7th days after the onset of fever she was delirious. On the 8th and 9th days she had more rigors. On the 10th day she was not delirious, but complained of severe pains in the legs and stomach. On the 14th day she had a rigor, and on the 15th nocturnal fever. On the 16th and 18th days she was delirious. On the 20th day she was in coma. On the 21st day she had pain in the left side, cough, sore throat and an acrid flux. She was still febrile on the 31st day but recovered completely on the 80th day.

(1st book of Epidemics, case 5).

The wife of Dromiades, on the 2nd day after giving birth to a daughter, was seized with a rigor and fever. She had nausea and pain in the hypochondrium, was restless and did not sleep. On the

3rd day after the onset of fever she had another rigor. On the 4th day she was somewhat comatose. On the 5th day she was delirious with lucid intervals. On the 6th day she had another rigor and was delirious. After convulsions she died.

(1st book of Epidemics, case 11).

A woman of the house of Pantimides was seized with fever on the first day after a miscarriage. On the 2nd day she had a rigor and was unable to sleep. On the 3rd day she was in pain. On the 4th day she was delirious, and died on the 7th day.

(3rd book of Epidemics, case 10).

The wife of Hicetas was seized with fever after a miscarriage in the 5th month. She had pain in the loins and alternating coma and insomnia. On day 4 she was anxious, depressed and delirious. She developed strabismus. On days 5 and 6 she was worse with much wandering and rapid recovery of reason. She died on day 7.

(3rd book of Epidemics, case 11).

A woman who lay sick by the Liar's Market, after a first, painful, delivery of a male child, was seized with fever. From the start there was nausea, abdominal pain and disordered bowels. On day 2 she had a rigor. On day 3 she was in pain with thin, copious diarrhoea. On day 4 she had another rigor, and was sleepless. On day 5 she was again in pain, and on day 6 she had more diarrhoea. On day 7 she had further rigors and slight delirium. On day 8 she was in coma part of the time. On days 9 and 10 she had rigors. On day 11 she vomited copiously and had further rigors. On days 12 and 13 she vomited black foetid matter and lost her speech. She died on the 14th day.

(3rd book of Epidemics, case 12).

The woman who lay sick by the cold water in Thasos had for a long time during her pregnancy suffered from fever, lost her appetite and stayed in bed. On day 3 after giving birth to a daughter, she was seized with a rigor and continuous fever with shivering. On day 8 and the following days she had diarrhoea and much delirium, quickly followed by recovery of reason. On day 11 she was comatose. On day 20 she had chills and slight wandering. On day 27 she had pain in the right hip. On day 40 she was coughing and had an irregular fever. On day 60 she had fever, shivering, convulsions of the right side of her jaw, coma and wandering. During all this time she was melancholy, despondent, irritable, sleepless, restless and averse to food. She died on the 80th day.

(3rd book of Epidemics, second series case 2).

In Cyzicus a woman gave birth with difficulty to two daughters. On the first day she suffered headache and a rigor. She was silent, sulky, refractory and sleepless. On the 6th night she was wandering. On day 11 she went out of her mind and then was rational again. On day 14 she had convulsions. On day 16 she was speechless, and she died on the 17th day.

(3rd book of Epidemics, second series case 14).

Puerperal fevers, with mental derangement, seem to have been common. When, therefore, in the 5th book of aphorisms (no. 40), he wrote:

when blood collects at the breasts of a woman, it indicates mania

he may have been referring to delirium complicating mastitis. In their account of diseases afflicting young women, the Hippocratic school also mentioned symptoms that occurred at the first eruption of the menses: in Littré's translation[18], they included *délire*, homicidal impulses, anxiety, terrible utterances and suicidal command hallucinations. Further progress had to wait for nearly 2,000 years.

The Sixteenth and Seventeenth Centuries

This literature is rather inaccessible. Writers had the advantage of a common language (mediaeval Latin). I owe to the scholarship of Imbert–Gourbeyre[19], Luiz de Mercado's discovery, in 1614, of a second childbearing organic psychosis, associated with seizures:

> A woman, who had two or three epileptic fits in the 4th month of pregnancy, suffered from severe headache as she went into labour. After the baby was born, she developed atrocious seizures, which continued for three whole days. She seemed near to death. When the seizures stopped, melancholia and mental alienation set in, which lasted seven days and then switched to mania.

About the same time Ioannis Hess[20] and Pieter van Foreest[21] (Forestus, the 'Dutch Hippocrates') reported mothers with recurrent puerperal insanity – the first long-term observations. Joannes Euthius[22] published a case of recurrent prepartum psychosis, with a hint of heredity.

The Eighteenth Century

This saw a great increase in accessible publication, starting with the *Miscellanea Curiosa sive Ephemeridum Medico-Physicarum Germanicarum Academiae Naturae Curiosorum* (ephemerides), which ran from 1670 until 1717.[a] There was a change from Latin to the vernacular languages, with the problem of language barriers.

On organic psychosis, Boenneken[23] described a second case of eclamptic psychosis. Behrens[24] wrote a scholarly thesis on labour during eclamptic coma, starting with this case:

> A 20-year old complained of headache at the end of her first pregnancy. She began to have involuntary movements of the hands and feet, and became inaccessible to questioning. This 'epilepsy' continued with facial grimacing and groaning, and foam issued from her mouth. Her tongue was severely bitten. The child was extracted, premature but alive. Seizures continued, and some hours later she died.

He cited a number of earlier reports of 'labour during profound sleep', and knew that this especially affected *primiparae*.

Kirkland[25], in his *Treatise on Child-bed Fevers*, described a third organic psychosis – transient delirium during labour; thus three organic psychoses were described before the first clear description of *puerperal mania*.

There were indications of severe disturbances during menstruation: Desmilleville[26] described monthly attacks of demonic possession in a 24-year old woman. A menstrual disorder was accepted as exoneration in this early medicolegal case[27]:

> A woman regularly lost her memory at the time of her periods, and was accused of hurling foul insults at a neighbour, which she denied on oath; it was accepted that her perjury was due to a menstrual disorder.

There were brief descriptions of non-organic psychoses of childbearing. De Berger[28] gave the first hint of post-abortion psychosis and Hoffmann[29] described late onset puerperal psychosis. To combat the theory that puerperal insanity was due to milk deposits in the brain[30–32], v. Battisti[33] and Abrahamson[34] remarked that it occurred in lactating and non-lactating mothers.

---

[a] A complete collection is to be found in the Ljubljana and Kremsmünster monastic libraries.

Up until the end of the eighteenth century, only eight nations had published cases – ancient Greece, the Netherlands, Austria, Spain, Switzerland, Germany, France and England.

Osiander's Description of Puerperal Mania

In his *Neue Denkwürdigkeiten für Ärzte und Geburtshelfer,*[b] he described two cases, the first an infective psychosis and the second probably non-organic[17]. *What Is Worth Knowing about 'Puerperal Psychosis'* contains a full translation of this gem of medical literature, which has been cited only 15 times. Here I will rehearse the psychiatric manifestations of the second case:

A 27-year old English woman, large, fine of skin and body-build, quiet, but emotional and irritable, was pregnant for the first time. On July 28th labour came on. Her husband asked me to supervise her delivery. Towards evening the contractions strengthened and by mid-night the cervix was fully dilated. The mobility of the head, its failure to engage and its slow progress through a good pelvis, made me fairly certain that the cord was wound round the neck. She longed to be delivered. The head was still high, and, when my Levret forceps arrived, I put them to use immediately. With about a dozen careful and moderate pulls, I successfully extracted a living female child. The umbilical cord was indeed wound round the neck and shoulders. The child was pale, but soon recovered and became lively. Just as her sensitivity and irritability had been raised during the strong pains, so was the mother's pleasure at the successful delivery excessive. The outpouring of her joy and gratitude, as earlier her anguish during labour, verged on convulsions. I recommended rest. But she felt so strong that she took advantage of my absence to get back on her feet, make her toilet and spend 15 minutes getting undressed; when she fainted, I was hurriedly called back. As I hastened to her bed, she was already so out-of-herself, and anxious, that it took half an hour to calm her down. Under these unsettling emotions, she began to bleed again, but not dangerously. After resting for another half hour, she was finally moved from the sofa to the bed, and by noon was as well as one could wish or expect. She intended to breast-feed, but neither the condition of her breasts, nor the whole birth process gave any optimism that, with her delicate constitution, this would be possible. But I considered it inadvisable completely to deny her this joy, at least once, and she tried to breast-feed the baby. On the second and third day she remained well. According to English custom she enjoyed her tea. She changed the linen more often than is the custom in Germany, and (secretly, without my agreement), soothed her haemorrhoids with linen soaked in cold water, placed in front of her anus.

On day 4 she became slightly delirious, which was put down to milk fever. On the 5th day this increased, and she talked nonsense all the time. The lochia flowed as normal, and the milk had come down. Because she was so extremely emotional, and her nervous system so disturbed, I prescribed infusion of Valerian root [a sedative], which powerfully restores a normal nervous system; it was beneficial, when taken on August 4th and 5th. But her delirium steadily increased, and she had a small rapid pulse. Scanty lochia flowed, and her milk gradually dwindled. She was nauseated, and her tongue coated, and, since bread and butter and caster oil failed to loosen her bowels, I prescribed an emetic – a half-skrupel [about 1.3 g] of Ipecacuanha and two grains of tartar emetic, which produced a glutinous vomit mixed with slime and bile.

At 11 am on day 7, immediately after vomiting, she broke out into such raving that it required four strong persons to keep her in bed. It was impossible to give her any medicine. We placed mustard poultices on her calves, but could not keep them on the soles of her feet because of her restlessness,

---

[b] I thank my friend Professor Anita Riecher-Rössler, who generously gave me a copy of this masterpiece, and corrected my translation.

which also made it impossible to give her an enema. After the raving and shouting had lasted four hours, and was increasing, I proposed the therapy that had been so effective in a previous case – cutting off her hair and applying icy water to her head. Her husband consented, and this was immediately put into effect. As far as her vigorous movements allowed, her hair was cut to 2½ inches – not without the worry that the loss of her beautiful long tresses might later cause a fresh emotional crisis. On her head we laid napkins soaked in cold water containing Salmiak [liquorice and ammonium chloride]; ice was brought up from the pit, crushed and wrapped into the cloths. Within a quarter of an hour her raving was reduced. Her pulse became fuller and softer, and it was possible to give her some oral medicine. I prescribed an emulsion of poppy seeds with camphor and Moschus [a homeopathic remedy], which achieved more sedation. Her pulse became fuller. The intervals between attacks of raving became longer, but application of ice to her head had the most effect. For five days she had 2–3 raving attacks each day. On one occasion she bled a little from her nose.

During these attacks this lady (a splendid singer) sang with a clear, elegant and melodic voice, and an expression of the highest enthusiasm. She sang or declaimed scenes from the time of her betrothal in self-composed verses with gestures of the finest and deepest emotion. Every movement of her facial muscles, eyes, arms, hands and fingers were the eloquent portrayal of the most ardent love under the finest veil of wistfulness. It was moving: everyone who heard her stirring songs was irresistibly moved to tears. No actress in the world, not even a Garrick, could have improved on her performance – on the fine nuances of muscular movement, on her indescribable originality, and the exaltation of her soul. But her peaceful mood would suddenly change to terror, and her tender nostalgia to fearful anger and the rage of a Medusa. She would hit out with arms of bronze, grasp whatever she could grab with an iron grip, let out heart-rending screams, bark and roar. A human being that had seemed, from her singing, to be a heavenly creature, sank to the level of a beast.

We achieved some control with ice packs, a cooling emulsion given by day, and, at night, a powder containing musk, camphor and opium, repeated, if she had no rest, the following morning; one night she received 8–10 grains of Moschus, 6–9 grains of camphor and 2–3 grains of opium. Three, sometimes four, grains of opium, given at night, were not enough for sleep, but they reduced the number of blows, and the frequency of anger attacks. Stroking and rubbing her arms and feet, which had been beneficial during labour, had a soothing effect. Before each paroxysm her pulse accelerated, and this gave a sure warning of the imminence of an attack. During and after the paroxysm, it became full and reached 130–140/minute. The end of the paroxysm coincided with sweating, especially on the face, breast and back. For the daily evacuation of her bowels, I used castor oil, Wienertränkchen [a laxative] and, as soon as possible, enemas; to prevent spasmodic holding back of excrement and gas in her full soft abdomen, we rubbed her with an ointment containing hyoscine and aniseed.

Her raving was particularly due to reduced pressure of blood to the haemorrhoids, so it seemed absolutely necessary to return the misdirected vital forces to the brain, by attracting blood to the haemorrhoidal region; so I sought to attach leeches to the anus. For several days her restlessness made this impossible. So, to stimulate haemorrhoidal blood flow through irritation, I bound sacks of mustard powder to the perineum, and put her feet in a warm mustard bath. On the 18th, her calmer behaviour allowed leeches to be attached to the anus and perineum. The effect of this powerful diverting treatment was large and salutary. From then on, her head was freer and the attacks milder and less frequent. We now stopped the ice packs, using them only during attacks. It is remarkable that they caused a burning sensation – she called them 'hot, scalding hot' – a feeling that cold water also brought to her half-frozen legs, by setting phlogiston and the stagnating blood in motion again. The patient liked above all the cold compresses on her head, and often, even in the utmost confusion of her mind, applied them to herself.

During her madness she showed an extraordinary acuteness and sensory sensitivity. She was kept in darkness as much as possible. Her sense of smell and hearing were acute, and loud noises, shouting, banging or music, anywhere near the house, had an unfavourable and distressing effect. As an example of her acute sense of smell, a visitor arrived with a small glass of Eau de Luce [a medicinal preparation of alcohol, ammonia and amber] in a leather case inside his pocket; when he was still at some distance from the sickbed, she told him to stay away. "It smells like an apothecary shop", she called out. No-one else had detected the hidden bottle of Eau de Luce. After its removal, the visitor could approach the bed without her complaining.

Attaching the leeches caused an astonishing frequency of micturition. On the 20th, to promote this, I prescribed a mould of Hb. Uvae ursi [extract of the bearberry leaf] and Rd. Altheae et Ononidis [roots of the common marshmallow and the spiny restharrow]; this sustained the urinary flow. The patient's consciousness and understanding had by this time improved. Delirium returned only at night, in the form of weeping, depression and lamentation.

Since, through her extraordinary and insane exertions, her strength was weakened, I sought to build her up, especially in the gut and renal system, and prescribed a saturated solution of boiled Fieberinde [Peruvian bark] and some rhubarb. From the 21st she took this every day, and, at night, a powder of musk, camphor and opium, with double the dose if she was restless, moaning or weeping. Her hysterical weeping and sensory sensitivity continued. So, instead of the musk, camphor and opium, I prescribed a half-Skrupel of Asafoetida and 3 grains of hyoscyamus extract, which she took before sleeping. During the day I gave her a vinous Cinchona preparation and aperient crocus of iron. Neither was successful, so I had to prescribe a watery solution of Fieberinde, and at night camphor, Castorium [a fungus] and opium. Her hysterical outbursts steadily dwindled. Her menstrual periods returned in mid-September. Most effective was the motion of driving, which I encouraged as soon and as often as possible. Bad weather was too often an obstacle. What I had gladly perceived as the completion of the treatment – a bath – was not possible in the circumstances. The continued use of Fieberinde, a nourishing diet, meat and wine, especially an old and tasty Nekkarwein had the desired effect, and her morale and strength came back. At the end of September she returned to her own country for convalescence, *mens sana in corpore sano*. She tolerated the sea trip, and I received good news from London. She had completely recovered from her puerperal illness, and was in good spirits.

This patient was said to have 'milk fever' following a forceps delivery, but the duration of six weeks is compatible with a non-organic psychosis.

The First Half of the Nineteenth Century

This epoch was dominated by the towering genius of Esquirol (1772–1840), who pioneered descriptive psychopathology. Marcé[35] paid this tribute to him:

His remarkable powers of observation, exquisite tact, kind and caring nature, dedication and vast experience, and the numerous students he attracted . . . gave him an authority and influence which he employed to make, in France, important improvements to the care of the insane.

In 1817 he taught the first French course of psychiatry, and this was the basis of his *Maladies Mentales considérées sous les Rapports Médicals, Hygiéniques et Médico-légales*[36]. His publications on the psychiatry of childbearing began with a dictionary annotation[37], followed by two papers[38,39], which described 20 cases and gave statistics on admissions to the Salpêtrière in 1811–1814:

In four years, 92/1,119 (8%) female in-patients became insane after childbirth: 37 had onset between the 1st and 15th day, 17 between the 16th and 60th days, and 19 during the rest of the first postpartum year. The diagnoses were mania in 49, melancholia or monomania in 35, and dementia in eight. The causes included heredity, previous episodes before any pregnancy, and previous postpartum episodes. Some women had attacks only after the birth of males, some every two births, and some 4–5 months after delivery. Emotional causes were the most important (46/92). 29 patients were single and 63 married. 55 were cured, compared with about 385/1,119 admitted to the Salpêtrière (a much higher proportion); but they were liable to relapses. Six died, but only one within six months; this compares with about 320 fatalities/1,119 women admitted.

His cases included two prepartum, one eclamptic, one delirium complicating a breast abscess, some cases of depression and 12 non-organic postpartum psychoses. They included day 1 onset, the first description of a relapse after an early postpartum episode and three unique recurrent cases (summarized in Section 4). His most important contribution was to pioneer long-term studies. His publications on puerperal psychosis have been cited more than 200 times by authors from 14 countries.

In this period, five more countries published cases – the United States, Scotland, Italy, Ireland and the Czech Republic. Friedreich[40] compiled a compendium of psychiatric publications.

Epidemics of puerperal fever were raging in the maternity hospitals[41], and it was gradually realized that this disease was contagious. Gordon[42] in Aberdeen, Wendell Holmes[43,44] and Kneeland[45] in the United States, and Semmelweiss[46] in Vienna knew about contagion and gave advice on its prevention. Burns[47] was perhaps the first to make a clinical distinction between puerperal mania and infective delirium.

Platner[48,49] lent his authority as a forensic pathologist to the eclamptic origin of unconscious delivery, and Gooch[50] first noticed the gap between seizures (lucid interval) and the onset of eclamptic psychosis. Montgomery[51] published six cases of parturient delirium, Barth[52] described postpartum delirium, and Kelso[53] and Tott[54] postpartum stupor. Kluge[55] described parturient rage and Albert[56] its fatal outcome for the newborn. Macdonald[57] published a large American survey, which included a case of puerperal mania with onset during labour. Révolat[58] described a mother with recurrent weaning psychosis.

On menstrual psychosis, Barbier[59] published the first case with substantial evidence. In 1825 a menstrual disorder was used successfully as a defence in law, when a mother was acquitted of infanticide[60]. Strecker and Wunsch[61] reported a postpartum filicide in a woman with a history of a phasic disorder that started at her menarche. Pritchard[62] gave this description of menstrual mood disorder:

> Many women who experience no interruption in the regular periodical return of the catamenia, display a degree of excitement and irritation in the system at the period of menstruation: these are chiefly females of very irritable habits . . . In such instances . . . an unusual vehemence of feeling and expression is observed . . . or there is torpor and dejection of mind with a despondent disposition, and often some melancholy hallucination.

He also described the menstrual relapse of postpartum psychosis. Brière de Boisment[63] surveyed 223 women and found that 43 complained of menstrual sadness, ill-humour or undue gaiety.

The Second Half of the Nineteenth Century

During this period, twelve more nations described cases – Turkey (the first from Asia), Canada, Poland, Russia, Croatia, Algeria (the first from Africa), Denmark, Hungary, Australia, Argentina (the first from South America), Norway and New Zealand.

Louis-Victor Marcé (1828–1864), in the prodigious output of his short and tragic career[64], wrote the first monograph giving a complete account of the insanity of childbearing, as then known[65]:

He covered the pre- and post-partum psychoses, the worries and fears of pregnant women (touching on tocophobia), and parturient insanity, together with its relevance to infanticide (for which he was criticised by Tardieu[66]), and discussed the legal responsibility of pregnant women. He recognized that some postpartum psychoses were organic, and his own cases included three with eclamptic psychoses and others with peritonitis or breast abscess. Excluding organic psychoses and depression, he described 49 cases of psychosis – 20 prepartum and 29 postpartum; they included some of the best cases of weaning psychosis. The summaries were brief, and none were followed long-term; 35 were his own, or borrowed from colleagues and 14 from the literature; this is much less than the 60 cases published by 1855 in the French literature, but it must have been difficult to access literature at that time; nevertheless, he failed to include Esquirol's cases.

He and several other mid-nineteenth-century authors reported that *multiparae*, not *primiparae* (as found in modern studies), were more at risk; a controlled study showed that advanced age was a factor. In his books[35,65] and an independent paper[67], he discussed the causes of pre- and postpartum insanity. He was the first to draw attention to the role of menstruation. Apart from a woman with seven menstrual episodes after weaning (see Section 4), he noticed that some of his postpartum psychoses started 5–6 weeks after delivery, at the first postpartum menses; in separate numerations he gave figures of 11/44 and 12/60. This promising clue is discussed in Section 5. Marcé's powers of observation were demonstrated by a paper on mental disorder in Sydenham's chorea, which includes a description of the hypnogogic and hypnopompic hallucinations that are a mark of this disease (see Section 2). Under the diagnosis of *affaiblissement intellectuelle passager*, he also described a case of Korsakow psychosis. In all, Marcé's publications have been cited 285 times by authors from 17 countries. This total has now been exceeded by two British authors, but his *Traité*[65] has the highest international recognition, with more than 150 non-French citations.

Five new organic psychoses were described – chorea psychosis complicating chorea gravidarum, Wernicke–Korsakow psychosis[68,69], cerebral venous thrombosis, Donkin psychosis and epileptic psychosis. In the field of eclamptic psychosis, Simpson established the link between postpartum psychosis and convulsions[70]; as a result, Donkin[71] described his eclamptic psychosis *sine* seizures, whose differential diagnosis is a matter of current interest. Later, when the clinical measurement of the blood pressure became possible with the Riva Rocci cuff[72], all the components of pre-eclamptic toxaemia were put together.

In this epoch, the causes of infectious disease were elucidated. Traube pioneered the clinical use of the mercury thermometer, and in 1870 the body temperature was first reported in a case of postpartum psychosis[74]. Pasteur[75], working on the fermentation of wine, discovered that infective agents were living organisms. From about 1870, more and more bacteria were identified. Lister[76] used creosote and carbolic acid to prevent surgical sepsis. In the next decade, antisepsis was replaced by strict cleanliness[77] and asepsis – the sterilization of dressings, instruments and gowns. The importance of infective psychosis was recognized, and exaggerated[78]. The introduction of antisepsis and asepsis had a modest effect in reducing the number of infective cases.

Little progress was made in the knowledge of non-organic psychosis. Fürstner[79] described his *hallucinatorische Irresein der Wöchnerinnen*, a syndrome that aroused great interest in German-speaking nations (with 100 citations), but has rarely been observed. There were two monographs – Ripping's[80] *Geistesstörungen der Schwangeren, Wöchnerinnen und Säugenden*, and Knauer's[81] *Über Puerperale Psychosen, für practische Ärzte*, which published a complete series of 70 cases, briefly described. French nosologists introduced the concept of *folie circulaire*[82] and *folie à double forme*[83] – the germ of the idea of manic depressive (bipolar) disorders. Chaslin[84] described the organic confusional state.

This was, however, the heyday of the study of menstrual psychosis. Brière de Boismont[85] described several cases. Two scholarly French monographs were published: Berthier[86] collected 242 cases, classified by symptoms (not timing), and related to dysmenorrhoea, menorrhagia, amenorrhoea and the menopause as well as the menstrual cycle. Icard[87] wrote a thesis, later published under the title *La Femme pendant la Période Menstruelle: Étude de Psychologie Morbide et de Médecine Légale*. In this work, whose humanity shines through its eloquent text, he gave evidence for *une sympathie génital*, that is, a connection between the reproductive organs and the central nervous system; he collected 261 cases. Both Berthier and Icard considered a wide range of psychiatric disorders, including kleptomania, pyromania, dipsomania, homicide, suicide, erotomania, religious insanity as well as *folies, manies* and *lypémanie* [depression]. In the German literature, v. Krafft–Ebing[14] reported 19 cases. An American, Ellen Powers, in her Zürich thesis[88], reviewed the early literature: she transcribed more than 50 cases, adding 9 of her own; she considered menstrual psychosis to be 'a new species in the family of periodic psychoses'. Wollenberg[89] described mid-cycle psychosis, and Schönthal[90] and Friedmann[91] periodic psychoses in adolescents, including episodes before the menarche.

The First 50 Years of the Twentieth Century

Eight nations published their first cases or surveys – El Salvador (the first from Central America), South Africa (a review), Brazil, Japan, Romania, Iraq, Chile and Cuba. There was a deluge of German works, including impressive studies of eclamptic psychosis[92–95], v. Hösslin's[96] monumental work on pregnancy paralysis (relevant to the Wernicke–Korsakow syndrome) and Bonhöffer's[97] description of symptomatische Psychosen.

Two rare causes of organic psychosis were described – hypopituitarism[98] and arterial occlusion[99]. Sheehan[100] fully explored pituitary necrosis as a complication of postpartum haemorrhage, and briefly described its early psychiatric effects. The proportion of organic psychoses, which had been just under 50 per cent throughout the nineteenth century, began to fall as better obstetrics brought pre-eclamptic toxaemia under control, and especially after the discovery of the bacteriostatic sulphonamides[101] and bacteriocidal antibiotics[102].

On menstrual psychosis, v. Krafft–Ebing, in the year of his death, published his *Psychosis Menstrualis*[15], after which interest in this disorder lapsed. One new variant was described – Runge's[103] periodic psychosis during pregnancy.

As for the non-organic psychoses of childbearing, Jolly[104] conducted a pioneering follow-up study. From the Netherlands, Engelhard[105] published a large obstetric survey, and in Norway Widerøe[106] the largest case series. The First World War had a severe effect on the quality and quantity of publication and there was a new factor – Kraepelinian blight: Kraepelin's two entities principle diverted attention to disorders defined by their prognosis. Nevertheless there were some impressive clinical studies: Edelberg and Galant[107] wrote a classic paper on post-abortion psychosis, and the quality of German descriptive studies remained high[108–110], some with full details and long follow-up[111,112] right up to the start of World War II. In spite of this conflict, two Dutch authors wrote exemplary theses with full description, many followed long term[113,114]. In France Delay[115] used serial uterine biopsies to study the menstrual process. Electro-convulsive therapy was introduced[116] and the therapeutic efficacy of chlorpromazine first noticed.

From 1950 until the Present Time

The last 65 years have been 'the age of biological psychiatry' with the introduction of radio-immune assays[117], neuro-imaging, and molecular genetics, as well as epidemi-ological studies using record linkage, and randomized double-blind controlled treatment trials. In-patient mother-&-baby units fostered the development of mother–infant psych-iatry. Additional cases or surveys were published by 27 nations – Israel, Portugal, Morocco, Tunisia, Sweden, Bulgaria, China, Saudi Arabia, Venezuela, Sudan, India, Senegal, Nigeria, Tanzania, the Isle of Réunion, Niger, Serbia, Singapore, Slovenia, Congo, Trinidad, Finland, Pakistan, the United Arab Emirates, Lithuania, Cameroon and Taiwan. This raises the total to 62 nations.

Eight new (but rare) organic causes of psychosis were described – subarachnoid haemor-rhage[118], water intoxication due to oxytocin[119], ethanol withdrawal[120], subdural haem-atoma[121], postpartum cerebral angiopathy[122], hyperammonaemic psychosis[123], HIV infection[124] and pre- and postpartum psychoses associated with N-methyl-D-aspartate recep-tor antibodies, often with ovarian teratomata[125]. After World War II, organic psychoses became uncommon, and began to be forgotten in the nations that conducted most of the research. The incidence should have fallen even lower, but for the shameful recurrence of a spate of Wernicke–Korsakow cases, due to the treatment of hyperemesis by intravenous glucose without vitamin B_1 (which had been available since 1936).

But, in spite of an increase in the number of publications, it is hard to identify any advances in our understanding of the causes of non-organic psychoses; there was consoli-dation of evidence that early onset puerperal psychosis was more common in *primiparae*[126], but there are no other confirmed findings (see Section 4). The most important advance was in nosology, when, in the 1970s, it was realized that the most characteristic symptoms of 'schizophrenia', such as 3rd person auditory hallucinations, disorders of the will and self, and catatonia, also occurred in mania. It then became apparent that puerperal mania, which is often 'schizomanic' in form, was linked to bipolar disorder. A new doctrine came into being – that puerperal psychoses belong to the bipolar spectrum – and led to attempts to prevent the disease by lithium and other 'mood stabilizers'.

Summary

This monograph reviews 2,450 publications on the psychoses of childbearing and 470 on menstrual psychosis. A personal series of 321 childbearing psychoses can be compared with the next largest (a Norwegian series[106]) of 66 cases, and includes 139 followed for at least ten years. A personal series of 60 menstrual psychoses is comparable with that of v. Krafft-Ebing's series[15].

A brief historical overview traces the discovery of more than twenty varieties of childbearing psychoses; it includes Hippocrates' eight cases and Osiander's pioneering description of puerperal mania. In the twentieth century, little was added to our knowledge of the causes of non-organic postpartum psychosis. The main contributions on menstrual psychosis were also made in the nineteenth century.

References

1 Brockington IF. *Motherhood and Mental Health*. Oxford: Oxford University Press; 1996.

2 Brockington IF. *Eileithyia's Mischief: the Organic Psychoses of Pregnancy, Parturition and the Puerperium*. Bredenbury: Eyry Press; 2006.

3 Brockington IF. *What is Worth Knowing about 'Puerperal Psychosis'*. Bredenbury: Eyry Press; 2014.

4 Brockington IF. *Menstrual Psychosis and the Catamenial Process*. Bredenbury: Eyry Press; 2008.

5 Hippocrates. (5th Century BC) *Epidemics*, books I and III, and *Aphorisms*, book 5, Translated by WHS Jones, 1931.

6 Brockington IF, Kendell RE, Leff JP. Definitions of schizophrenia: concordance and prediction of outcome. *Psychological Medicine*. 1978;8:387–398.

7 Brockington IF, Leff JP. Schizoaffective psychosis: definitions and incidence. *Psychological Medicine*. 1979;9:91–99.

8 Feighner JP, Robins E, Guze SB. Diagnostic criteria for use in psychiatric research. *Archives of General Psychiatry*. 1972;26:57–63.

9 Haub C. 1911. Available from: www.prb.org/publications/articles/2002/HowManyPeopleHaveEverLivedonEarth.aspx.

10 Brockington IF. Menstrual psychosis. In: Nomura J, editor, *Neurobiology of Depression and Related Disorders*. Mie: Mie Academic Press; 1998. p. 31–67.

11 Brockington IF. Menstrual psychosis. *Archives of Women's Mental Health*. 1998;1:3–13.

12 Brockington IF. Menstrual psychosis. *World Psychiatry*. 2005;4:9–17.

13 Brockington IF, Cernik KF, Schofield EM, Downing AR, Francis AF, Keelan C.

Puerperal psychosis: phenomena and diagnosis. *Archives of General Psychiatry*. 1981;38:829–833.

14 v. Krafft–Ebing R. Untersuchungen über Irresein zur Zeit der Menstruation. *Archiv für Psychiatrie*. 1878;8:65–107.

15 v. Krafft–Ebing R. *Psychosis Menstrualis: eine klinisch-forensische Studie*. Stuttgart: Enke, 1902.

16 Brockington IF, Kelly A, Hall P, Deakin W. Premenstrual relapse of puerperal psychosis. *Journal of Affective Disorders*. 1988;14:287–292.

17 Osiander FB. *Neue Denkwürdigkeiten für Ärzte und Geburtshelfer*. Volume 1. Göttingen: Rosenbusch; 1797. p. 52–89 and 90–128.

18 Hippocrates. *Des Maladies des Jeunes Filles*. Volume 8. Translated by Littré E. Paris: Baillière; 1852. p. 467–469.

19 Imbert–Gourbeyer. Des paralyses puerpérales. *Mémoirs de l'Académie Impériale de Médecine*. 1861;25: 46–53.

20 Hesso Norico J. (16th century) Quoted by Schenck (reference 73).

21 van Foreest P. *Puerperas nonnunquam phreniticas fierit et sineglectim habeantur, sibi ipsis vim inferre*. 1609; *Observationes, scholio* 7, lib. 10 (summarized by Schenck, reference 73).

22 Euthius JA. *De muliere alias mente sana, gravida demente. Miscellanea Curiosa sive Ephemeridum Medico-Physicarum Germanicarum Academiae Naturae Curiosorum*. *Decuriae* III;II; 1694 observation 4, p. 10–11.

23 Boenneken JFW. *Biga casuum medicorum* etc., Werthemiae,. In: Haller A editor, 1757, *Disputationes ad morborum, historiam et curationem facientes*, Lausanne: Bousquet; 1744.

24 Behrens JBH. *De partu mirabili foetus vivi in somno matris profundo.* Inaugural-Dissertation, Helmstedt; 1751.

25 Kirkland T. *A treatise on childbed fevers and on the methods of preventing them,* London: Baldwin & Dawson; 1774. p. 56–63, 72–73 and 92–95.

26 Desmilleville. Observation addressée à M. Vandermonde. *Journal de Médecine et de Chirurgie.* 1795;10:408–415.

27 Pyl JT. *Aussätze und Beobachtungen aus der gerichtlichen Arztneiwissenschaft.* Berlin: Malins; 1791. p. 232–241.

28 de Berger, J. *Puerperarum mania et melancholia.* Thesis, Göttingen; 1745.

29 Hoffmann, F. *De primipara ex terrore facta maniaca et feliciter restituta.* In his *Medicinae Rationalis Systematicae, Dec III, casus III,* Venice, Colltei, 1721

30 Puzos M. *Traité des Accouchemens, contenant des Observations Importantes etc,* Paris: Deslandes, Desaint and Saillant; 1759. p. 387–394.

31 Levret A. *L'Art des Accouchemens etc,* Paris: Osmont; 1753.

32 Williardts JCF. *Dissertatio de metastasi lactea.* Inaugural-Dissertation, Tübingen; 1770.

33 Bartholomaeo de Battista a St Georgio. Von der Tollsucht den Kindbetterinnen. In: *Abhandlung von den Krankheiten des schönen Geschlechtes.* Vienna: Sonnleithner; 1784. p. 113–114 in the 1819 edition.

34 Abrahamson M. Von dem Wahnsinn bey Kindbetterinnen. *Meckels Neues Archiv der Praktischen Arzneykunst für Ärzte.* 1789;1:47–49.

35 Marcé LV. *Traité Pratique des Maladies Mentales.* Paris: Baillière; 1862. p. 143–147.

36 Esquirol JED. *Des Maladies Mentales considérées sous les Rapports Médicals, Hygiéniques et Médico-Légals.* Paris: Baillière; 1838. Translated into English in 1845.

37 Esquirol JED. Folies. In: Panckoucke CLF, editor, *Dictionaire des Sciences Médicales.* Paris; 1816. p. 192–193.

38 Esquirol JED. Observations sur l'aliénation mentale à la suite de couches. *Journal Général de Médecine, de Chirurgie et de Pharmacie Français et Étrangères.* 1818;62:629–648.

39 Esquirol JED. De l'aliénation mentale des nouvelles accouchées et des nourrices. *Annuaires Médicales-chirurgiques des Hôpitaux de Paris.* 1819;1:600–632.

40 Friedreich JB. *Systematische Literature der ärztlichen und gerichtlichen Psychologie.* Berlin; 1833. Reproduced: Amsterdam: Bonset;1968.

41 Loudon I. *The tragedy of childbed fever.* Oxford: Oxford University Press; 2000.

42 Gordon A. *A treatise on the epidemic puerperal fever of Aberdeen.* London: Robinson; 1795. p. 22–27.

43 Holmes OW. Dr Holmes reported his observations on an outbreak of puerperal fever to the Boston Society for Medical Improvement on February 13th (1843). In: Loudon (2000) ref 41.

44 Holmes OW. *Puerperal fever as a private pestilence.* Boston: Ticknor; 1855.

45 Kneeland S. On the contagiousness of puerperal fever. *American Journal of the Medical Sciences.* 1846;11:45–63.

46 Semmelweiss I P. *Die Aetiologie, der Begriff und die Prophylaxis der Kindbettfiebers.* Pest, Wien & Leipzig, Hartleben, 1861.

47 Burns J. *The principles of midwifery including the diseases of women and children.* London: Longman, Hurst, Rees, Orme & Brown; 1809. p. 275–279 and 319–321.

48 Platner E, Tilesius WT. *Quaestiones medicinae forensis XIV: de lipothymia parturentium, quantum ad excusationem infanticidii.* Inaugural-Dissertation, Leipzig; 1801.

49 Platner J. *De lipothimia parturentium quantum ad excusationem infanticidii. Medizinische Zeitung.* 1817;30:56.

50 Gooch R. *An account of some of the most important diseases peculiar to women.* London: Murray; 1829. p. 108–175.

51 Montgomery WF. On the occasional occurrence of mental incoherence during

natural labour. *Dublin Journal of Medical and Chemical Science.* 1834;5:52–69.

52 Barth. Ein Fall von plötzlich nach der Entbindung entstandener *Mania transitoria. Henke's Zeitschrift für der Staatsarzneikunde.* 1828;16:108–110.

53 Kelso J. Nervous exhaustion dependent on and complicating the puerperal state with cases. *Lancet.* 1840;i:945–948.

54 Tott CA. Fälle von *Melancholia attonita* bei Neuentbundenen. *Neue Zeitschrift für Geburtskunde.* 1844;16:187–190.

55 Kluge. *Mania parturientium transitoria. Medizinische Zeitung.* 1833;2:97–98.

56 Albert of Euerdorf. Wut der Gebärenden und Wöchnerinnen. *Medizinisches Correspondenz-Blatt Bayerische Ärzte.* 1850;11:737–738.

57 Macdonald J. Puerperal insanity. *American Journal of Insanity.* 1847;4:113–163.

58 Révolat, père. Mania puerpérale intermittente. *Annales Médico-psychologiques.* 1847;9:310–311.

59 Barbier MV. *De l'influence de la menstruation sur les maladies mentales.* Thèse, Paris; 1848.

60 Hitzig JE. Mord in einem durch Eintreten des Monatsflusses herbeigeführten unfreien Zustande. *Henke's Zeitschrift für der Staatsarzneikunde.* 1827;12:239–331.

61 Strecker of Dingelstädt, Wunsch of Heiligenstadt. Gutachten über eine *Mania transitoria* einer Wöchnerin. *Henke's Zeitschrift für der Staatsarzneikunde.* 1830;20:115–135.

62 Prichard JC. *A treatise on diseases of the nervous system: part the first, comprising convulsive and maniacal affections.* London: Underwood;1822. p. 203–208.

63 Brière de Boismont A. *De la Menstruation considérée dans les Rapports Physiologiques et Psychologiques.* Paris: Baillière; 1842.

64 Luauté JP, Lempérière T. *La Vie et l'Oeuvre Pionnière de Louis-Victor Marcé.* Paris: Glyph; 2011.

65 Marcé LV. *Traité de la Folie des Femmes Enceintes, des Nouvelles Accouchées et des Nourrices, et*

Considérations Médico- légales qui se rattachent à ce Sujet. Paris: Baillière; 1858.

66 Tardieu A. (1859)In a review of Marcé (1858). Annales Médico-psychologiques.

67 Marcé LV. Études sur les causes de la folie puerpérale. *Annales Médico-psycholologiques.* 3rd series 1857;3: 562–584.

68 Wernicke C. *Lehrbuch der Gehirnkrankheiten für Ärzte und Studirende.* Volume 2. Kassel and Berlin: Fischer; 1881. p. 229–242.

69 Korsakow SS. Über eine besondere Form psychischer Störung, combinirt mit multipler Neuritis. *Archiv für Psychiatrie und Nervenkrankheiten.* 1890;21:669–704.

70 Simpson JY. On the causation of puerperal mania by albuminuria. *Edinburgh Medical Journal.* 1857;2:761 only.

71 Donkin AS. On the pathological relation between albuminuria and puerperal mania. *Edinburgh Medical Journal.* 1863;8: 994–1004.

72 Riva Rocci S. Un sfigmomanometro nuovo. *Gazetta Medica di Torino.* 1896;47:981–996 and 1001–1017.

73 Schenck J. of Grafenberg. *Observationum medicarum, rararum, novarum, admirabilum, et monstrosarum,* published by his son JG Schenck after his death; 1609.

74 Fritz CL. *Quelques considérations sur la pathogénie de l'eclampsie et ses rapports avec la manie puerpérale.* Thèse, Strasbourg; 1870.

75 Pasteur L. *Sur les corpuscules organisés qui existent dans l'atmosphère.* Paris: Hachette; 1861.

76 Lister J. An address on the antiseptic system of treatment in surgery. *British Medical Journal.* 1868;ii:53–56.

77 Lawson Tait R. *An Essay on Hospital Mortality Based on the Statistics of the Hospitals of Great Britain for Fifteen Years* (1877). Republished in Charleston, SC: Bibliolife; 2009.

78 Hansen T. *Om forholdet mellem puerperal Sindssygdom og puerperal Infection.* Thesis, Kopenhaagen; 1888.

79 Fürstner C. Über Schwangerschafts- und Puerperalpsychosen. *Archiv für Psychiatrie und Nervenkrankheiten.* 1875;5:505–543.

80 Ripping LH. *Die Geistersstörungen der Schwangeren, Wöchnerinnen und Säugenden.* Stüttgart, Enke; 1877.

81 Knauer O. *Über Puerperale Psychosen, für practische Ärzte.* Berlin: Karger; 1897.

82 Falret JP. Mémoire sur la folie circulaire, forme de maladie mentale caractérisée par la reproduction successive et régulière de l'état maniaque, de l'état mélancolique, et d'un intervalle lucide plus ou moins prolongé. *Bullétin de l'Académie Impériale de Médecine.* 1853;19:382–400.

83 Baillarger M. De la folie à double forme. *Annales Médico-psychologiques.* 1854;6:367–391.

84 Chaslin P. La confusion mentale primitive. *Annales Médico-psychologiques.* 7th series 1892;16:225–273.

85 Brière de Boismont A. Recherches bibliographiques et cliniques sur la folie puerpérale, précédées d'un aperçu sur les rapports de la menstruation et de l'aliénation mentale. *Annales Médico-psychologiques.* 2nd series 1851;3:574–610.

86 Berthier P. *Les Névroses Menstruelles ou la Menstruation dans ses Rapports avec les Maladies Nerveuses et Mentales.* Paris: Delahaye; 1874.

87 Icard S. *La Femme pendant la Période Menstruelle.* Paris: Alcan; 1890.

88 Powers EF. *Beitrag zur Kenntniss der menstrualen Psychosen.* Inaugural-Dissertation, Zürich; 1883.

89 Wollenberg R. Drei Fälle von periodisch auftretender Geistesstörung. *Charité-Annalen.* 1891;16:427–476.

90 Schönthal, of Heidelberg. Beiträge zur Kenntnis der in frühem Lebensalter auftretenden Psychosen. *Archiv für Psychiatrie und Nervenkrankheiten.* 1892;23:815–833.

91 Friedmann M. Über die primordiale menstruelle Psychose (die menstruale Entwicklungspsychose). *Münchener Medizinische Wochenschrift.* 1894;41:4–7, 27–31, 50–53 and 69–71.

92 Kutzinski A. Über eklamptische Psychosen. *Charité-Annalen.* 1909;33:216–260.

93 Kleinknecht F. *Die posteklamptischen psychosen.* Inaugural-Dissertation, Leipzig; 1914.

94 Sioli F. Eklamptische und post-eklamptische Psychosen. In: Hinselmann H, editor, *Die Eklampsie.* Bonn: Cohen; 1924. p. 597–524.

95 Herrmann E. *Die Eklampsie und ihre Prophylaxie.* Berlin and Vienna: Urban & Schwarzenberg; 1929. p. 150–159.

96 v. Hösslin R. Die Schwangerschaftslähmungen der Mütter. *Archiv für Psychiatrie.* 1904;38:730–861 and 40:446–576.

97 Bonhöffer K. *Die Symptomatische Psychosen.* Leipzig and Vienna: Deuticke; 1910.

98 Verga P. Contributo allo studio dell'infarto della ipofisi. *Pathologica.* 1930;22:4–15.

99 Rangell L. Cerebral air embolism. *Journal of Nervous and Mental Disease.* 1942;96:542–555.

100 Sheehan HL. Post-partum necrosis of the anterior pituitary. *Journal of Pathology & Bacteriology.* 1937;45:189–214.

101 Domagk G. Ein Beitrag zur Chemotherapie der bakteriellen Infektionen. *Deutsche Medizinische Wochenschrift.* 1935;61: 250–253.

102 Fleming A. On the antibacterial action of cultures of a Penicillium with special reference to their use in the isolation of B. Influenzae. *Journal of Experimental Pathology.* 1929;10:226–236.

103 Runge W. Die Generationspsychosen des Weibes. *Archiv für Psychiatrie und Nervenkrankheiten.* 1911;48:545–690.

104 Jolly P. Zur Prognose der Puerperalpsychosen. *Münchener Medizinische Wochenschrift.* 1911; 58:130–133.

105 Engelhard JLB. Über Generationspsychosen und den Einflus des Gestationsperiode auf schon bestehende psychische und neurologische Krankheiten. *Zeitschrift für Geburtshülfe und Gynäkologie.* 1912;70:727–812.

106 Widerøe J. Puerperale Psykoser. *Saertryk av Tidschrift f Nordisk Retsmedesin og Psykiatri*; 1903. p. 1–103.

107 Edelberg H, Galant. Über psychotische Zustände nach künstlichem Abort. *Zeitschrift für die Gesamte Neurologie und Psychiatrie.* 1925;97:106–128.

108 Steinmann I. Die Verursachung der Wochenbettpsychosen. *Archiv für Psychiatrie und Nervenkrankheiten.* 1935;103:552–579.

109 Römer H Jr. Zur nosologischen und erbbiologischen Beurteilung der Puerperalpsychosen. *Zeitschrift für die Gesamte Neurologie und Psychiatrie.* 1936;155:555–591.

110 Schröder P. Über Wochenbettpsychosen und unsere heutige Diagnostik. *Allgemeine Zeitschrift für Psychiatrie.* 1936;104:177–207.

111 Daseking JGW. *Verlauf und Prognose der im Puerperium entstandenen Schizophrenien und schizophrenieartigen Erkrankungen: eine katamnestische Untersuchung.* Inaugural-Dissertation, Berlin; 1931.

112 Beckmann E. Über Zustandsbilder und Verläufe von Puerperal-Psychosen. *Allgemeine Zeitschrift für Psychiatrie.* 1939;113:239–293.

113 Van Steenbergen–van der Noordaa MC. *Generatie-psychosen.* Amsterdam: Academisch Proefschrift; 1941.

114 Visscher GRA. *Generatie-psychoses en hersenstam. Een katamnestisch onderzoek.* Thesis, Groningen; 1949.

115 Delay J, Boitelle G, Corteel A. Les psychoses du postpartum: étude cyto-hormonale. *Semaines des Hôpitaux de Paris.* 1948;24:2891–2901.

116 Cerletti U. L'Elettroschock. *Rivista Sperimentale di Freniatria.* 1940;1:209–310.

117 Berson SA, Yalow RS, Bauman A, Rothschild MA, Newerly K. Insulin-I_{131} metabolism in human subjects: demonstration of insulin-binding globulin in the circulation of insulin-treated subjects. *Journal of Clinical Investigation.* 1956;35:170–189.

118 Luzzatto A. Rilieve su taluni quadri neurologici e psicotici osservati durante il puerperio. *Rivista di Patologia Nervosa.* 1955;76:856–960.

119 Liggins GC. The treatment of missed abortion by high dosage syntocinon intravenous infusion. *Journal of Obstetrics & Gynaecology of the British Commonwealth.* 1962;69:277–281.

120 Nichols MM. Acute alcohol withdrawal syndrome in a new-born. *American Journal of Diseases of Childhood.* 1967;113:714–715.

121 Jack TM. Post-partum intracranial subdural haematoma. *Anaesthesia.* 1979;34:176–180.

122 Rascol A, Guiraud B, Manelfe C, Clanet M. Accidents vasculaires cérébraux de la grossesse et du postpartum. In: *2-ème conference de la Salpêtrière sur les Maladies Vasculaires Cérébrales.* Paris: Baillière; 1979. p. 84–127.

123 Yamada N, Fukui M, Ishii K, et al. [Adult hypercitrullinaemia with consciousness disturbance and marked hypertransaminasemia after delivery]. *Nihon Shokakibuyo Gakkai Zasshi.* 1980;77:1655–1660.

124 Birnbach DJ, Bourlier RA, Choi R, Thys DM. Anaesthetic management of Caesarean section in a patient with recurrent genital herpes and AIDS-related dementia. *British Journal of Anaesthesia.* 1995;75:639–641.

125 Yu AYX, Moore FGA. Paraneoplastic encephalitis presenting as postpartum psychosis. *Psychosomatics.* 2011;52:568–580.

126 Kendell RE, Chalmers JC, Platz C. Epidemiology of puerperal psychoses. *British Journal of Psychiatry.* 1987;150:662–673.

2

The Organic Psychoses of Pregnancy and the Puerperium

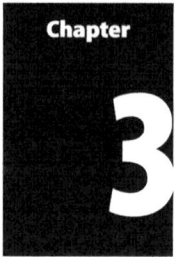

Chapter

Infective Delirium

This is an abridgement and updating of chapter 5 of *Eileithyia's Mischief*[1].

The uterus is liable to infection whenever childbirth occurs in unhygienic conditions, and the lactating breast is also vulnerable. Infective delirium is not only the first to be described, but it is the most common organic psychosis.

The account of the history in Section 1 detailed Hippocrates,[2] cases of delirium complicating infections. Osiander[3] described a 'benign fever in a puerperal woman with rhyming madness, and fatal erysipelas in the newborn child', a finely observed and meticulous account by a scholarly and observant clinician; the diagnosis of infective delirium is based on fever (headache, heat and sweating), contact with a newborn infant who died from erysipelas, and recovery in two weeks with amnesia for the illness. *What Is Worth Knowing*[4] contains a complete translation of this case.

Throughout the eighteenth and nineteenth centuries there was a mounting toll from puerperal fever, aided by the foundation of the great maternity hospitals, the increasing use of instrumental delivery and the practice of attending necropsies. As Loudon[5] has explained, these 'lying-in hospitals' were subject to epidemics; for example, in Dublin's Rotunda Hospital, the mortality reached 7.3 per cent in the 1860s. It is certain that many mothers, desperately ill with streptococcal septicaemia and peritonitis, became delirious, but there have been difficulties from the beginning, right up to the present, in the differential diagnosis. A few perceptive clinicians recognized a distinct form of puerperal psychosis associated with inflammation – Burns[6] and Conolly[7] in Britain, Neumann[8] and Leubuscher[9] in Germany, Berndt[10] in Austria, Kiwisch von Rotterau[11] in the Czech Republic, Guislain[12] in Belgium, Grant[13] in Canada, and Holm[14] in Denmark – but most could not make the distinction, until it was clarified by Chaslin's *confusion mentale*[15] and Bonhöffler's *symptomatische Psychosen*[16]. There was, and is, much uncertainty about the forms and degrees of puerperal sepsis that cause delirium, and the time relationships between fever and cognitive disorder.

Eileithyia's Mischief[1] reported an analysis of 67 British and American cases, all with fatal or severe infections (septicaemia, pyaemia, peritonitis, meningitis, pneumonia or multiple infections) and a clinical picture of delirium. This clarified the timing – in 41 the onset of psychosis was simultaneous with signs of infection, and, in the rest, up to a week later. Only four mothers had signs of psychosis before infection. These data, applied to 600 cases with some evidence of infection, were used to identify 84 probable and 184 possible infective psychoses. When, writing *What Is Worth Knowing*[4], I reviewed more than 4,000 published cases of puerperal psychosis, and obtained a very different result: 559 cases of infective delirium. There are three reasons for this enormous increase:

- In *Eileithyia's Mischief*, the aim was to explore the clinical features of infective delirium, and the conditions under which it developed. For this purpose the focus was on the most convincing cases, setting a high threshold and excluding any that were doubtful. In *What Is Worth Knowing* the focus was on non-organic psychoses, excluding any that might have an organic cause. If, therefore, there was substantial evidence of infection with compatible timing, and nothing else in the course, personal history or family history to suggest a bipolar disorder, the provisional diagnosis was infective delirium.

- One of the inclusion criteria in *Eileithyia's Mischief* was 'a clinical picture compatible with delirium'. But there is much evidence that infective psychoses can present with manic features. In *Motherhood and Mental Health*[17] I wrote:

> It is not only a question of excitement – thrashing around, kicking and screaming. There are also states of exaltation and exhilaration[18]. A few hours before death the patient can show 'the greatest gaiety and vivacity – singing, joking and laughing'[19]. A woman suffering from scarlet fever three days postpartum had a constant desire to talk, contradict and compose rhymes[13]. A woman dying of puerperal sepsis was in a fever of excitement with exalted delusions[20]. Another with foetid lochia and a fever of 103.8° was 'foolishly talkative and erotic, singing, swearing and using obscene language'[21].

In *Eileithyia's Mischief* I gave two examples[22,23]:

> A mother suffering from abdominal pain with a fever of 105° had a protracted laughing fit. She was in the wildest state of excitement. She had little sleep for four nights and was talking, laughing, crying or singing most of the time.

> A mother with pelvic inflammation and pyaemia was extremely excited, absurdly singing, talking and crying by turns, repeating names in a meaningless way, accompanied by incessant bantering talk and interrogation.

Here are two more[24,25]:

> A mother gave birth to her first child, the placenta being removed manually. On day 5 she complained of headache and abdominal pain; her face was flushed and her eyes were wild. She seemed happy, and laughed, saying her pain was over and she would soon be in Heaven. For a day and a night she raved, talking loudly and incessantly about devils, angels and dead friends; her words became gibberish, with continual repetition of the same phrases. She looked cheerful, and was beating time to music playing under the window. She died a few hours later.

> A 27-year old gave birth to her 2nd child. On day 2 she had a rigor, and developed a high fever that lasted for three weeks. She was sleepless for eight nights. On day 9 her mood was high, and she was planning to buy beautiful clothes. On day 12 she ran out of the house, threatened to kill her child (already dead), and bit her husband on the hand. On day 16, admitted to hospital, she claimed she was God, and had special powers of healing – she could make all the patients well; she was a millionaire and would donate 50,000 thalers to the hospital. On day 19 she began to recover.

Recognition that infective delirium could present with excitement, and typical manic symptoms, not just delirium, considerably increased the number of eligible cases.

- In *Eileithyia's Mischief*, I drew attention to the perplexing mismatch between the proportion of infective cases, published within each 25-year period, and the development of infection control. In 1901–1925 infection was thoroughly understood and asepsis widely used. It made no sense that the proportion of infective psychoses should be higher in that generation (8.5 per cent) than in 1851–1875 (6 per cent) when epidemics of puerperal fever were raging. There must have been many more cases lurking in the obscurity of the early 19th century. The duration of illness could be a guide. In the 19th century there were 41 cases with a surprisingly short duration – less than two weeks. In my series (see Section 4), only 18 bipolar episodes, with all the power of modern therapy, recovered in such a short time. Psychoses that cleared up rapidly in the absence of any effective treatment could not be the 'puerperal psychosis' we struggle to control with a panoply of therapies including neuroleptics and ECT. In addition, there were 28 fatal cases, in which the cause of death was unknown. It used to be thought that puerperal mania could result in death by exhaustion, but it seems more likely that these patients died from an organic disease that was not diagnosable at the time. In addition there were 27 symptomatic psychoses, with visual hallucinations, misidentification of persons and/or disorientation, together with memory loss or other cognitive defects, myoclonic jerking or seizures, or evidence of somatic disease, such as haemorrhage, neurological lesions or disordered metabolism. These must have been organic psychoses, mainly infective or eclamptic.

For these reasons I transferred nearly 300 cases from non-organic to infective psychosis. The pendulum may have swung too far, but the numbers in both groups are so large that a misclassification of 100 cases would not alter the conclusions.

Clinical Features

- Of those with known parity, 46 per cent were *primiparae*. This is only slightly less than recent surveys of non-organic psychosis.
- The onset of fever was rarely prepartum (eight cases) or during labour[26,27]. In two-thirds it was during the first postpartum week, and in 90 per cent during the first three weeks. Thus infective psychosis occupies the same time space as non-organic psychosis of early puerperal onset. A few cases develop later in the puerperium.
- Onsets of infection and psychosis are closely related, rarely more than a few days apart – either simultaneous (48 per cent) or with infection first and psychosis second (42 per cent, usually within two weeks).
- Of the patients 28 per cent died. In those who survived, the duration was evenly spread, with approximately equal numbers recovering within a week, during the second week, during the rest of the 1st month, in the 2nd month and in the 3rd month, while, in 90/322 with data, it lasted more than three months. Thus the median duration was two months – shorter than non-affective psychosis (6.8 months before 1940, see Section 4), but longer than eclamptic psychosis (two weeks, see page 32). Very short episodes, therefore, are more likely to be eclamptic or Donkin psychosis. About one-quarter became chronic, either because the infection was chronic, or because the psychosis outlasted it. Chronicity, outlasting the infection, implies structural brain damage, which gradually heals, as in stroke.
- It is rare for infective delirium to recur after subsequent births, but a few women suffered more than one symptomatic psychosis. There is only one instance of a mother who suffered two postpartum infective episodes[28].

As for frequency, there is a difference between obstetric and asylum surveys, because many mothers died or recovered before transfer. In asylum surveys, the peak, in Western Europe and North America, of 18 per cent of admissions, was reached in 1876–1900. It remained high (14 per cent) in 1901–1925, well after the introduction of asepsis. It fell dramatically after the introduction of sulphonamides and antibiotics. The last case in the literature was reported in 1972[29].

Personal Experience

Two mothers in my series may have suffered from infective delirium:

A woman with no family history of mental illness lost her mother at the age of two, and was sexually abused, but became a stable married woman, who held a responsible job, supervising 50 people. After a period of infertility, she conceived at the age of 30. The pregnancy was complicated by placenta praevia, and she was delivered by Caesarean section. She developed a staphylococcal wound infection, and the organism was grown from the blood. In the maternity hospital she became over-active and over-talkative. At home she was on 'an absolute high', had music blasting all night, visited the hospital in her wedding dress, was 'desperate for sex', pestered colleagues and friends with telephone calls, invited many to visit her, and bought 40 pairs of knickers from an itinerant salesman. Food tasted delicious, and everything looked clear and vivid. On day 15 she was admitted to hospital: there were signs of delirium, and curious physical signs: she could not hold up her head, control her head muscles or walk. She had lost 2½ stones in weight. She recovered promptly and was discharged on day 19, after only four days in hospital. Interviewed 13 years later she had remained well and given birth to a second child.

A woman with a family history of 'postnatal depression' had a stable background and a good marriage. At the age of 24, after a 30-hour labour, she was delivered by emergency Caesarean section of her 1st child. She developed a wound infection, with "terrific" pelvic pain. On day 3 she became euphoric. Although she could neither eat nor sleep, she had 'boundless energy'. She had difficulty in speaking, but scribbled notes. She began to believe her baby was dead, and, looking out of the window, heard a voice say, "Go on, jump!" After three weeks she was transferred to a psychiatric hospital, where she seemed confused. It was discovered that she had septicaemia. Critically ill, she was transferred to a medical ward. The infection was brought under control, and, four weeks later, she was returned to the psychiatric hospital, very weak and thin. She took six months to recover completely.

Although both these mothers had a typical manic syndrome, it would be unwise to diagnose bipolar disorder in the presence of such severe infection.

Puerperal sepsis is still prevalent, as shown by a number of recent reports. It accounted for 46/571 maternal deaths in Bangladesh[30] and 7/39 in Northern Nigeria[31]. In Zambia, it was the cause of 35 per cent of postpartum hospitalizations[32]. It has occasionally resulted in maternal death, usually with septic shock, in the United States[33], Germany[34,35], France[36] and Britain[37]. Although the susceptibility of *Streptococcus pyogenes* (the usual infective agent) to antibiotics has greatly reduced the risk of cerebral complications, it is important to remember this cause of organic psychosis.

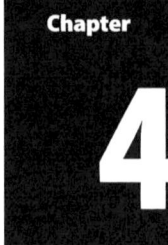

Chapter

4

Eclamptic and Donkin Psychoses

This is an abridgement and updating of chapter 4 of *Eileithyia's Mischief*[1].

Eclampsia and Pre-Eclamptic Toxaemia

The word 'eclampsia' means 'flashing forth' and refers to the sudden eruption of convulsions in a pregnant woman, usually around the time of delivery. These resemble epilepsy, but occur in women who have no history of the 'falling sickness'. In the nineteenth century, it was gradually realized that there was a prodromal state – pre-eclamptic toxaemia (PET) or gestosis. In a recent survey of more than 275,000 women in 24 nations, pre-eclampsia had a prevalence of 4 per cent[38]. The syndrome includes:

- Atrocious headache and transient blindness[39]
- Massive oedema, extending to the hands, labia, jaws, face or eyelids
- Albuminuria
- Hypertension
- (As recent additions), haemolysis, raised liver transaminases and low platelet count (HELLP syndrome)[40]

At the beginning of the twentieth century, eclampsia complicated 2–3 per cent of pregnancies[41]. Better diagnosis and antenatal care have reduced this to about 1/500–1/1,000 pregnancies[42]. But the frequency is still high in the developing world, for example, India[43], Nepal[44] and Nigeria[45]. Indeed, in Kolkata, the astonishing rate of 7.4 per cent was reported in 70,000 *primigravidae*[46]. In Brazil, Gabon, Mexico and South Africa it is the most common cause of maternal death[47–50], and in Bangladesh the second highest after haemorrhage[30]. Most of these reports do not mention psychosis, but small series were reported from Delhi[43] and Maiduguri[45].

Pre-eclamptic toxaemia is still a disease of unknown cause. There are widespread renal and hepatic lesions. In the brain, they are found in 60 per cent, ranging from microscopic haemorrhages and petechiae to large cerebral bleeds together with white matter oedema[51], especially in the posterior parietal, temporal and occipital regions ('reversible posterior leukoencephalopathy syndrome'). The vasomotor disturbance that underlies seizures and coma usually leaves no residue. Thus, 'toxaemia' or gestosis appears to be a widespread arterial disease, with ischaemic lesions due to a transient but profound vasoconstriction.

Eclampsia is uniquely related to pregnancy and cured only by delivery of the placenta. Its increased frequency in hydatidiform mole show that the foetus is not responsible. Page[52] suggested that the placenta – 'a ruthless parasitic organ' – was the agent, secreting a pressor in response to ischaemia. Its role was demonstrated by a case of abdominal pregnancy, where the infant was surgically removed, leaving part of the placenta, and the mother experienced a worsening of pre-eclampsia for two weeks[53]. Recent papers[54,55] have assembled the evidence of placental dysfunction: various placental anomalies predispose – multiple pregnancy, excessive placental size or abnormal implantation. Roberts has suggested that the placental pressor targets the endothelium, which is not, like cellophane, a barrier between blood and the collagen of the vessel wall, but a complex organ with numerous functions; the consequences include arteriolar spasm and activation of the coagulation cascade, causing microthrombosis. He has also[56] suggested that the primary abnormality is a failure to remodel the spiral arteries in early pregnancy. There are biochemical changes (discussed later).

The neuropsychiatric complications of this endothelial disease include parturient coma (see Section 3), seizures and psychoses. Eclamptic psychosis is the second most common neuropsychiatric disorder related to childbearing.

Frequency

There have been many studies of its frequency. Some have been based on psychiatric surveys, with a denominator of female admissions or puerperal psychosis; others on obstetric surveys, again with alternative denominators – births or cases of eclampsia.

- Three surveys related its frequency to all female mental hospital admissions: eclamptic psychosis accounted for less than 1 per cent. Bourson's study[57] has the merit of reporting a complete series of cases from Strasbourg in the years 1945–1957; he found 81 cases among 9,000 female admissions (0.9 per cent).
- In 31 surveys from eleven nations in 1847–1997, eclamptic psychosis was related to puerperal psychosis. The total is 110 eclamptic psychoses among 4,000 puerperal psychoses (2.7 per cent). Since puerperal psychosis affects about 1/1,000 mothers, this suggests a frequency of about 1/40,000 births.
- These two estimates will be low because only a small fraction require admission to psychiatric hospitals. The frequency in obstetric surveys, related to the number of births, shows a wide variation – from .06 to 1.7/1,000 births – but even the lowest estimate is much higher than that based on psychiatric admissions. In some obstetric studies, the number of eclamptic psychoses can be related to other psychoses seen on the maternity wards. Engelhard's[58] classic study found 10 cases among 29 psychoses seen on a Dutch academic unit. Hohmann's[59] survey found that 11/24 psychoses were eclamptic. Feldman[60] in Venezuela found 4 cases of eclampsia among 10 confusional or manic states. Ndosi[61] in Tanzania reported that 15/86 psychoses had gestosis.
- Eleven surveys have related eclamptic psychoses to eclampsia. In total there were 259 psychoses among 8,467 eclampsias (3 per cent). The range is from 1 per cent to nearly 8 per cent. Other reviewers, who had access to unobtainable papers, gave higher figures: Anton[62] amalgamated 8 studies, finding 49 psychoses in 757 cases of eclampsia (6 per cent). Kleinknecht[41] evaluated 14 studies, finding 169 psychoses in 3,418 eclampsias (5 per cent). Sioli[63] also drew on 14 studies published before 1914: he found 185 psychoses among 3,427 eclampsias (5.2 per cent). It would be fair to conclude that about 5 per cent of eclampsias develop psychosis. Guzman[64] conducted a detailed analysis in Venezuela: among 4,617 cases of pre-eclamptic toxaemia seen in 1965–1973, 54 (just above 1 per cent) had psychiatric complications; this suggests that the decline in high-income nations may not apply to the countries where most children are born.

The Spread of Knowledge

Eclamptic psychosis is suitable for studying the dissemination and decay of knowledge, because both elements – seizures and psychosis – are easy to recognize. It is a striking example of the failure of scientific advances to cross language barriers. French and German studies considerably extended our knowledge. In France, Wieger's paper[65] on eclampsia is a classic, and Bidon's article[66] drew attention to severe disorders of memory; francophone nations have contributed 70 cases. Most of the major analyses were German[41,59,63,67], and German-speaking writers contributed 86 cases. Dutch and Italian authors, who contributed 16 cases, cited major papers and recognized the concept. But British and American writers not only failed to assimilate continental works, but seem not to have acknowledged its existence. The British published 26 cases, but misdiagnosed them, for example, as anaemic psychosis[68] or cerebral venous thrombosis[69]; they were even unaware of Donkin's landmark observation[70] from Newcastle (discussed later). The Americans published 18 cases, and the depth of their ignorance is illustrated by this case conference in 1964[71]:

> A 17-year old single woman in Louisville, Kentucky, who had denied her pregnancy, was admitted after suffering two convulsions about six weeks before her expected delivery. She was in coma. Her blood pressure was 170/110, and she had periorbital oedema and albuminuria. Labour was induced and she had three more seizures. After the birth she had four more fits and her blood pressure rose to 190/130. Three days after delivery she became confused and disorientated, then withdrawn and unresponsive. She was admitted to a psychiatric unit, treated with ECT, and recovered after an illness lasting 18 days. This typical eclamptic psychosis was given a diagnosis of 'undifferentiated schizophrenia'.

Onset of Seizures and Psychosis

Eclampsia began during pregnancy in 48 cases of eclamptic psychosis. In 22 mothers the psychosis also began before delivery (17 in the 3rd trimester and five in the 2nd trimester), as in this case[72]:

> A 24-year old had an eclamptic seizure at six months gestation. She had eleven further fits in two hours, and there was albumin in the urine. Two days later she could not see. In the week before her delivery, she began to ramble and sing, became incoherent and violently excited and developed the idea that she was a princess awaiting her prince and her mother was the Queen of Hungary; she made the whole world happy. A foetal hand appeared at the vulva. The foetus was turned and extracted. Excitation continued and five days postpartum she had nocturnal hallucinations, was loquacious, frightened, excited and assaultive. She recovered after three weeks.

In 121 cases eclampsia was prepartum or intrapartum, but the psychosis continued or started soon after the birth, as in this example[73]:

> A 39-year old, with a history of eclampsia when she gave birth to her 5th child, had a recurrence at eight months gestation of her next pregnancy. The doctor arrived to find her unconscious and convulsing. She had albumin in the urine. Fits recurred more and more frequently, at shorter intervals and with greater intensity. A dead child was removed by breech extraction. She remained in deep stupor. The next day she became blind and knew no-one. On day 2 she awoke with no memory of the previous days. That evening she had hallucinations of devils and thought the room was full of smoke. She developed delusions of surveillance, believed she heard guns and cannons, and searched for hidden weapons. On day 5 she fled the house, scantily clad and barefoot in freezing weather, to take refuge with a neighbour, believing that she was escaping threats to her life. Two days later, after an illness lasting only 6–7 days, she recovered.

In 64 cases eclampsia started after delivery, as first described by Esquirol[74]:

> His laconic account stated that a woman gave birth on April 22nd, had seizures for 24 hours and on the 24th developed a psychosis that lasted 21 days.

Considering that eclampsia and gestosis rapidly subside after delivery of the placenta, this is a high proportion. Thaler[75] quantified the increased risk after postpartum seizures: psychosis complicated 14/391 (3.6 per cent) of prepartum and 13/81 (16 per cent) of postpartum eclampsias.

After the seizures there is, in the majority, a period of stupor, lasting from hours to several days, with an average of two to three days[76]. In many, the psychosis begins as the patient comes out of this period of impaired consciousness. This may be identical to the post-ictal confusional states that follow epilepsy[77].

Onset of Psychosis after a Gap

Gooch[18] was the first to notice that some patients had a lucid interval between post-convulsive unconsciousness and the onset of psychosis.

> A *primipara* was seized with convulsions during labour. The child was delivered by perforating the head. The convulsions ceased and for several days she seemed to be doing well. But a few days after the birth, she became maniacal and died on day 8.

Kutzinski[76] found that in 10 cases the psychosis started immediately after recovery from the seizures, in 18 after an interval of 1–6 days, in three a week or more afterwards, and in one case 20 days after the last seizure. Herrmann[78] stated that most psychoses began 2–3 days after the onset of eclampsia; only 10 of his 60 cases started more than 6 days later – after intervals of 7–16 days. The literature contains 15 cases with a gap of just one day (or of a short uncertain duration), 9 of 2 days, 12 of 3 days, and three of 4 days; gaps longer than 4 days were reported by Fellner[79] (5–6 days), Jahnel[80] (8 days), Clauser[81] (11 days), Marzotko[82] (15 days), Lértora[83] (16 days) and Franchini[84] (20 days). Thus there is much evidence for a lucid interval. These gaps are too long for post-epileptic confusion.

Donkin Psychoses

In 1863, Arthur Donkin[70], Lecturer in Medical Jurisprudence at Newcastle, described a related disorder:

> A 23-year old gave birth to twins. Her face was puffy and oedematous, and her urine contained albumin. On day 1 she became agitated and complained of uneasiness and lightness in the head, photophobia, drumming in the ears, noise intolerance and insomnia. On day 3 she became excited, violent and maniacal, and required restraint. She insisted there was another baby to come, and it would be necessary to cut open her womb. With brief remissions, delirium and excitement continued until day 12. She then recovered.

This is eclamptic psychosis without seizures. Although one can, with hindsight, identify earlier cases[85,86], Donkin recognized its eclamptic origin; this was because Simpson in Edinburgh (where he trained) had started to measure albumin in the urine. Donkin psychoses are the best evidence of the independence of seizures and psychosis. Other evidence includes the eruption of psychosis before the first seizure, as in this case[87]:

> A Maryland woman complained of headache at term. Immediately after the birth, when the placenta was lying in the vagina, she became 'a complete maniac'. Potassium bromide and five hours of anaesthesia with chloroform had no effect on her raving and mental excitement.

It required two attendants to keep her in bed. Two days after the birth and onset of mania, she had a convulsion, after which she lay perfectly quiet. She had further fits at intervals of about an hour, until, 12 hours after the first, she had her last and most violent fit. She then recovered.

Donkin psychoses and the onset of psychosis before seizures establish that gestosis results not only in seizures (with post-epileptic confusion), but independently in a symptomatic psychosis.

Since writing *Eileithyia's Mischief*, I have pondered the relationship between Donkin psychoses and the curiously delayed onset of some eclamptic psychoses. These delayed episodes may be Donkin psychoses, occurring after a lucid interval in mothers who also suffered seizures. With this adjustment, I have identified 46 Donkin cases. A study of their distribution by generation showed that there were 230 eclamptic and only 35 Donkin psychoses before 1950 and 10 eclamptic and 11 Donkin psychoses after 1950 – an approximately equal number. If this is the true ratio, at least 100 Donkin psychoses are concealed in the early literature.

Some Features of Eclamptic and Donkin Psychoses

- All authorities agree on the preponderance of first time pregnancies. For example, Kleinknecht[41] had 26/37 *primiparae*, and in the literature the ratio was 76/128.
- Eclampsia that progresses to psychosis is more severe, with an average of eighteen seizures compared with eight[41], longer stupors and more renal dysfunction[63].
- In postpartum cases, the onset of psychosis is early (median day 3). This is also true of Donkin psychoses, except for those with a lucid interval (median day 7).
- Most episodes are brief, with a modal duration of 3–4 days. The median for eclamptic psychosis was 8 days, and for Donkin psychoses 14 days.

Onset and duration are important elements; Table 4.1 shows data in patients with sufficient information:

Table 4.1 Onset and duration of eclamptic and Donkin psychoses

Diagnosis	Onset				Duration[a]		
	Pregnancy	Labour	Days 1–10	>10 days	<14 days	14–28 days	>1 month
Eclamptic psychosis	21	9	133	3	107	25	34
Donkin psychosis	6	2	26	8	17	2	14

[a] This is duration in survivors; 23 mothers with eclamptic psychosis and 7 with Donkin psychoses died.

Onset after day 11 is unusual, but there are seven cases in the literature with later onset, as in these examples[84,88]:

A 26-year old had eclamptic fits in the 8th month of her 1st pregnancy. On day 15 after the birth she presented with aphasia, confusion, retardation and ideas of ruin. She had heavy albuminuria. She recovered and was discharged after eight days.

A 27-year old, in the 7th month of her 1st pregnancy, developed headache, dyspnoea and albuminuria. After the birth, the placenta was noted to have infarcts. On day 4 she became agitated and clouded and believed she would die, but this was transitory. On day 41 she developed *délire*, with confusion, retardation, hallucinations of coffins, paraesthesiae and loss of memory. She recovered after five months.

These cases suggest that these psychoses can present later than the second week.

As for duration, brevity is one of the hallmarks of these psychoses, with 74/138 episodes lasting no more than a week. But there is no doubt that a minority last longer – 48 (21 per cent) lasted more than a month, and 18 (10 per cent) more than three months, up to a maximum of nine months. In five mothers, this was partly due to a second psychotic episode following the same birth, as in these two examples[89,90]:

A 28-year old developed oedema and albuminuria in the last month of her 1st pregnancy. After the birth she had eclamptic seizures for 24 hours. She was well for three days, then developed auditory and visual hallucinations, became disorientated and misidentified people. After two weeks she recovered. Three weeks later she again became anxious, thought she was going to die, and 'saw visions'. Readmitted, she was restless and disorientated. *Her albuminuria had returned!* She lay still, staring in front of her. After seven months she recovered her memory and her health, and a year later had a normal delivery.

A 21-year old suffered from headache, oedema and albuminuria four days before the onset of labour. On the day of the birth she suffered the first of ten seizures. On day 3 she had her 11th seizure, then recovered consciousness. After a 2-day gap she became agitated, misidentified people and her surroundings, and tried to escape through a barred window. After 13 days she recovered. She had no memory of the delivery, and thought she had given birth to twins. But seven days later, without further fits, she relapsed, and remained ill for two months.

Psychopathology

With the exception of Kutzinski's analysis[76], accounts of the symptomatology in the literature are poor. The most common symptoms were agitation, excitement, raving, restlessness and violence, with the need for restraint. Many were disorientated and misidentified relatives or staff. Delusions, backed by hallucinations, of fire seem common. Speech was incoherent, irrational or nonsensical. As in all psychoses, some patients had ideas of persecution or poisoning, usually with food refusal. Five showed catalepsy. Other symptoms were occasionally seen, such as perseveration (five cases), incontinence of faeces (four cases) or dysphasia (three cases). Command hallucinations, or disorders of will and self have never been reported. Sioli[63] claimed that the majority had organic features – delirium, twilight states, hallucinatory confusion or stupor, with frequent and rapid changes between these phases, as in Bonhöffer's[16] description of exogenous reactions. But manic features, amnesia and signs of cognitive damage require special mention.

Manic Features

As in infective delirium, some patients showed manic features such as extreme loquaciousness (13 cases), singing (15), excessive mirth (6), euphoria (3), grandiose delusions (3), disrobing or sexual coquetry. Kleinknecht[41] misdiagnosed mania in 17/34 cases. Garcia Rijo's[72] prepartum case has been summarized previously. Here are two more examples[63,91]:

A 31-year old had 23 seizures in two days and was in stupor for one day. After a period of clear consciousness she developed hallucinations, anxiety and ideas of guilt. This changed to mania with cheerfulness, pressure of speech, flight of ideas and erotic behaviour together with amnesia, confabulation, perseveration and incoherent speech. After a few days of euphoria, she returned to normal.

A 22-year old developed eclampsia, then coma, in the 8th month of her 2nd pregnancy. A live child was skillfully extracted. Within an hour she had four more seizures. On day 2 she became manic, with exhausting loquacity, ideas followed each other with astonishing rapidity; during the night she did not stop talking for an instant. She recovered after two days, and was astonished to see her infant, because she could not believe she had given birth.

Amnesia

Loss of memory, obliterating the illness and the birth, was often present. In the seventeenth century, Segeri[92] was the first to draw attention to this complication:

> A patient from Bratislava had convulsions during and after delivery. She was lethargic, lost her sight, and did not know what was happening. She denied the child was hers.

Bidon[66] devoted a paper to this symptom, after which it was often reported and came to be accepted as one of the main features. Occasional cases had no other psychotic signs, but the majority had a typical post-eclamptic psychosis, with amnesia as a sequel. One must distinguish between anterograde and retrograde amnesia. In many, amnesia for the birth and illness was inevitable because of confusion, stupor or coma between seizures. A few, however, had retrograde amnesia, as in 3/13 of Kutzinski's[76] series. There are at least nine with a striking retrograde loss, as in these impressive examples[66,76]:

> A 26-year old eloped with a watch-maker. He soon gambled away her dowry and they lived in poverty. After developing facial oedema and albuminuria, she had 14 seizures, and was in a state of hebetude and delirium. After recovery she looked at her baby with incomprehension. She had forgotten her marriage and, although she recognized her husband, addressed him formally. She believed she was still living with her parents, who were resisting her marriage to the watch-maker.

> A single woman concealed her pregnancy with the help of her brother who, when she was having the baby, arranged to have postcards sent from Leipzig, pretending she was on a visit there. She suffered eight eclamptic seizures before and after the birth. On day 4 she became confused. She recovered a week later, but had no memory for the birth and the preceding two weeks, and had forgotten the subterfuge perpetrated by her brother.

Other Cerebral Lesions

Long-term memory deficits presumably result from focal cerebral damage. There are other such manifestations, including dysphasia, hemiplegia and blindness. A mother who had frightful convulsions during pregnancy and labour remained in coma for 12 days and lost her memory even for writing, counting and marking her lingerie[93]. One of Bidon's patients[66] forgot the topography of Paris. Another mother lost the ability to make simple calculations[41]. Westphal[94] described this case at enormous length:

> A 19-year old had swollen feet, headache, vomiting and albuminuria. Some hours after the birth she had over 30 seizures. She lost consciousness for three days, during which time she developed a pressure sore and pneumonia. On day 4 she became delirious, and was repeating nonsensical words in a monotonous stereotyped fashion. She gradually recovered and two weeks later was in a twilight state – disorientated in time and space and showing perseveration. Three months later, she still had cognitive deficits, including aphasia for the names of everyday objects like firewood, knives and wallets. More than that, she did not know that a hen-house was a place where fowls lay eggs. She had forgotten how to use numbers and the alphabet, and did not know how to write, nor when to use capital letters. This lasted many weeks, with eventual recovery.

Recurrences

Sioli[63] maintained that there were no unequivocal examples of recurrent eclamptic psychosis, although eclampsia itself recurs in 1–2 per cent of patients. I found six possible recurrences[95–98], including three of van Steenbergen-van der Nordaa[98] (nos. 14, 19 and 30); but all had psychotic episodes after other pregnancies without eclampsia. There are many examples of normal pregnancies after eclamptic psychosis. This, and the lack of a family history of psychosis, is in marked contrast to puerperal bipolar/cycloid disorder.

Personal Experience

I have encountered only one case of eclamptic psychosis, recounted by one of my nursing colleagues (see *What Is Worth Knowing*[4], page 77); but my series contains a considerable number of mothers who *may* have suffered from a Donkin psychosis. In all, 26 mothers had PET or severe hypertension; this is 8 per cent, not much higher than the general population. After excluding those with mild PET, depression or recurrent puerperal psychosis, there remained 13 patients in whom Donkin psychosis was possible, although none was typical. This is one of them:

> A 30-year old was pregnant for the first time. She developed a high blood pressure (140/90) and was admitted to hospital five weeks before the expected date of delivery because the baby was small; a Doppler test showed a grossly abnormal placenta. She said she had swelling of the face (not recorded in the records). A few days later, at 37 weeks gestation, she was delivered by Caesarean section of an infant weighing 4 lb 8 oz. Three weeks after the birth she became sleepless and irrationally anxious; for example, she was afraid of drowning in the shower. She woke up, convinced the baby was dead, screamed and tried to escape. She believed she was dying, was living in another world and had various and multiple illnesses; her parents and sister were dead. She accused a friend of having an affair with her father, and thought the house was haunted and on fire. She attacked her husband and believed she had killed him. On admission to hospital, she thought the ambulance men were police and she was being imprisoned. She appeared anxious, perplexed and confused, but was fully orientated. She had various auditory hallucinations. She could smell the hospital ward on fire and hear the crackling. She soon recovered and was discharged three weeks after the onset of the psychosis.

Although the onset was at the limit for Donkin psychoses, the duration was short for a bipolar/cycloid puerperal disorder. There was no personal or family history of manic depression and she remained well during the next 19 years.

Conclusion

The difficulty with Donkin psychosis, as with other nosological concepts in psychiatry (including mania), is that the intension (essence) is clear, but the extension (boundary) is not clear at all. This problem may not be soluble at the clinical level – it may require electro-encephalograms and laboratory tests. In the last 20 years biochemists have demonstrated the presence of a number of pressor substances in PET and an increase in anti-angiogenic proteins secreted by the placenta[99–107]. This is a complex and rapidly developing field of study, and there will probably be new developments before the ink is dry on this monograph. It would be wise to consult with experts before planning a prospective investigation. But, after consultation, it may be possible to use laboratory tests to confirm the diagnosis and indicate the severity of the gestosis, helping to define the mental disorder Donkin discovered. Until the differential diagnosis has been clarified, it would be unwise to assume that any of the 13 patients in my series with severe gestosis suffered from puerperal bipolar disorder.

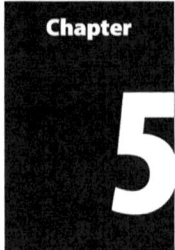

Wernicke-Korsakow Syndrome Complicating Pernicious Vomiting

This is an abridgement and updating of chapter 2 of *Eileithyia's Mischief*[1].

Hyperemesis Gravidarum and Its Complications

'Morning sickness' is common, but intractable vomiting is a dangerous disease. The incidence, carefully measured in the United States, is 3–4/1,000 pregnancies[108]. It can lead to rupture of the oesophagus, liver failure, hyponatraemia, hypokalaemia, rhabdomyolysis, renal failure, disseminated intravascular coagulation, and vitamin K deficiency. In addition it can cause two brain lesions: central pontine myelinolysis and the Wernicke–Korsakow syndrome. The first is symmetrical destruction of the pons, causing quadriparesis, eye palsies, dysphagia, dysarthria and facial weakness; the second has eye palsies and memory loss but also leads to psychosis.

Dubois[109] was the first to describe psychiatric symptoms complicating hyperemesis. He drew attention to the mortality risk in an address to the Académie de Médecine, describing 17 cases of which 13 were fatal; 4 of his fatal cases, all with headache and visual disturbance, suffered from mental changes – two had 'wandering of the mind' and two somnolence, coma and hallucinations. The British physicians Boulton[110] and Madge[111] also provided early descriptions. Wernicke[112] described *polio-encephalitis haemorrhagica superior*. He had three cases – a woman who developed a pyloric stricture after swallowing sulphuric acid, and two men who abused cognac and schnapps; they shared a fatal acute inflammation causing ophthalmoplegia, ataxia and impairment of consciousness (Wernicke's triad). Korsakow[113], in a series of papers, reported 38 cases, many of whom were ethanol addicts, with a combination of polyneuritis and mental changes that included chronic retrograde amnesia and confabulation. It was later realized that they were the same disease[114–116] with the same morbid anatomy and histology, and following the same course. Amnesic psychosis is present in almost all cases of Wernicke's disease that live long enough, provided that loss of memory is not masked by confusion. The term 'Wernicke–Korsakoff syndrome' is used for this group of disorders with a wide range of clinical pictures and degrees of severity[117]. It can now be diagnosed, with high sensitivity, by MRI scanning[118]. Recently visual loss due to papilloedema and retinal haemorrhages has been added to the syndrome[119,120].

The Wernicke-Korsakow Syndrome

There are lesions in the thalamus, mamillary bodies, central grey matter of the midbrain, hypothalamus, floor of the 4th ventricle and cerebellum but no cortical lesions. Memory disturbance is due to lesions in the walls of the 3rd ventricle, as shown by the occurrence of

Korsakow psychosis in tumours in this brain region; in the series of Victor and his colleagues[117], only the five patients without a lesion in the medial dorsal thalamic nuclei were spared memory loss. The majority of patients are ethanol addicts, but others suffer from gastric carcinoma or other diseases causing intractable vomiting. The study of the associated peripheral neuropathy[121,122] led to the concept of 'vitamins' and the identification of vitamin B_1 (thiamine), which was synthesized[137], and became available for therapy, in 1936.

Thiamine, compounded with pyrophosphoric acid, acts as a co-enzyme for at least 24 enzymes including pyruvate dehydrogenase and α-ketoglutamate dehydrogenase in the Krebs cycle, and transketolase in the pentose phosphate pathway. Patients with Wernicke–Korsakow syndrome have a low blood thiamine level (<3 µg/100 ml) and raised fasting pyruvate level. Anyone at risk should have oral thiamine 50 mg/day, and anyone with signs of deficiency intravenous thiamine 200–300 mg/day[123].

Wernicke-Korsakow Syndrome Due to Hyperemesis Gravidarum

A pregnant woman has an increased need for thiamine, not only for the growing foetus, but also because of a 20 per cent increase in her metabolic rate[124]. The requirement for B vitamins is increased threefold[125]. The recommended daily allowance during pregnancy is 1.5 mg[118]. Infection may be an additional factor in puerperal and post-abortion cases. Hyperthyroidism is another factor[126–131]. Many cases illustrate the iatrogenic risk of giving intravenous dextrose therapy without vitamins.

There are about 150 published cases of the Wernicke–Korsakow syndrome in pregnant or puerperal women.

Causes Other than Hyperemesis

In four mothers, ethanol addiction was responsible[72,132–134]; one of them also had hyperemesis[132]. This is Garcia Rijo's[72] case:

> A 31-year old alcoholic, during her 9th pregnancy, was drinking anisette and cassis. She developed cramps in the legs and difficulty in speaking. She became apathetic and disorientated, with weak memory and enfeebled mental powers. She made many mistakes and got lost for two days on her way home from hospital. She developed a delusional system that included ambitious ideas, ideas of poisoning and imaginary childbirths.

Seven other patients developed the syndrome in association with severe postpartum or post-abortion infections[135,136,138–141], one of whom had hyperemesis as well[139]. This accords with Bonhöffer's contention[16] that Korsakow psychosis is an occasional sequel to infective delirium, as in this early example, published before the Wernicke–Korsakow syndrome was described[142]:

> A 32-year old had given birth eleven times, most of the deliveries complicated by convulsions. After the 11th birth, she had a haemorrhage and seizures. On day 5 she developed fever, and became delirious. She had moments of complete loss of consciousness, chattered non-stop, had visions, and disrobed shamelessly. On day 12 her face became bloated, and she was unable to remember the slightest thing she did or said a few minutes earlier. She had paraesthesiae in the right ankle, lost the feeling of the right side of her head and complained of pain in the thigh, hips and arms. Impairment of memory became chronic.

In another case with no mention of hyperemesis, Korsakow psychosis developed in association with severe hypertension[143]:

A 40-year old gave premature birth to her 4th child at five months gestation. Immediately afterwards she complained of headache, and showed apathy, disorientation and loss of memory. One month later she suffered a left hemiparesis and was found to have a blood pressure of 220/140. She was unable to stand upright, tending to fall backwards. She had a typical Korsakow syndrome with retrograde amnesia and confabulation, from which she made a complete and rapid recovery.

Prepartum Onset

The great majority, however, developed Wernicke–Korsakow syndrome during pregnancy in association with pernicious vomiting. Usually termination of pregnancy or delivery cures the vomiting. Foetal death *in utero* has the same effect: Dubois[109] gave a striking example of hyperemesis that cleared up immediately after the cessation of foetal movements:

> His 12th case was a woman in the 6th month of her 2nd pregnancy. Six weeks of obstinate vomiting had reduced her to a state of extreme feebleness and emaciation. Her tongue was dry and red, her skin hot, her pulse rapid, and her breath exuded an acid foetor. The following day lively foetal movements weakened and ceased. This was the signal for a notable improvement, soon followed by complete cure.

Nevertheless, seven cases developed after, and in spite of, foetal death[113,130,144–147]. Before leaving the prepartum cases, one should note that a woman may present with a 'postpartum psychosis' after suffering from a prepartum Wernicke–Korsakow syndrome that escaped diagnosis and treatment. When the following case was presented at a medical meeting in Bordeaux, one of the audience recognized the patient and filled in the details at the next meeting[148,149]:

> The patient vomited continuously from the 3rd month and lost more than two kilograms per week. She sank into torpor and delirium. The pregnancy was terminated. Vomiting ceased, but her mental condition deteriorated. She no longer recognized anyone and cried out day and night. Later she presented at another mental hospital in a state of puerperal confusion. She was completely disorientated, and did not know she had given birth. She was unable to stand, because of muscular atrophy and hypotonia, and complained of headache and pain in the limbs. She had loss of memory with confabulation.

Post-Abortion Onset

Early in the nineteenth century, termination of pregnancy became an established treatment. Dubois[109] reported one death among four women aborted, and ten deaths in all the patients managed conservatively. Abortion continued to be an accepted treatment until the introduction of vitamin therapy. But the disease sometimes advanced after abortion, as in this case[150]:

> A 28-year old, who had recently suffered from malaria and pneumonia, had hyperemesis in her 2nd pregnancy, with increasing weakness, exhaustion and paralysis of the legs. In the 4th month she became confused, and the pregnancy was terminated. She remained confused, sang and talked nonsense in a loud voice. Some days later she stopped speaking and became sleepy and almost unconscious. She developed retrograde amnesia and loss of short-term memory. There was a slow improvement, but a year later she still had a considerable memory disorder.

There are also patients whose first symptoms developed after termination[151–157], as in this example[152]:

A 32-year old developed hyperemesis in the 2nd month of her 1st pregnancy. Vomiting ceased immediately at termination. Three days later she had a rigor and fever of 39.5°. She ate voraciously and her condition improved, but lost her voice for three days. After another week she had forgotten all recent events and believed she was engaged to be married. She became doubly incontinent and suffered pain in the legs. Her mind cleared, but she still could not walk.

Four cases followed miscarriage[158–161]. In this case, chronic amnesia developed after delayed thiamine treatment[161]:

An 18-year old developed hyperemesis in the 2nd month of pregnancy. She was treated with intravenous fluids without thiamine. She developed nystagmus, ataxia, coma and weakness of the legs. CT and MRI imaging showed bilateral caudate lesions as well as thalamic, hypothalamic and periaqueductal lesions. She miscarried. After thiamine treatment, she developed severe amnesia. Seven months later she was discharged with amnesia and weakness of the legs.

Postpartum Onset

Ten patients developed the first signs of mental illness after the birth[58,162–170]. Marcé's patient[162] is of interest because the disorder ran through two pregnancies:

A 29-year old vomited everything she ate and became extremely thin during her 9th pregnancy. She also had a prolonged haemorrhage. Her intelligence was impaired: she lost her way in the streets, and could no longer work. She became pregnant for a 10th time, and again had a serious haemorrhage. Her intellectual disorder increased and her ideas became incoherent. She recovered with a good diet.

The following patient suffered a return of vomiting after delivery[164]:

A woman developed hyperemesis in the 8th month of her 7th pregnancy. At the birth, vomiting ceased for two days, then returned. On day 4 she was sleepless, and began to complain that the neighbours were spying on her through holes in the walls. On day 10 she rushed out of the house naked with her baby, demanding instant baptism. On day 12 she developed weakness in the legs, progressing to paralysis by day 20. She lost all memory for the last few months – her new domicile and husband's occupation, names of the staff, visits of her husband and family. At night she disturbed other patients by singing at the top of her voice, and was surprised to be admonished, saying she had spent the night at home, or away on a trip. She would often ask why people wanted to kill her, and why she was accused of killing her children. After five months she recovered her sanity and memory, but not her full motor function.

The Clinical Picture of Wernicke–Korsakow Syndrome Associated with Hyperemesis Gravidarum

This shows the same wide range reported in ethanol addicts[117,171]. In six patients, memory loss lasted at least 12 months, as in this case[172]:

A 24-year old had hyperemesis from the beginning of her first pregnancy. She became dehydrated and developed ataxia, nystagmus and disorientation. She was treated with intravenous glucose and deteriorated. She could no longer stand, and developed ophthalmoplegia, dysarthria, dysphagia, pyramidal signs and coma. With vitamin therapy, her mental state improved within 24 hours, but she still had anterograde amnesia, anosognosia, misidentifications and confabulation. Vomiting persisted, so the pregnancy was terminated. Memory deficit remained 18 months later.

Almost all patients had the neurological symptoms of Wernicke's encephalopathy, peripheral neuropathy or both. Only six had no neurological signs[162,169,173–176]; they presented with a prepartum or postpartum psychosis, without neurological clues. This is an example of a patient who presented with stupor and delirium during pregnancy[175]:

> A 23-year old presented with vomiting and malnutrition in the 3rd month of pregnancy. She was bed-ridden and hardly slept, and, within a few days, became completely immobile, mute and stuporose. She developed hallucinations of animals and people threatening her, and was disorientated. The family pressed for a termination, having seen a neighbour cured by this intervention, but in 4th month the vomiting stopped and her confusion disappeared. She gave birth and recovered.

Another patient presented with memory loss in pregnancy, continuing into the puerperium[173]:

> A 37-year old suffered hyperemesis in her 4th pregnancy and, by the 5th month, had lost 60–70 pounds in spite of rectal feeding. For two months before delivery she had difficulty in remembering things from day to day. After the birth, she was apathetic and did not seem to realize she had a child. She had visual hallucinations, and a marked impairment of memory, with confabulation. She had forgotten most of her pregnancy, including the rectal feeding.

Recurrence of the Disease

The cause has long been established, prevention is cheap and readily available, diagnosis not too difficult, and treatment rapidly effective. This disease should, therefore, be extinct.

There are certainly signs of an improvement in its clinical features and course – since World War II (coinciding approximately with the ready availability of vitamin therapy), there have been only four published postpartum or post-abortion cases[159–161,170] and two of these had no mental changes[160,170]. Patients now usually present with Wernicke's triad (or variants, such as blindness[120,177]) rather than Korsakow psychosis. But severe cases continue to be described to the present day. During the last 15 years, five patients have died[178–182] and at least six suffered from lasting memory loss[131,172,183–186]. There has in fact been a spate of new cases, related to rehydration without vitamin supplements, the majority treated in Western Europe, Australia, the United States or Japan. In the last five years, seven mothers have developed Wernicke's encephalopathy in these circumstances[131,184,185,187–190], all from France, Belgium, Italy, Spain or the United States – nations that claim to have high medical standards. The flood of recent cases of a disease that should have been eliminated 75 years ago requires explanation, so I conducted a citation analysis (See Table 5.1).

This showed that 80 cases were published between 1868 and 1941 ('the old series'); there was much cross-referencing, each paper being cited an average of five times. The syndrome then disappeared from the literature for 27 years. Chaturachinda's paper[191] was followed (after a further gap of 14 years) by a flood of at least 70 cases, which has continued up to the present time ('the new series'). Many resulted from rehydration by intravenous glucose without vitamin supplements. There may be under-reporting, because some authors will have been ashamed to publish such flagrant malpractice. There has been some cross-referencing of these modern cases (with an average of four citations/paper), but cases from the old series have hardly ever been mentioned. Recent reviews illustrate this: Chiossi[118], who used the National Library of Medicine database, cited almost all the recent cases but none earlier than Chaturachinda's[191] paper. Another Italian review[131] built on this, adding 11 more cases published between 2005 and 2011. Scalzo[192], in an article entitled 'Wernicke–Korsakoff syndrome not related to alcohol use: a systematic review', used the Index Medicus to search for cases reported since 1888 and claimed 115 cases associated with hyperemesis; but it was limited to the English language, and, since the majority of the 'old series' were published in other languages, he missed a great deal; he referenced no article published before 1973.

Table 5.1 Date chart on Wernicke-Korsakow syndrome related to childbearing

Generation	Number of cases	Events
1826–1850	1	1st description by Fischer (1841)[142]
1851–1875	5	Cases preceding Korsakow's description (1890)[113]
1876–1900	16	
1901–1925	33	The old series
1926–1950	25	
1932	1st use of intravenous glucose in treatment[155]	
1936	Thiamine became available	
1937	Vitamin B$_1$ first used in treatment[156]	
1951–1975	1	Chaturachinda's paper[191]
1976–2000	27	
After 2000	48	The new series

There are, therefore, two separate literatures on Wernicke–Korsakow syndrome complicating hyperemesis gravidarum. Is it possible that the scandalous return of this preventable disease is due to the loss of the old knowledge – that the medical profession *forgot* that women with pernicious vomiting can develop Wernicke-Korsakow syndrome, and require urgent treatment with thiamine? Forgetting would explain the new cases in the 1970–1980s, but many other cases reported in the 21st century have not stemmed the flow. It seems incredible that a failure of 'scholarship' should be the sole cause of the return of an extinct disease, but those who do not accept this explanation will have to find another.

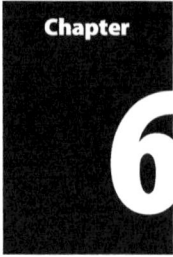

Chapter

Chorea Psychosis Complicating *Chorea Gravidarum*

6

This is an abridgement and updating of chapter 1 of *Eileithyia's Mischief*[1].

Sydenham's Chorea (St Vitus' Dance)

Sydenham[193]wrote:

> This disorder is a kind of convulsion, which chiefly attacks children of both sexes, from ten to
> fourteen years of age. It first shows itself by a certain lameness, or rather unsteadiness of one leg,
> which the patient draws after him like a fool, and afterwards affects the hand of the same side,
> which, being brought to the breast . . . cannot be held in the same position for a moment, but is
> distorted, or snatched away into a different posture and place, notwithstanding all his efforts to the
> contrary. If a drink is put in his hand, he uses a thousand odd gestures, like a juggler, to get it to his
> mouth – as soon as it has happily reached his lips, he flings it suddenly into his mouth, and drinks
> it very hastily, as if the poor wretch only meant to make sport.

Many of these patients died of rheumatic heart disease, and an immunological link between
cardiac tissue and *Streptococcus pyogenes* was established. Chorea is a late complication of
streptococcal infection, setting in several months after migratory polyarthritis, when the
titre of streptococcal antibodies is falling. At necropsy, endarteritis of small vessels and
perivascular lesions are widespread in the brain, with the greatest damage to the caudate
nucleus. At the biochemical level, heightened dopaminergic action in the striatum is
postulated, and supported by the adverse effects of dopamine agonists such as l-DOPA
and amphetamines.

The streptococcus is highly susceptible to penicillin and other antibiotics, and (unlike the
staphylococcus) does not readily become resistant. Prophylactic penicillin has greatly reduced
the cardiac complications of rheumatic fever. One might, therefore, expect that this other
complication should be much less frequent, and it is. But it still occurs[194] and chorea is also a
complication of other diseases – systemic lupus erythematosus (SLE) and anti-phospholipid
syndrome; they can also cause childbearing psychoses, as in this case[195]:

> A 23-year old became irritable, rash and hesitant in the 3rd month of pregnancy. She had
> albuminuria and hypertension and, four days before delivery, renal function deteriorated. On
> day 4 her thought processes were confused. On day 6 she was screaming, refusing to eat and
> reported auditory hallucinations. A diagnosis of SLE was made. She was treated with steroids and
> recovered after 22 weeks.

A review of 323 patients with systemic lupus[196], of whom 127 had anti-phospholipid
antibodies, found that 25 had a psychosis (no details) and another 12 an acute confusional
state; neuropsychiatric symptoms were strongly associated with anti-phospholipid
antibodies.

Chorea Gravidarum

This is a more severe variety, with a higher mortality rate – 33 per cent in the 19th and 13 per cent in the 20th century – and more frequent psychiatric complications. It usually starts in the first half of pregnancy and often clears up rapidly when the uterus is emptied. At one time it was an indication for termination of pregnancy, indeed the strongest of all reasons. It can be recurrent: Buist[197] found that 31/214 patients had recurrent attacks, up to a maximum of five. There is a close association with childhood chorea: more than half suffered earlier attacks, and one-quarter of girls with childhood chorea later suffered a recurrence during pregnancy[198]. The frequency has declined. In 1899 it was 1/1,000[199] and in 1932 1/3,000 pregnancies[198]. In 1958–1965 a Strasbourg study of 32,000 deliveries found no cases[200]. But, in the 21st century, it still occurs[201–203].

Chorea can start after delivery. Horstius[204] described this case:

> A peculiar thing happened to Ludimoderator's wife after childbirth, I have no idea why. For 12 years or more, when she is awake, her whole left side is affected by continuous involuntary movements – her eye winking, her lips opening and closing, her arm jumping about, her fingers gesticulating and her foot never still, all without sensation or pain. When she is asleep, everything settles down.

It can follow abortion. It is affected by menstruation, and may be associated with amenorrhoea and oestrogen-containing oral contraceptives.

The Psychiatric Complications of Sydenham's Chorea

Breton's[205] thesis gave a full account, with historical quotations and many descriptive cases. In addition to depression, which is common in disabling and life-threatening illness, there are five mental disorders associated with chorea:

(1) A change of character, with irritability and waywardness. Breton devoted a chapter to this subject with 38 illustrative cases. Diefendorf[206] described his young patients as fretful, peevish, fault-finding, passing rapidly and without provocation from one mood to another, with tears and passionate outbursts when they would rip up books and break toys. These changes may precede chorea by a week or two and survive it by many weeks.

(2) Tourette's syndrome. Sandras and Bourgignon[297] described this case:[a]

> A seven-year old was seized with convulsive contractions of the hands and arms, especially when she was trying to write. These involuntary movements spread to her shoulders, neck and face, resulting in extraordinary contortions and grimaces. When they spread to the voice, she uttered bizarre cries and nonsensical words, even though her mind was clear. There was no improvement at puberty. After her marriage she rapidly deteriorated. Among the continual and disorganized movements, those affecting the organs of voice and speech were particularly worthy of attention. They presented a rare and disagreeable phenomenon that deprived her of all the delights of company. In the middle of a lively conversation, suddenly and irresistibly, she would interrupt her speech or that of her companion with bizarre exclamations, or extraordinary utterances that formed a deplorable contrast with her refined manners and good will. Most were foul-mouthed oaths or obscene epithets, but no less embarrassing for her and her hearers were frank and unfavourable opinions on those present.

> This description of coprolalia antedates that of Gilles de la Tourette by some decades.

---

[a] I cut the relevant pages in the library of l'Académie de Médecine, the whole book being in a pristine state.

(3) <u>Hypnagogic and hypnopompic hallucinations</u>. We owe to Marcé[208] the description of these symptoms, which in their flamboyant severity seem unique to chorea:

> A 22-year old congenital syphilitic presented with a 15-day history of chorea. Her sleep was interrupted by 'dreams'. Before falling asleep she saw devils, headless corpses, ravens, bats and other terrifying objects. She believed they were going to strangle her, and found it hard to breathe. These hallucinations also occurred at the moment of waking, when she would cry out and disturb other patients. She believed her food was poisoned and heard voices telling her she was damned. She recovered after a few weeks.

Although other authors mention visual hallucinations, only Breton[205] has provided descriptions of the same quality:

> An 11-year old became irritable, morose and forgetful during her 3rd attack of chorea. Every night, at the moment of falling asleep, she had the same visions – of burglars round her bed, men dressed in black with black faces, red noses, round hats and fingers covered in rings. She heard them say they were going to cut her throat. Another robber cut open the head of her sister. As soon as she closed her eyes, the visions would reappear, and she would hide under the bed-clothes. Terrified, she would search under the bed. She undressed slowly and silently, hoping the robbers would not hear.

I do not know the explanation of these symptoms, which seem more vivid than the classic accounts of hypnagogic hallucinations[209-211]. They may simply result from intense REM pressure in patients completely sleep-deprived. Alternatively they may arise from lesions in the dorsolateral pons, from which the ponto-geniculo-occipital spikes –presumably the source of hypnagogic and dream phenomena – originate.

(4) <u>Acute psychosis</u>. Frank[212] may have been the first to mention this:

> Most have a disorder of intelligence and memory, and some epilepsy and madness.

There are difficulties in the recognition of psychotic signs when speech and behaviour are disorganized by violent muscular spasms, which can mimic agitation and thought disorder. Arndt[213] and Lehmann[214], in an authoritative discussion of the evidence, argued that a spurious appearance of mania could result from extreme involuntary movements. Nevertheless, there is overwhelming evidence that an independent psychosis can also be present, especially the dissociation between the timing and severity of the two cerebral disorders. According to Willson and Preece[198] this is the most common major complication; they found 51 cases among 951 choreic pregnancies in 797 women (16 per cent of choreic pregnancies). Psychosis is a bad prognostic sign. As for the form of the illness, this was mainly delirium, although stupor was also seen.

(5) <u>Intellectual deficits or chronic organic brain syndrome</u>. These can be transient[215] but chronic deficits occur.

Psychosis in *Chorea Gravidarum*

Many cases have been described. The crude total is greater than 50, but the data are often scanty. One must subtract patients with alternative causes of delirium, such as terminal heart disease or infection. The following case has been claimed as the first description, but sepsis was an alternative cause:

A prostitute was admitted after an abortion. Seven days earlier, following a fright, she was seized by a fit, after which her legs were agitated by chorea. Her whole body became affected by jerking motions. She became delirious or maniacal and died a month later. She had an abscess of the left scapula[216].

In Marcé's[208] patient, with postpartum onset, the hallucinations were hypnagogic:

Chorea started six weeks after delivery, interrupting sleep. For the first time, she was troubled by dreams with visual hallucinations. She saw her daughter falling, threatened by her father with a stick. As she closed her eyes to fall asleep, she saw animals in her bedroom and on her bed. This nightly experience began to wane *pari passu* with the recovery of the chorea.

Another patient with postpartum chorea and hallucinations also had Tourette's syndrome[217]:

A woman developed chorea four months after her 1st delivery. Her intellectual faculties were in disorder: she saw dogs with their throats cut, blood pouring out, all in living tableaux, but silent. She also put her hand before her mouth when speaking, to prevent shameful words escaping.

Most chorea psychoses present during pregnancy, but some present as postpartum or post-abortion psychoses, even when chorea started before delivery.

Prepartum Onset

This is the usual manifestation, with at least 40 cases in the literature: there are 15 fatal cases and at least 18 with single episodes and early recovery. In some the psychosis came to an end before the birth. In others, it cleared up promptly after delivery or termination, as in this example[218]:

An 18-year old gave birth to her first child in January. She became pregnant again in April. In September she suddenly became disturbed. She threw things around the room and expressed ideas of persecution involving her landlady, who was serving her tainted tea. She was poorly orientated and had choreiform movements. Two weeks later (long before the end of the pregnancy) the movements disappeared and her psychic state changed to a prolonged 'exhaustion state', in which she was mute, perplexed, hallucinated and would only feed with assistance. In January she gave birth and rapidly recovered. She had no memory for her illness.

In others, it continued into the puerperium, as in this case[219]:

In the 6th month of her first pregnancy, a 26-year old developed slight involuntary movements and auditory hallucinations. She became agitated and incoherent. She believed she was being poisoned. Her chorea worsened, and she had albuminuria. She gave birth to a premature infant weighing 2 kg. After the birth she remained agitated. She believed it was a cousin who had given birth and did not wish to see the infant. She still had auditory hallucinations. The chorea disappeared, but she became depressed and lost weight. Two months after the birth she recovered, but without remembering anything.

This patient remained ill for several weeks after termination of the pregnancy[220]:

A 20-year old became pregnant in February. In March she became nervous and irritable. In April she developed twitching of her right arm; delirium and abnormal movements were marked. Her uterus was evacuated. She remained noisy, disorientated and irrational. She saw Field Marshall Hindenburg standing outside the door disguised as a doctor (it was 1918). She thought all women were murderers and saw eels and snakes. She was incontinent of faeces. In May choreiform movements ceased, but she still failed to recognize her husband and rambled incoherently. Two months after the abortion she recovered.

Eight patients suffered from recurrent *chorea gravidarum*. Two with prepartum chorea developed psychosis only during the first choreic episode. One had postpartum chorea without psychosis, and relapsed, with chorea and psychosis, during her next pregnancy[221]. The other five developed psychosis each time[222-226]. This patient had three episodes[224]:

> In the 6th month of her first pregnancy, a 21-year old, with no history of rheumatic fever or chorea, suddenly became restless and overtalkative. She heard voices, saw things in her bed, struck out and refused food. In January 1906 she gave birth five weeks early. She recovered several weeks afterwards [a prepartum psychosis with no mention of chorea]. In June she conceived again. In September she developed abnormal mouth movements, neglected her work and lay in bed all day. Chorea was diagnosed. After a night of raving she was admitted to an asylum. Chorea was so severe that she had to be held down by four attendants. The pregnancy was terminated. She remained clouded and delirious, had delusions of fire, robbery and her husband's death, and hallucinations of black faces. In October the choreiform movements ceased; within a week she recovered from psychosis and was discharged. She remained well until December 1909 when she became pregnant for the 3rd time and suffered a relapse: admitted to hospital in March she had severe chorea and a marked mood disorder – lability, irritability, euphoria and frequent bursts of laughter. The pregnancy was terminated, but she died the next day. Necropsy showed endocarditis.

Postpartum Psychosis

There are eight cases of postpartum psychosis following prepartum chorea[227-234]. The following patient is unusual because she had recurrent prepartum chorea, with no psychosis the first time, and a postpartum episode the second time, with fatal outcome[231]:

> In the 8th month of her second pregnancy, a woman developed chorea. In the 5th month of her 3rd pregnancy she became irritable and absent-minded, and said queer things. In the 6th month she developed such violent chorea that it required four nurses to keep her in bed and prevent self-injury; only chloroform stopped them, and when she came round they were worse than ever. Labour was induced, but the birth had no effect – her eyes developed a wild look, she no longer recognized her husband and became excessively violent. She gradually changed from agitation and loss of control to acute mania and was transferred to an asylum, where she died one week later.

The next patient had two distinct episodes of chorea psychosis, one before and one after delivery[233]:

> A 24-year old, whose mother committed suicide, had three pregnancies without chorea. Soon afterwards she became pregnant for the fourth time. In the third or fourth month, she became depressed, spoke little, and believed people were talking about her. At about the same time she developed chorea. At night she feared attack by people and animals. She was admitted to an asylum. Within two months, her chorea and depression cleared up. In the last days of pregnancy, chorea returned, improved, then worsened three weeks after the birth of a stillborn child. She heard voices, and believed the house was on fire, and she would be poisoned by her husband. After two months both chorea and psychosis cleared up simultaneously.

Three patients developed a post-abortion psychosis following prepartum chorea[230,235,236] and five developed both chorea and psychosis after childbirth[214,237,239-241].

Outcome

There is a wide range of outcome, including recovery before the end of pregnancy, recovery immediately after the uterus is emptied, continuation into the puerperium, chronic psychosis and early death. Four patients developed a defect state[242–245]. This is an example of a patient whose delirium continued after delivery, with loss of memory[245]:

> A woman developed chorea in the first month of her first pregnancy. She was depressed with hallucinations and complete insomnia. At seven months she gave birth to a stillborn child. Two weeks later, her chorea improved, but she remained disorientated with no memory for her hospitalization.

Antibiotics have almost, but not quite, eliminated the psychosis associated with *chorea gravidarum*. Piña[246] reported a case from Mexico, although details were scanty. It is, therefore almost extinct. Nevertheless it is important to remember this cause of childbearing psychosis, and the facts established from the study of many published cases. It may return if the streptococcus evades antibiotic control or becomes more virulent.

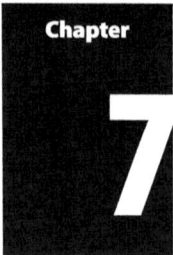

Chapter

Vascular Disorders

This is an abridgement and updating of chapter 6 of *Eileithyia's Mischief*[1].

Cerebral Venous Thrombosis

Anatomy

The brain is drained by cerebral veins that open into valve-less sinuses lying between the two layers of the dura mater. The largest is the superior sagittal (longitudinal) sinus, which runs in the margins of the falx cerebri; the arachnoid granulations (Pacchionian bodies), which drain cerebro-spinal fluid into the venous system, project into the lateral diverticula of this sinus. The superior sagittal sinus anastomoses with the straight sinus and continues as one of the lateral (transverse) sinuses; the lateral sinus becomes the sigmoid, which drains into the jugular vein. At the base of the brain are the cavernous sinuses that drain into the superior and inferior petrosal sinuses. The great vein of Galen joins the basilar vein, which enters the inferior sagittal and right transverse sinuses.

These sinuses can become thrombosed through infection. Cavernous sinus thrombosis is a notorious complication of facial infections. Lateral sinus thrombosis is almost exclusively caused by otitis media. Septic thrombosis of the superior sagittal sinus is associated with meningitis and sinusitis. Septic thrombophlebitis has become rare since the introduction of antibiotics.

They can also become thrombosed for other reasons, especially after childbirth. The first indication that puerperal women were liable to thrombotic complications is the description of leg vein thrombosis (*phlegmasia alba dolens*) in the seventeenth century[247]. Another is the frequency of pulmonary embolism, which, if multiple, can cause thromboembolic pulmonary hypertension[238]. As for thrombosis of the cerebral veins, Morgagni[248] described a woman who died of apoplexy after childbirth, and was found to have the dural veins thickened and hardened, and the left cerebral ventricle filled with blood. Abercrombie[249] described this case:

> A 24-year old suffered from violent headache at the beginning of the 2nd week after her 2nd delivery. Several days later, she complained of uneasiness in the head and a peculiar numbness in the back of the head and neck. She lost sensation and movement in her right arm and leg, then her speech with twisting of her mouth. She had a convulsion, stronger on the left, then three more, then seizures every half hour. She lost consciousness and died two days later. Necropsy showed an ecchymosis on the surface of the left hemisphere. The veins were turgid and distended with firm fleshy blood. There was a thrombus in the longitudinal sinus, and two areas of softening, the larger in the left hemisphere.

Cruveiller[250], in one of his beautifully illustrated pamphlets on pathological anatomy, described headache and hemiplegia starting 15 days after childbirth, leading to death in coma 6 days later; necropsy showed thrombosis in the superior longitudinal sinus, right lateral sinus and superior cerebral veins. Ducrest[251] described 5 cases found among 259 obstetric necropsies. Hauser[252] has an historical anecdote about Hughlings Jackson: he first observed his eponymous focal epilepsy in his own wife, who died from a puerperal sinus thrombosis. Kalbag and Woolf[253] wrote a masterly review, based on 500 references and their experience at the Midland Centre for Neurosurgery in Smethwick: they gathered more than 25 cases from the literature, but not all were women. Sheehan and Lynch[254] found 6 cases in their series of more than 500 obstetric necropsies, and 396 postpartum cases in the literature, of which 107 had necropsy proof; symptoms began later than day 4 of the puerperium, and resembled eclampsia, which is, however, rare at that stage.

Frequency

Cerebral venous thrombosis can also occur during pregnancy[255]. Sheehan and Lynch[254] found 16 cases in the literature, of which 5 were in the 2nd and 3rd trimesters. It can occur after abortion[256]. Puerperal cases make up only a small proportion – about 3 per cent. Lanska and Kryscio[257] tabulated fifteen studies, of which six were population-based: the range was huge – 0 to $39.4/10^5$ births in Europe and North America and $196/10^5$ in India, where there is much evidence of an increased incidence. Banerjee and colleagues[258] collected 8 cases from 880 consecutive necropsies conducted over a two-year period, and cited five earlier reports going back to 1957. Bansal and colleagues[259] found 12 patients in two years on the medical wards. Chopra and Prabhakar[260] collected 41 cases in seven years among 251 strokes in young persons: 37 presented after delivery and 4 during pregnancy. Srinavasan has published several papers[261–263] and is frequently cited for his figure of $296/10^5$ births, or even $450/10^5$ births. By 1984 he had collected 145 patients from a city with a catchment of one million. Prasad[264] collected another 145 patients in Bangalore. The frequency of cerebral venous thrombosis may result from the custom of secluding newly delivered women in overheated rooms, with insufficient fluids. The high figures from India occur in other countries: 13 cases were reported in two years from a general hospital in Cuauhtemoc, Mexico[265].

Recurrences can occur after another pregnancy[266]. Huhn[267] drew attention to their frequency, citing 7 in the literature; in his series of 23 Köln patients, 12 had further pregnancies, and 3 a recurrence, while one had another episode after her 3rd child was born. He recommended termination of pregnancy and sterilization in recurrent cases.

Pathogenesis

There have been several suggestions explaining the frequency of this remote form of thrombophlebitis after the pelvic events of childbirth. Batson's hypothesis of retrograde venous embolization *via* the vertebral veins has been much criticized[253,268]. The other explanations are:

- An increased tendency to thrombosis. Cerebral venous thrombosis is associated with pulmonary embolism, and thrombophlebitis in the pelvic or leg veins. Nearly all patients have evidence of venous thrombosis somewhere else in the body[266]. This suggests an enhanced clotting tendency. There seem to be many candidates, but no consensus on the reason for increased thrombosis in the puerperium.

• The anatomy of the cerebral venous sinuses. Various factors favour stasis and obstruction in these sinuses – the absence of valves, the low pressure and the angle of entry into other sinuses.

Clinical Features

Cerebral venous thrombosis is more common in first time mothers. The usual history is of a sudden onset in the first fortnight after a normal delivery free from sepsis. The course of the illness may involve relapses, as the thrombosis spreads in the sinuses and into the cerebral veins[269]. At least two-thirds present with the neurological triad of headache, seizures and focal cortical damage. Headache is present in almost all cases, due to involvement of the pain-sensitive dural sinuses; it is sometimes accompanied by nausea and vomiting. The majority have seizures – 29/47 in Dubois' series[270]. About half have impairment of consciousness in the form of stupor or coma. Unless the motor cortex is affected, there may be no other neurological symptoms, but a few have hemiparesis, dysphasia or other focal signs. Papilloedema is usually present. Transitory blindness, due to venous congestion of the fundi, sometimes occurs. The scalp veins, which communicate with the superior longitudinal sinus, may be dilated. Exophthalmos can occur. The cerebro-spinal fluid is usually under pressure with raised protein and often a certain amount of blood. The diagnosis can be confirmed during life by angiography or MRI scanning. Relating symptoms to pathology, there are two factors[266]:

• Obstruction of the arachnoid granulations raises intracranial pressure. This causes headache, vomiting, photophobia, papilloedema and lethargy, torpor or confusion progressing to coma. These patients often show anxiety, aggression or apathy and may develop delirium; such cases can simulate puerperal psychosis.

• Sinus thrombosis increases resistance in the cerebral circulation, resulting in dysfunction of the cortex drained by that vein. Extension of the thrombus, obstructing the superior cerebral veins, causes softening about two inches in diameter around the vein, leading to cortical deficits, and, in many cases, convulsions.

Sheehan and Lynch[254] also stated that involvement of the straight sinus interfering with drainage along the great vein of Galen causes a generalized disturbance including vomiting, papilloedema and torpor progressing to coma and early death. In addition, involvement of the veins over the frontal lobe can lead to stupor or psychological disturbances.

The differential diagnosis includes cerebro-vascular accidents due to arterial embolism, and eclampsia. Cerebral venous thrombosis accounts for nearly all cases diagnosed as 'late eclampsia'[270].

Heparin has reduced the mortality to about 10 per cent.

Psychiatric Presentations

The great majority present with neurological symptoms, but there are mechanisms by which psychiatric symptoms can occur. Motet[272] published the first case with a psychiatric presentation:

A 28-year old was upset by a casual visit from an inebriated stranger eight days after childbirth. She spoke of the incident all night and could not sleep. The following day, her ideas were disordered and she had terrifying visions. She tried to jump out of the window. Her agitation increased, and within three days she was in a state of continual mania. She died 24 days after delivery. Necropsy showed clots in the cerebral veins, but not the sinuses.

Dubois[270] promoted the idea that cerebral venous thrombosis was a cause of postpartum psychosis. A few patients present with confusion, delirium, clouding of consciousness, disorientation or a psychosis mimicking puerperal psychosis[253,273–279]. These are sufficiently frequent to be numbered in asylum surveys: Skottow[275] had one case among 26 admitted to Buckinghamshire Mental Hospital in 1936–1940, Visscher[280] 2 cases among 106 admitted in Groningen in 1928–1945, Combs[281] one case among 50 admissions in Atlanta, and Drenk[29] one case among 131 admitted in Köln 1951–1966. Huhn[267] stated that the clinical picture included disturbances of affect and drive, memory and consciousness as a primary manifestation in 13 per cent, and secondarily in 22 per cent. Koek and Schreuder[282] described a patient who recovered from cerebral phlebitis and then relapsed with acute delirium, resulting in a four-week admission to hospital. Some cases supporting these claims will now be summarized.

Two had onset during pregnancy. The first patient had delirium with some neurological features[253]. In the other, neurological symptoms were minimal and a diagnosis of catatonia was favoured[283].

A 29-year old tried to induce an abortion with wormwood, and suffered seizures in the 3rd month of pregnancy. She became drowsy and confused, then comatose. She had focal fits involving the left face and arm, and a left hemiplegia. Three days later she miscarried, and died within a week. Necropsy showed thrombosis of superior longitudinal and left lateral sinuses and the jugular vein (case 14).

A 20-year old became forgetful and disorganized, and then disorientated in the 8th month of her 2nd pregnancy. After six days she was admitted and gave birth to a premature child. She showed no sign of pain, had no memory of the birth and believed the child belonged to someone else. She had visual hallucinations of fire and of her husband. She was incontinent, and had some jerking movements and stiffening of the body. The following day she was restless with clouding of consciousness. She sang incoherently. Disorientation and hallucinations continued for five days, when she became mute and resisted any passive movements. She failed to recognize people and refused food, which she believed was poisoned. After a month she suddenly died. Necropsy showed thrombosis in the superior longitudinal sinus, both transverse sinuses, the sigmoid sinus and the jugular vein, as well as some cerebral veins.

There is one post-abortion case[274], but this woman developed a psychogenic psychosis after a criminal abortion and, as a second complication, died from cerebral venous thrombosis five months later (see Section 4).

Fifteen had postpartum onset. One, with clots in the veins (not sinuses) has already been summarized[272]. Schröder[284] briefly described catatonia and delirium after childbirth, and extensive sinus thrombosis at necropsy. In six, delirium, raving, stupor or memory disorder was a minor feature in a neurological disorder[75,280,285–288]. Two had no necropsy proof[289,290]. These are the others:

A 21-year old developed headache, vomiting and convulsions 20 days after her 1st delivery. A week later she became excited, restless, noisy and violent, and needed restraint. There was clouding of consciousness. She had aphasia and right-sided Jacksonan fits. She died a few days later. Necropsy showed extensive thrombosis of the cerebral sinuses and veins[291].

A 35-year old had a brief attack of agitation after giving birth to her 3rd child. On day 7 after her 4th delivery she developed agitation and mental confusion. On day 15 she had a seizure, then a right facial palsy and left hemiparesis. Her temperature rose to 39°. On day 20 she sank into coma and died. Necropsy showed thrombophlebitis of the longitudinal and right lateral sinuses[292].

A 25-year old became pregnant for the 5th time and gave birth to twins. On day 11 she became confused, disorientated and hallucinated. She had a pelvic infection and high fever. She died, and necropsy showed thrombi in the sagittal and right transverse sinuses (case 12594)[280].

A 33-year old became confused five days after a normal pregnancy and delivery. She was thought to be suffering from 'puerperal psychosis'. Ten days later she developed a fever (104°) and right hemiplegia. The erythrocyte sedimentation rate was 75 mm in the 1st hour and she had a leucocytosis of 14,000/mm³. The EEG showed excess slow waves. An angiogram showed a right fronto-temporal mass and absent filling of the veins. She died and necropsy showed massive sinus thrombosis[293].

A 39-year old developed headache in the 38th week of her 2nd pregnancy. She had seizures, a blood pressure of 140/90, oedema and albuminuria, suggesting eclampsia. The infant was delivered by Caesarean section. Sixteen days later she developed headache, vomiting and *status epilepticus*. Her temperature was 102° and she had pus in the eye. She was drowsy and disorientated. Lumbar puncture showed purulent meningitis. Necropsy showed thrombus in the superior longitudinal sinus and pelvic veins (case 19)[253].

A 44-year old developed pleurisy and leg vein thrombosis (involving the vena cava) soon after childbirth. Admitted to hospital she was confused and disorientated, rambling and talking incessantly. Several weeks later she showed alternating periods of lucidity and incoherence. After treatment with penicillin she improved, but was still depressed and hallucinated with 'hysterical' outbursts. She suffered pulmonary infarcts and swelling of the left arm. The phlebitis diminished but she remained noisy, restless and difficult at night, and began to express delusional ideas. She died eleven months after admission. Necropsy showed pulmonary embolism, haemorrhagic pericarditis and dilatation of the veins in the fissure of Rolando, with softening of the white matter. There was no information about thrombi in the sinuses, so this may have been thrombophlebitis migrans with involvement of the cerebral veins (case 21)[253].

The following recent case had no necropsy proof, but the diagnosis was established by an MRI scan[294]:

A 28-year old suffered from hyperemesis during pregnancy. Eight days after the birth she presented with euphoria, repetitive hair-brushing, aggressive tendencies and (later) mutism. She expressed the idea that her infant had special powers, and wished to harm it and herself. She complained of left-sided retro-orbital headache, but had no neurological symptoms. Blood tests showed a raised platelet count, fibrinogen and C-reactive protein. Lumbar puncture showed raised protein with nine red cells/cubic mm. An MRI scan showed a left transverse sinus thrombosis. She rapidly responded to heparin.

The psychiatric features were prominent, but all had some signs of an organic disorder.

Other Vascular Lesions

Stroke

There is an increased risk of stroke in pregnancy and the puerperium[257,295–297]. Arterial occlusions cause circumscribed lesions with mainly local effects, but they sometimes lead to impairment of consciousness. Milder cases will occasionally present with confusion in addition to hemiplegia and other neurological signs, as in this basilar artery thrombosis[298]:

A 37-year old was admitted about eight weeks into her 2nd pregnancy. She was lethargic, incoherent, disorientated, irrational and had impairment of memory for recent and remote events. She had motor paralysis of the right 5th nerve, nystagmus, an enlarged right pupil, ankle clonus and sensory impairment on the right side. She died five days later and necropsy showed a basilar artery thrombosis with encephalomalacia of the left cerebellar hemisphere.

Amniotic Fluid Embolism

Pulmonary embolism by vernix, meconium or placental fragments contained in amniotic fluid[299] may be quite common[300,301]. King[302] stated that it could cause confusion and convulsions during labour or immediately afterwards.

Air Embolism

Air embolism is recognized as a rare cause of maternal death. Churchill[303] described this case:

> A 26-year old gave birth to her 4th child. Seven days later she suddenly became insensible, with twitching of the face. On recovery after a few days she had a right hemiplegia and difficulty in speaking. Later that day she had another attack of more complete paralysis. She continued to improve until, a month after the birth, laughing heartily at some remark of her sister's, she suddenly said, "Oh dear!" and died. On opening the dura mater every blood vessel contained bubbles of air.

The authority is Rangell[304], who cited several cases from the nineteenth century. The circumstances include:

- Criminal abortion
- Investigations using air under pressure
- Surgical treatment of placenta praevia
- The use of a uterine douche to free an adherent placenta
- Postpartum knee-chest exercises, resulting in an inrush of air under pressure

He collected 17 cases that occurred in an apparently normal puerperium. In multiparous women, the uterus could be atonic, or its sinuses held open by retained products. Most of these patients died suddenly or rapidly. Embolization of the cerebral vessels can occur; air has sometimes been found in the cerebral arteries, and even the cerebral veins or the longitudinal sinus. Some patients have seizures and a few had a brief period of delirium. It is possible that those with a favourable outcome would show a mild cerebral disturbance. He described this unique case:

> A 24-year old gave birth to her 2nd child. On day 6 she commenced knee-chest exercises. She immediately let out a moan and cried for help. She was lying rigid with all limbs extended, hands supinated and feet plantar-flexed. She screamed through clenched teeth. Her pupils became dilated and she lapsed into coma. The following day she was febrile (104°). A diagnosis of subarachnoid haemorrhage was made, but the CSF was clear, with a raised protein (78 mg/100 ml). She had a Jacksonian convulsion, beginning in the right leg, then developed *status epilepticus*. On day 10 she became confused and apprehensive, screamed with fright, and became so noisy, overactive and unmanageable that she was transferred to a psychiatric hospital. Her mood changed rapidly from a facetious euphoria with giggling and laughing to tearfulness and fear. She would beg to be pulled down on to the bed, so that her 'floating' would stop – the entire room was swinging back and forth. Everything was rotated through 90°, so that she seemed to be standing up, with the ceiling directly in front, and other people lying on their backs. She saw a non-existent clock on the wall, spoke about a man in the room who vanished, and complained of green and grey sticky fluid on

the sheet that she tried to brush away. She asked for a baby to be removed from the foot of her bed, saying that it might be her husband. She believed she was still in the obstetric hospital, and had lost all recall of the week following her first seizure. This mental state continued for four days. She improved rapidly with patchy memories of her illness.

This appears to be the only well documented case of arterial embolism resulting in a postpartum psychosis – and some of the symptoms were atypical of delirium.

Postpartum Cerebral Angiopathy

In 1979, Rascol[305] described a new puerperal arteriopathy, of which about 30 cases have been described. The disorder had already been reported in cocaine or amphetamine addicts. A few days after a normal pregnancy, these mothers present with headache, vomiting, seizures and focal neurological signs. The CAT scan may show cerebral oedema, especially in the posterior brain. The symptoms clear up completely after a few days. The defining investigation is a cerebral angiogram, which shows multiple segmental stenoses and dilatations in the medium-calibre cerebral arteries – like a string of sausages. When the angiograms were repeated after recovery, the vessels had returned to normal – thus the disorder is vasospastic. In some puerperal cases, sympathomimetic agents, ergot derivatives or bromocriptine[306] have been implicated. The manifestations are mainly neurological, but include disturbances of consciousness.

Subarachnoid Haemorrhage

Apart from ruptured aneurysm (the most common cause), this can result from eclampsia[307,308] or cerebral venous thrombosis[309]. It usually presents with the sudden onset of headache and nuchal pain. The following patients developed a postpartum confusional state at some stage in the evolution of their illness[143,310]:

> A 32-year old gave birth to her 4th child. Eight days later she complained of headache and difficulties in balance. After four weeks she fell and was unconscious for some hours. She then lay in a state of torpor and was disorientated. She had a fever up to 39.5°. She improved but, eleven weeks later, again complained of headache and lost consciousness. When she came round she was excited and euphoric and had absurd ideas of persecution. Three months after the birth, she lost consciousness and died.

> Thirty-six hours after her 3rd child was born, a 27-year old appeared drowsy, and responded neither to her husband nor the baby. She vomited, and remained mute throughout the day, refusing to eat or drink. The following morning she was still mute, and maintained uncomfortable postures. On admission to a psychiatric ward she had a fever of 100° and was in stupor. She had a stiff neck. The CSF contained blood, and the EEG showed slow waves. She recovered during the next seven weeks, although she had a seizure nine months later.

Subdural Haematoma

Epidural anaesthesia gives the best pain relief during labour. Serious complications are rare – 1 in 4,000 cases. They include direct trauma to the cord or nerve roots, toxic venous injection, meningitis or epidural abscess, anaphylactic shock, spinal cord infarction and epidural or subdural haematoma. Jack[311] described this case:

> A 29-year old presented with hypertension at 36 weeks gestation in her 3rd pregnancy. At 38 weeks, labour was induced. The Tuohy needle became filled with blood. Since the baby was

promptly delivered, the procedure was abandoned. On day 4 she was awakened by headache and neck pain. On day 5 she had dizziness and vomiting that persisted for several days. On day 12 she improved, but headache returned. From day 18 she became drowsy, weak and disorientated, with a poor memory. She was unable to stand, her left eyelid drooped, and she was found to have ophthalmoplegia and haemorrhagic papilloedema. She lapsed into coma. Carotid angiography showed large bilateral subdural haematomas, which were evacuated. She made a gradual but complete recovery.

Jack reviewed 11 earlier cases, and at least 19 others have since been described; they are often bilateral. Although the full syndrome usually takes days to evolve, the onset has occurred as early as the second day. Post-epidural headache or persistent leakage of cerebrospinal fluid can be treated by an epidural blood patch, but this does not always prevent the complication. The salient symptom is headache dating from the dural puncture, with a gradual onset of vomiting, photophobia and neurological symptoms such as convulsions, paraesthesiae, ataxia, dysphasia, blurred vision, ptosis, ophthalmoplegia, papilloedema, neck stiffness or hemiparesis. Drowsiness and somnolence are common, and confusion has been reported. Two of Jack's patients were confused. Here are two others with psychiatric presentations[312,313]:

A 33-year was delivered of her first child by Caesarean section, performed under lumbar-subarachnoid anaesthesia. On day 4 she complained of headache, worse in the erect position. She improved and was discharged on day 9. One week later she presented with headache, vomiting and disorientation. She opened her eyes in response to her name, but did not react to commands. A CAT scan showed a left fronto-temporal haematoma, which was drained by a burr-hole, and she recovered.

A 21-year old gave birth to her first child under epidural anaesthesia. The following day she developed severe headache. In the next 10 days she had mood swings and erratic disorganized behaviour towards the infant. On day 11 she made a suicide attempt and assaulted her son. A diagnosis of puerperal psychosis was made. She began to vomit, and complained of intolerable headache and blurred vision. She was found to have papilloedema. A CAT scan showed subdural haematomata. She was cured by burr hole drainage 5–6 weeks after delivery.

In addition there is this patient, who developed vasospasm in the branches of the middle cerebral artery that (unlike postpartum cerebral angiopathy) persisted for three months[314]:

A 30-year old gave birth to her second child under epidural anaesthesia. Seven hours later, she complained of headache that was not relieved by a blood patch. After a second blood patch on day 3 she developed mental confusion and agitation. A CAT scan was normal. On day 9 she developed seizures and a right hemiparesis. Transcranial Doppler ultrasonography and an MRI scan showed ischaemia in the left middle cerebral territory. Right arm weakness was still present three months later. Homonymous hemianopia persisted for at least 12 months.

The authors considered that the dural puncture or blood patch had caused cerebral vasospasm.

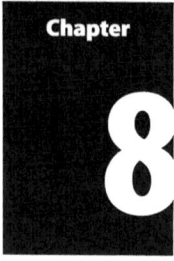

Other Specific Neuropsychiatric Disorders

8

This is an abridgement and updating of chapter 7 of *Eileithyia's Mischief*[1].

Epilepsy

Eclampsia and epilepsy are different disorders, but women with a lifelong epileptic history and without evidence of gestosis are also liable to convulsions in pregnancy, childbirth and the puerperium.

There are at least two forms of psychosis in patients with centrencephalic epilepsy.

- In close relationship to seizures, acute, transient psychoses can occur. The most common is the post-ictal psychosis, which may take the form of delirium, twilight states, or psychoses with mood disorder, delusions, visual and auditory hallucinations or catatonia[77,315]. As in eclampsia, there is often a lucid interval between the seizures and psychosis, ranging from one to six days.

- In the absence of seizures, patients with *petit mal* status may present with a transient recurrent confusional or twilight state, or an illness dominated by mood disorder and delusions, and are found to have electro-encephalographic signs of seizures without the motor phenomena. These psychoses have an abrupt onset and sometimes a sudden recovery[316–318].

It was established long ago that epilepsy is influenced by menstruation (see Section 5). One would therefore expect some effect of pregnancy. Seizures can be reduced or abolished in pregnancy, but also increased[319,320]. Epilepsy can develop for the first time, or return after a long interval. Fits can occur during labour[321]. Thus, the childbearing process has a variable and complex influence on epilepsy.

In the literature there are 31 cases in which epileptic seizures (probably not eclamptic) were a possible factor in the pathogenesis of childbearing psychoses. These are of a bewildering variety in onset, context and form. They include menstrual epilepsy[322], nocturnal seizures[323], absence states[324,325], twilight states[326] and hystero-epilepsy[327]. The onset of psychosis occurred throughout pregnancy and the postpartum period – in the 3rd month of gestation, in the 9th month, immediately before the onset of labour, during parturition, on day 1, on days 2–10, three weeks later, five weeks later and at eight months.

Prepartum Psychoses

Three mothers had onset during pregnancy[325,328,329] as in this example[325]:

A 24-year old was considered lazy, and had "attacks" at work every day or so, lasting up to a minute, when she would go blank and stare. She became pregnant, and in the 9th month took to her bed, mute and incontinent of urine. She was grimacing and making stereotyped movements, had to be fed and made strange remarks – "My sister has been burnt". She was transferred to the obstetric hospital for the birth, and returned after a fortnight in the same state. She knew nothing about her admission. Two weeks later she improved, and her relatives took her home.

Parturient Psychoses

These four mothers had onset during labour:

A woman with a history of epilepsy became depressed after her marriage, but recovered when pregnancy was diagnosed. When she went into labour she had a fit, followed by a 'violent maniacal disturbance' ('delirious excitement'). A live baby was extracted. She had no further fits and recovered uneventfully[330].

An 18-year old was subject to 'hystero-epilepsy' related to marital squabbles. When she became pregnant she had fewer attacks. At term she had another attack, and lost consciousness for 36 hours. During this time she gave birth without her knowledge, and without the knowledge of her household. When a midwife and doctor arrived, she was agitated and delirious, cried out, swore and fought. When she awoke (rather abruptly) she did not know where she was, and at first would not believe she had given birth[327].

In the other two cases it resulted in filicide:

A patient suffered from seizures in childhood and then menstrual epilepsy. After giving birth to her first child she had fits and *Tobsucht*; on the first night she threw her child into the yard, where it was eaten by dogs[322].

An epileptic woman had several similar attacks of *Dämmerzuständen* [twilight states] immediately after delivery; in the last of these she threw her two children out of a 4th storey window[331].

Postpartum Psychosis

Twelve patients had onset after the birth[59,95,223,225,310,324,326,332,334–336], as in this example[323]:

A patient had suffered from mainly nocturnal seizures since her menarche. When she became pregnant, they increased in severity and frequency. In the final week she had 20–25 nocturnal attacks. Her intelligence seemed clouded, with slow responses and difficulty in accomplishing simple acts. When she went into labour she suffered violent seizures, and needed six people to hold her down. In the first two days after delivery, she had no fits, but they then reappeared. Her appetite was insatiable. She became febrile (39°). She had violent crises, in which she became rigid, with staring eyes and clonic convulsions. Nineteen days after the birth psychiatric symptoms appeared – she spoke to herself, made piercing cries, had to be restrained, sang at the top of her voice and believed she was being electrocuted. Her temperature rose to 41.2° and she was found to have albuminuria. This lasted for three days, and two weeks later she was discharged well.

The next case was mentioned to me by a colleague. Although the episodes were brief, the case is unique because there was a recurrence after the next delivery:

A 42-year old had a history of temporal lobe and grand mal epilepsy, possibly related to her menses. She had two children. After each birth she suddenly ('like turning on a switch') developed ideas of poisoning. The 1st time the duration was 2–3 hours, the 2nd time 24 hours. In each case recovery was sudden. Later she had four attacks of panic and agitation with persecutory ideas, with some evidence of premenstrual onset.

As for frequency, Gregory[337] diagnosed three epileptic psychoses among 118 cases of puerperal psychosis; all had suffered from epilepsy for years, with post-epileptic excitement or confusion. Sivadon[225] had one among his 145 puerperal psychoses.

Mothers with No History of Epilepsy

Another seven patients had no seizures before the first child was born, but developed epilepsy and psychosis as a sequel to pregnancy[88,324,338–341]. Three had prepartum onset[88,326,340], and the rest postpartum episodes. This patient had a prepartum episode after several postpartum attacks[326]:

> A mother had her first epileptic fit three days after giving birth to her 1st child, then suffered fits every 2–4 weeks. After her 4th infant was born, she was briefly confused. Five weeks after her 5th birth, she had a seizure followed by a severe hallucinatory disturbance; three weeks later; after many more fits, she was discharged well. Five weeks after her next birth she was in the same state. Since then she suffered many seizures, absences and twilight states. After two normal births, she had a third episode of hallucinatory confusion starting shortly before the birth, lasting four weeks.

In my series, a mother with evidence of brain damage and epilepsy suffered an atypical episodic psychosis, with one early onset puerperal episode:

> A 7-year old was referred to a child guidance clinic with a conduct disorder. At 24 she gave birth to her 1st child and remained well for a year. Fourteen months after the birth she developed a psychosis with various delusions and auditory and visual hallucinations; during an 18-month hospital admission she set fire to herself. The infant was removed and adopted away. She was married and divorced, then at 35 had another child that lived only an hour. At 37, after several miscarriages, she gave birth to her 3rd child. On day 10 she developed a psychosis with delusions and visual hallucinations. She was admitted to the Queen Elizabeth mother & baby unit for diagnosis and a trial of mothering, and remained there for most of the next two years. She was a devoted mother, but was subject to brief bouts of agitation associated with unusual delusions – for example that her baby had been exchanged for another child, or his eyes had changed colour – together with confusion and disorientation. She had an abnormal EEG with frontal and generalized sharp waves. Magnetic resonance imaging showed cortical atrophy with metallic deposits in the pallidum and thalamus. Lamotrigine shortened episodes and reduced their frequency. After a prolonged battle in the courts, she was allowed to keep her child, and mothered him successfully for some years, in spite of continued episodes.

The 'epileptic psychoses' associated with childbearing defy classification, because no two cases are alike.

Withdrawal of Ethanol and Other Sedative Drugs

The story of foetal alcohol syndrome[333,342] testifies to the severity of ethanol abuse during pregnancy. The infant's blood level may be so high that an alcoholic foetor surrounds the incubator[343]. Ethanol has many effects on mental health, and one must distinguish between alcoholic intoxication and withdrawal syndromes (especially *delirium tremens*). Ethanol has been used as an anaesthetic during labour (see Section 3).

Ethanol Withdrawal during Parturition

Several reviews have made general statements, or mentioned cases without giving a convincing description[88,162,337,344,345,347–349]. Herzer[350], analysing 25 years experience of

221 puerperal illnesses in Basel, claimed that four patients had *delirium tremens* in the puerperium and two in the lactation phase. It is, however, hard to find a convincing case description. There are several mothers in whom *delirium tremens* seemed likely, though not beyond doubt[344,351–355]. The following case unequivocally exemplifies puerperal (and post-operative) *delirium tremens*[356]:

> A 37-year old presented at the end of her 7th pregnancy. She had a strong odour of alcohol on her breath, slurred speech and generalized tremor, which was thought to be early *delirium tremens*. During labour she was irrational, and gave birth with one violent push, causing a cervical laceration extending into the uterus. She had an emergency hysterectomy. Her postpartum course was complicated by hallucinations, agitation and generalized tremors. On day 4 she became aware of her surroundings. The infant also had withdrawal symptoms.

Alcoholic Hallucinosis

Dupouy[223] described two cases in the first postpartum year. This is one of them:

> A 25-year old drank wine, rum and absinthe. She gave birth to two infants, the second in August 1903. In March 1904 she began to hear voices – a neighbour said her feet smelt, she had lice, battered her infants, had erotic ideas, was a prostitute, thought her husband was a murderer and that she and her children would die. She responded angrily to these voices, and, to escape them, tried to jump out of the window. She tried to hang herself, then recovered (case 25).

Other Sedative Drugs

In the literature there are two cases related to other drugs of addiction. This fatality occurred in an opium addict[357]:

> A 21-year old gave birth to her 1st child. On the 3rd night she was sleepless and, next morning, had a fever of 102°. By noon she was violently insane. She asked for a laudanum bottle. Her husband said, "That is the first sane remark she has made for three days. She is an opium eater". She consumed laudanum by the pint before her confinement; she could not sleep without it and drank from the bottle. The doctor gave her an injection of 30 mg morphine. She slept an hour. Her temperature rose to 106°, and she died.

This mother suffered from barbiturate withdrawal[358]:

> A woman had been taking barbiturates in increasing doses for years, and latterly 30 grains of sodium amytal daily. Two days after admission to the maternity unit she became restless, sleepless and excited. She was wandering up and down the ward at night, and screamed abuse at the night nurse. The next morning she was confused, disorientated and visually hallucinated. A few hours later she had several seizures. She remained confused for several days, then gradually recovered.

Hypopituitarism

Pituitary Necrosis from Postpartum Haemorrhage

The anterior pituitary produces follicle-stimulating hormone, luteinising hormone, adrenal corticotrophic hormone, growth hormone and thyroid stimulating hormone. Loss of these hormones causes the failure of lactation and menstruation, genital atrophy, shrinkage of the breasts, loss of pubic and axillary hair, and of libido. Simpson[359] was aware of wasting constitutional diseases that followed parturition, although it was not until 30 years later that the pituitary lesion was identified. Glinski[361] observed two fatal postpartum cases and found the pituitary lesion in both. Simmonds[362] published this case:

> A 35-year old had severe puerperal sepsis after the birth of her 5th child. She remained weak, emaciated and amenorrhoeic. Eleven years later she lapsed into coma and died. Necropsy showed atrophy of her pituitary, especially the anterior lobe.

Sheehan[363] described 11 early cases, dying between 14 hours and 30 days post partum. There was necrosis of the anterior pituitary, with the appearance of an infarct, which he considered to be due to thrombosis, not embolism. He[271] defined the syndrome after a clinico-pathological analysis of more than 120 cases – 54 of his own, and the rest from the literature; he included 32 who survived at least a year, and had necropsy confirmation. The most common cause was severe postpartum haemorrhage or circulatory collapse. The pituitary is vulnerable because, in pregnancy, it becomes vascular and doubles in size. But pituitary destruction has many other causes, including surgery, tumours, gummata, tuberculosis and other granulomas. In a third paper[364] he focused on 95 cases with necropsy proof. More than 50 per cent pituitary loss was necessary for symptoms, and 95 per cent for severe symptoms. The incidence was about 0.2/1,000 for severe cases, plus 0.7/1,000 milder cases. His contribution was completed by a monograph[365]. The thoroughness of the work led many to rename the puerperal disorder 'Sheehan's syndrome'. Diagnosis is often delayed for years[366]. There seem to be limited data on worldwide distribution, but recent papers have reported large series from Anatolia and South Eastern Turkey – a hint that this disease may be more common in countries with high birth rates[367–369].

Psychiatric Complications

In hypopituitarism there are general symptoms, such as weakness, apathy and sensitivity to cold resembling myxoedema, to which Addisonian crisis, with hypoglycaemia, hyponatraemia and hypochloraemia, may also contribute[370–371]. In addition the literature contains at least 20 cases of chronic psychoses (confusional, depressive or delusional) starting 3–30 years after the postpartum crisis, often developing insidiously after a long delay. These are irrelevant to puerperal mental disorders. Many of Sheehan's own patients, in whom the diagnosis was made the day after delivery, remained remarkably well in the early stages. This suggests that the cerebral effects of hypothyroidism, hypoglycaemia or hyponatraemia take a long time to develop.

But there are also, less commonly, acute psychoses[372–378]. Most have been associated with hypoglycaemia, but two had hypothermia[376], and one also had hyponatraemia[378]; in one patient, recurrent hypoglycaemia led to nine attacks of delirium[373]. The conditions for psychosis exist in the early stages. Several mothers, within 10 days of a severe postpartum haemorrhage, have developed hyponatraemia[379–382]. One developed hypoglycaemic coma 14 hours after delivery and emergency hysterectomy[383] and one had both hyponatraemia and hypoglycaemia[366].

Against this background, there are ten cases in which acute pituitary necrosis has possibly caused a postpartum psychosis. The first two had onset within a few days of the birth, but infection may have contributed:

> A 41-year old had a severe haemorrhage after her 9th child was born. On day 4 she developed fever, and on day 5 agitation and mental confusion. On day 11 she was transferred to a psychiatric clinic

with disorientation, logorrhoea and hallucinations (visual & auditory). She was profoundly anaemic. She died 15 days after the birth. Necropsy showed necrosis of the pituitary[384].

A 30-year old collapsed 36 hours after the birth of the first twin in her first delivery. She became delirious, lapsed into coma and died. Necropsy showed widespread bronchopneumonia, in addition to a large retroplacental blood clot and necrosis of the anterior pituitary (case 4)[363].

This case, however, with onset on day 1, had no other factor:

A 41-year old gave rapid birth for the 8th time. The placenta was retained and she had a severe haemorrhage with collapse. Later that day she became mentally confused and died 27 hours post partum. Nearly the whole of the anterior lobe of the pituitary was in a state of early necrosis (case 2)[363].

In four mothers the onset was later, but within three weeks. The first was mild, but she was treated promptly. In all the diagnosis was established by CAT scanning:

A 27-year old gave birth to a healthy infant, after which she had a 2-litre haemorrhage, with shock. One week later, she complained of headache and weakness, paraesthesia, slurred speech and somnolence; she was 'obtunded'. Her serum sodium was 111 mE/L and blood sugar 5.5 mMol/L. She had low corticotropin and cortisol levels, and very low prolactin, but normal thyroid hormones. A CAT scan showed pituitary infarction[385].

A 23-year old gave birth to her 1st child, with unspecified 'complications'; lactation failed and she remained amenorrhoeic. After 15–20 days she became apathetic, and some days later fearful, complaining that people were out to harm her; she heard voices and had delusions of infidelity. Investigations showed low levels of cortisol, thyroid hormones, LH and FSH. A CAT scan showed an empty *sella turcica*. All symptoms responded to prednisolone and thyroxin[386].

A 25-year old was admitted with confusion two weeks after childbirth. She was hypotensive (BP 80/40) with bradycardia (40–50/min). A CAT scan showed patchy pituitary necrosis[387].

A 31-year old gave birth to her 1st child, and suffered a postpartum haemorrhage. Within 16–18 days she became fearful and expressed the idea that her friends and family were spying on her; she could hear them conspiring to harm her. She slept only a few hours/day, talked to herself, neglected her hygiene and dressed in unusual clothes. She failed to lactate or menstruate. When she was brought to the hospital four months later, she had signs of myxoedema. She was unkempt and apathetic, her speech irrelevant and incoherent. She had low levels of FSH, LH, thyroid hormones and cortisol. A CAT scan showed a partly empty *sella turcica*. She improved with thyroid and steroid hormones[388].

The others had later or uncertain onset within the first postpartum year:

A woman presented with a confused and dream-like puerperal psychosis associated with an adrenal syndrome - cachexia, asthenia, pallor, extreme hypotension and large plaques of brown pigmentation over the whole abdomen. She responded to hormonal therapy[389].

A 32-year old had a severe post-partum haemorrhage, with retention of the placenta and shock. Her haemoglobin fell to 5.5 g/100 ml. She failed to lactate, and her periods failed to return. Three months later she had an attack of confusion and drowsiness, from which she recovered spontaneously. Two weeks later she was readmitted in stupor. Her blood sugar was 41 mg/100 ml. She responded to treatment by glucose and steroids, but her blood sugar continued to fluctuate between 24 and 76 mg/100 ml[373].

A 40-year old suffered postpartum haemorrhage and shock, after which she became indifferent and laconic, neglected her household, lost track of events and had bouts of confusion and disorientation. Four years later she lapsed into coma with a temperature of 35.5°. She responded to hormone treatment (case 1)[376].

One can conclude that conditions exist for the development of a psychosis as an early complication of postpartum pituitary necrosis.

Water Intoxication

Sheehan's syndrome is one cause of hyponatraemia after childbirth. Another is water intoxication. This was described by Rowntree[390]. Its manifestations include polyuria and pollakiuria (frequent urination), salivation, nausea and vomiting, restlessness, tremor and muscular twitching, ataxia, seizures, coma and death. There is an increase in intracranial pressure. Postpartum water intoxication can be due to the antidiuretic action of oxytocin, or to polydipsia.

Du Vigneaud discovered oxytocin in 1954, and synthesized it a year later. Its main action is on the myometrium and breasts. It was introduced into clinical practice in 1959, in the treatment of postpartum haemorrhage, to accelerate normal labour or to evacuate the uterus in abortion, hydatidiform mole, mid-trimester pregnancy or foetal death *in utero*. But it is structurally similar to vasopressin, another octopeptide produced by the posterior pituitary, whose main effect is anti-diuretic. Water intoxication due to the therapeutic use of oxytocin was first described in 1962[391]:

> A single woman became pregnant, but foetal movements ceased at 22 weeks. She presented at 30 weeks with a missed abortion. In order to evacuate the uterus, she was given 820 units of oxytocin with 4.5 litres of 5% dextrose in ten hours. She had a seizure, and became irritable, drowsy and confused. Her serum sodium eleven hours after the seizure was 124 mEq/litre. She recovered within 24 hours.

By 1975, 23 cases had been reported[392]. At least two were fatal[393,394], and one mother, who survived, could no longer read or write[395]. Necropsy has shown generalized oedema including the brain. Usually these patients have a seizure, and lapse into coma. They may pass through a phase of delirium as they recover. The following three patients presented with delirium, although other signs soon appeared:

> A 15-year old concealed her pregnancy. She developed hypertension (BP 155/100) and albumin-uria. She gave birth to a live child but, to treat haemorrhage, was given an infusion of 80 units of oxytocin in four litres of 5% dextrose. She became excitable and incoherent. Soon afterwards she had a seizure, and lapsed into stupor. Her serum sodium was 110 mEq/l. With the infusion of 5% sodium chloride she recovered within 24 hours[396].

> An 18-year old was given an infusion of oxytocin and dextrose to induce an abortion. After she had received 140 units and 3½ litres of dextrose, she had a seizure and vomited. She was stuporose and disorientated with widely dilated pupils. Serum sodium was 112 mEq/l. The EEG showed bilateral slowing. Treated by diuretics and 3% sodium chloride solution, she remained disorientated for two days, then recovered[394].

> A 24-year old was given an infusion of oxytocin and dextrose (10 units/litre) to induce an abortion. While the 4th and 5th litres were being infused, she became restless, drowsy and confused. She vomited twice, and was found on the floor in coma. Her serum sodium was only 100 mEq/l. She was discharged well five days later, with amnesia for the period of coma[392].

The introduction of prostaglandins has reduced the need for prolonged oxytocin infusion.

Other women have developed hyponatraemia from drinking too much water. One woman in labour drank seven litres of water in less than 12 hours, and also received a small dose of oxytocin: her serum sodium was 118 mEq/litre; her symptoms were drowsiness and unintelligible responses[397]. As in other cases, the infant was also hyponatraemic. One of my colleagues saw this case:

> A 26-year old fitness instructor was referred with a provisional diagnosis of puerperal psychosis five days after childbirth. She had been drinking excessive quantities of water – 16 pints in a day – on instruction from the midwife, to aid breast-feeding. She had a serum sodium of 121 mM/L. She was restless and agitated, mimicked contractions and said she needed to get the baby out. She thought it was September (actually April). She was reliving her mother's birth. With fluid restriction she became lucid in two hours, and recovered the following day.

Hyperammonaemia

About 80 per cent of nitrogen is excreted as urea in the liver, through a series of reactions called the Krebs–Henseleit urea cycle. Six enzymes are involved – two in the formation of carbamoyl phosphate (carbamoyl phosphate synthetase 1, and N-acetyl glutamate synthetase), and four in the generation of citrulline from ornithine (ornithine transcarbamoylase), arginosuccinate from citrulline (arginosuccinate synthetase), arginine from arginosuccinate (arginine succinate lyase) and ornithine plus urea from arginine (arginase). Deficiency of each of these enzymes results in hyperammonaemia. These inborn errors of metabolism usually result in symptoms from birth, and are rapidly fatal unless steps are taken to reduce protein intake, remove ammonia or replace intermediates in the urea cycle. But adult disorders can develop in the milder variants, and in heterozygotes. The overall incidence of urea cycle disorders is about 1/8,000[398]. Those at risk can be identified by various metabolic challenges or by pedigree and mutation analysis. Hyperammonaemic encephalopathy presents with lethargy, vomiting and coma. The cause of death is cerebral oedema, with flattened gyri and herniation of the cerebellar tonsils. It can be treated by haemodialysis, and with sodium benzoate, sodium phenylacetate or arginine hydrochloride.

Arginosuccinate Synthetase Deficiency

This is an autosomal recessive disorder. Yamada[399] described the first case of postpartum psychosis due to a urea cycle disorder.[a] This and two others are summarized in the following:

> A 24-year old developed fever, headache and fatigue, and lost consciousness for a week. She was 13 weeks pregnant. In September, at 36 weeks gestation, she gave birth to a son. On day 3 she became drowsy and almost mute with impaired consciousness. Hepatic encephalopathy was suspected. Her blood citrulline was 50 times normal[399].

> A 24-year old Bolivian woman developed occasional headache, dizziness and confusion. In the 19th week of her 1st pregnancy she lost 10 kg, and developed restlessness, abnormal behaviour and a disturbance of consciousness. She had hyperammonaemia. The pregnancy was terminated, but she had brain atrophy and died eight months later. Arginosuccinate synthetase was undetectable in her liver[400,401].

---

[a] I thank Yumi Okumura for translating this article.

After her 1st (Caesarean) delivery, a woman developed speech and gait abnormalities lasting several days. After giving birth to her 2nd child, she was admitted to a psychiatric ward with memory loss, aggressive behaviour, agitation, incoherent speech and disorientation; she lapsed into coma for three days, thought to be due to hepatic encephalopathy. On the day following her 3rd birth she developed confusion, disorientation and lethargy. Her blood ammonia was 422 μmol/L (normal 37). A diagnosis of acute yellow atrophy of the liver was made. Plasma citrulline was 594 μmol/L (normal 47), glutamine 936 μmol/L (normal 832) and urine orotic acid 4.28 μmol/L (normal 0.98). She was found to be suffering from arginosuccinate synthetase deficiency[398].

Another article reported three more postpartum cases, with scanty clinical details[402].

Ornithine Carbamoyltransferase Deficiency

In 1962, this inborn error of metabolism was described in two cousins with learning disability[403]. It proved to be an X-linked disorder, the most common of the enzyme disorders involved in urea synthesis, with an incidence of 1/30,000. Asymptomatic female carriers have raised plasma glutamine and alanine, and reduced arginine and citrulline. They are at risk of hyperammonaemic encephalopathy[404,405], especially in the puerperium. In addition to the following four cases, there may be three others: two died after childbirth and the third had nervous symptoms on day 3, thought to be due to emotional maladjustment[406].

A 21-year old gave birth at 38 weeks. Eight days later she developed headache and confusion. She became uncommunicative and was admitted to a psychiatric hospital. The initial diagnosis was postpartum depression. Within 24 hours (11 days postpartum) she became comatose and developed seizures. She had decorticate posturing, bilateral Babinski signs, dilated pupils and papilloedema. A diagnosis of subarachnoid haemorrhage was made, but the cerebro-spinal fluid did not contain blood. Her plasma ammonium was 411 μmol/L (normal <40), and glutamine 1097 μmol/L (normal 337–673). Urinary orotate level was 84 μmol/mmol creatinine (normal <2). She died and necropsy showed flattening of the gyri and herniation of the cerebellar tonsils (case 1)[407].

A 22-year old was known to be a carrier of this inborn metabolic error. Three days after childbirth she developed vomiting, diplopia, ataxia and somnolence. She was admitted to hospital 12 days after the birth. Her symptoms were attributed to postpartum emotional adjustment. She was found to have a plasma ammonium of 211 μmol/L. Treated with sodium benzoate and sodium phenylacetate, she recovered in six days (case 2)[407].

A 28-year old *multipara*, who had childhood seizures and disliked meat, developed pyelonephritis in the 31st week of pregnancy and went into labour. An infant was delivered by Caesarean section under spinal anaesthesia. On day 3 she developed vomiting, headache, fever (103°), confusion, lethargy and delirium, progressing to coma in six hours. The EEG showed diffuse slow waves. The infant became ill; a diagnosis of ornithine transcarbamylase deficiency was made, and he was treated by liver transplantation. The patient was also found to have a high serum ammonia level (180 μmol/L). A tomogram showed cerebral oedema. Treated with lactulose, her serum ammonia returned to normal in two days. She regained consciousness with amnesia for the postpartum period[408].

A 24-year old, heterozygous for ornithine transcarbamoylase deficiency, had one normal pregnancy leading to the birth of an unaffected girl, then, after the birth of unaffected boys, two more births complicated by mental state changes on day 3. In her 4th delivery (also of an unaffected boy) her blood ammonia rose alarmingly, but she was stabilised by sodium benzoate[406].

Several reasons have been suggested for the timing of these episodes. One theory, based on the birth of normal boys, is that the unaffected foetal liver detoxifies maternal ammonia until delivery. Another emphasizes the metabolic load imposed by the involution of the uterus. The risk of postpartum psychosis is not high: an 18-year study of 76 asymptomatic carriers who had 260 pregnancies showed that only 3 experienced episodes of coma as adults – one following surgery for a leg fracture, one following a traffic accident and one (at 19) for no known reason; none had a postpartum episode[404].

Carbamoyl Phosphate Synthetase I Deficiency

This is an autosomal recessive disorder. Wong[409] described this case:

> A 26-year old, who had a self-selected vegetarian diet, had a history of occasional bouts of confusion and disorientation. At the end of her 1st pregnancy she had another just before the onset of labour. Ten hours after delivery she became disorientated and agitated. Within a few hours she was in coma, and 24 hours later had generalized seizures. Her blood ammonia was 1,000 μmol/l (normal 35). The EEG showed diffuse encephalopathy. She developed diabetes insipidus. Her glutamine level was 857 μmol/l (normal 578), glutamic acid 507 μmol/l (normal 24), alanine μmol/l 1,065 μmol/L (normal 373) and urine orotic acid 62 μmol/l (normal 60). Citrulline was normal. She died and necropsy showed cerebral oedema. The liver contained virtually no carbamoyl phosphate synthetase I.

This enzyme deficiency, and a fourth enzyme deficiency in this cycle (liver arginase deficiency[410]), have also been associated with possible cases of menstrual psychosis[411] (see Section 5).

Disorders of Calcium Metabolism

It is known that tetany can be associated with psychosis[412,413] and can occur during pregnancy and the puerperium[234,414]. Frankl–Hochwart[415] studied 55 cases, mainly in men, but a few started in pregnancy or the puerperium; one of his patients had her first attack in the 9th month of her 4th pregnancy, and further attacks in several other pregnancies. There is a conceivable connection between this obscure literature and hyperventilation (which can cause tetany): hyperventilation leads to respiratory alkalosis, cerebral vasoconstriction, hallucinations[416,417] and absence spells with retrograde amnesia[418]; during vigorous over-breathing the dominant EEG frequency can fall from 10 to 3[419], associated with impaired consciousness. There are two cases of postpartum psychosis associated with tetany[335,420]:

> A 36-year old was depressed and worried about the future of her only child during her second pregnancy. She sat for hours doing nothing, or spent days in bed. She suddenly fell off her chair in a fainting fit. She was vomiting continuously. She was admitted and delivered by forceps. The next day she became stuporous, disorientated and cataleptic, but recovered on the second day. Ten days later she had a seizure, after which she was restless, incoherent, disorientated and catatonic for 10 days. She had recurrent tetany. She took her own discharge against medical advice and there was no follow-up.

> A 30-year old was delivered by Caesarean section. Two months later she presented with 'depression', which included apathy, somnolence and faecal incontinence. She had at least one seizure. She had bilateral cataract, and low serum calcium, magnesium and parathyroid hormone. A diagnosis of 1° hypo-parathyroidism was made. On correction of her serum calcium, her psychosis improved.

Human Immunodeficiency Virus (HIV) Infection

In *Eileithyia's Mischief*[1] (page 303), I predicted that acquired immunodeficiency syndrome (AIDS) encephalitis would present in pregnancy or the puerperium and this has been claimed[421]:

> A 30-year old Haitian woman, 28 weeks pregnant and HIV-positive with herpes simplex vaginitis, was admitted with acute psychosis: she was disorientated, with auditory hallucinations. A diagnosis of AIDS-related dementia was made. A male infant weighing 1.7 kg was delivered by Caesarean section.

Anaemia

Pregnancy is a time of increased demand for iron and vitamins, and blood loss (often heavy) is an inevitable consequence of delivery; many puerperal women are significantly anaemic. From time to time, it has been claimed that the resulting anaemia is a cause of psychosis[68,422,423]; all cases had other causes for psychosis, or no psychosis at all. Iron deficiency anaemia does not in itself cause delirium, even when severe. Cyanocobalamin (vitamin B_{12}) deficiency can cause organic brain syndromes, even without anaemia[424–428], but this vitamin deficiency is not a puerperal problem. Folic acid deficiency does occur in pregnancy, and its association with puerperal psychosis in this case was supported by the response to treatment[429]:

> A 17-year old became depressed three months after her 1st delivery. She had episodes of confusion and disorientation, and frightening visual hallucinations of ugly threatening figures. In the next 19 months she was hospitalised and treated with ECT, with transitory benefit, and neuroleptic drugs. She was frequently placed in seclusion, took two overdoses and cut her wrists. She was found to have a macrocytic anaemia (haemoglobin 10.8 g/100 ml), with normal vitamin B_{12} but no detectable folic acid. Treated with intramuscular folic acid, she began to improve after seven days and recovered after ten days, remaining well.

Other Possible Causes

In the literature there are two interesting disorders that have been described only once. The first is a mysterious recurrent catatonia in the mother, which also affected the baby:

> A 44-year old lost six children from bowel disorders, one recently. In the 7th month of her 11th pregnancy, she was found unconscious. She had fever, but no other physical signs except dilated pupils and stiff cataleptic limbs. With chloroform she lost the stiffness, and slept peacefully for four hours. On waking she was unaware of what had happened. That evening she had another attack that continued for two hours, and four further attacks that day. Neither chloroform nor bromides had any effect. Two days later, attacks returned, and continued every day. Pilocarpine had a temporary effect, but atropine gave the best result, and was continued until she gave birth to a large healthy boy. For four days she remained well. On day 5, while breast-feeding, she suddenly became cataleptic. She had another attack two days later, then remained well during a 12-week follow-up period. The child developed the same cataleptic cramps as the mother, and died a few days later[430].

The second is a prepartum behavioural disturbance associated with hypersomnia.

> A single woman in her early 20s suddenly went berserk and caused extensive damage to her place of work. At home she threatened to stab family members and drown herself. Admitted to an asylum four days later, she had no symptoms and little memory of the incident. Two

months later she had another attack, threatened suicide, refused to eat and said she would be burnt; again, on admission, she appeared well. Two months afterwards she suddenly fell off her chair, unconscious with jerking of the arms and legs. When she came round, she cried out in fear that she would be killed, spoke with her mother (not present), and said she saw fire, blood and water into which she wanted to jump. This state lasted three days, after which she had no memory of it. Two months later she suddenly fell off her chair. She appeared to be in a state of natural sleep, but did not react to loud noises or needle pricks. After six hours she woke up, and was astonished to find herself in bed. In the next two months she had 13 similar attacks, when she would suddenly fall asleep: they occurred at any time, without any connection to events, and lasted five minutes to six hours, with an average of 15–20 minutes. The last attack occurred eight months after the first. She then gave birth to a healthy boy, and never had another attack[431].

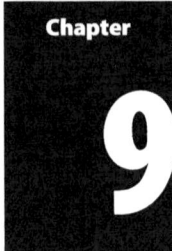

Chapter

9

Incidental Organic Psychoses

This is an abridgement and updating of chapter 8 of *Eileithyia's Mischief*[1].

Introduction

During the nine months of pregnancy and the first year after childbirth, a woman can develop organic psychoses with no known relation to the reproductive process. These are 'incidental psychoses'. The distinction between specific and incidental psychoses is illustrated by the venereal diseases. Any venereal disease can have a specific link with childbearing psychoses if it causes neuropsychiatric symptoms within 21 months of the sexual contact responsible for both infection and conception. But there have so far been no reports of prepartum or puerperal delirium resulting from gonococcal meningitis or temporal lobe encephalitis due to herpes simplex. The same is true of meningeal or meningo-vascular syphilis, which can cause CNS effects within a year of infection. So far, the only venereal disease with a specific link is AIDS encephalitis.

The incidental psychoses include neurosyphilis, meningitis, encephalitis, heart disease; respiratory, renal and hepatic failure; tumours and presenile dementia.

Neurosyphilis

There is a considerable literature on neurosyphilis (resulting from infection in the distant past) in pregnancy and the puerperium. These late effects include gummata and general paresis. At a time when syphilis was rife, several surveys found cases in the asylums[134,350,432–435]. Cristiani[436] gathered 23 puerperal cases from the world literature.

This mother, who denied a history of venereal disease (and it was not known when she became infected), had an illness that ran a fulminating course[437]:

> A 25-year old gave birth to her first child. On day 1 she became restless, and the next day disorientated with muddled speech. That afternoon she had a seizure, and then ten more, after which she was found to have a left hemiparesis. On day 3 she became doubly incontinent. On days 5–6 she developed pneumonia and died. She had a strongly positive Wassermann reaction. Necropsy showed acute meningo-encephalitis.

This woman developed her terminal illness during pregnancy[438]:

> A 42-year old had two children by her 1st marriage and four by her 2nd husband, who was treated for syphilis. During her 7th pregnancy, she became vague and confused, and had difficulty in walking. She was looking for objects she held in her hand, and called her husband when he was standing beside her. She was disorientated in time and place, and after hospitalisation, thought she was still at home; she said she had been at the theatre that evening and gave details of the play and

the people she had met. She seemed very happy. Two weeks later she died. She had a gumma in the right frontal lobe.

This mother presented in the puerperium[439]:

A 35-year old gave birth to her first child. On day 13 she left the clinic and was found, two days later, 30 kilometres away. She was somnolent, and did not remember the fugue. Three months later she was admitted to the asylum with a diagnosis of puerperal psychosis. She was confused, disorientated, passive and inert. She responded to all questions with, "I don't know." Her affect was of 'passive joy'. She had grandiose ideas about her wealth. She had severe defects of memory and knew neither the date of birth, nor the sex of her infant. She had dysarthria and unequal pupils. Her Wassermann reaction was positive.

This was reported recently from the United States[440]:

A 30-year old, 18 weeks pregnant with her 3rd child, suddenly started expressing ideas that she had several adult children, and could hear her unborn child crying. She was receiving messages from the television telling her to hurt herself. She was frightened and feared strangers would harm her. She was briefly admitted to hospital with a diagnosis of 'schizophrenia'. She became agitated, and said men were coming to take her baby away "the way they took my other babies away." On admission she was smiling and 'giddy'. Neuropsychiatric testing showed evidence of frontal lobe damage, and she had serum and CSF evidence of untreated syphilis. She recovered with penicillin.

Pre- and Postpartum Meningitis

Meningitis occasionally develops during pregnancy[441–444]. Commandeur[445] collected eight cases from the literature, and added one of his own:

A 29-year old nursed her husband and children with a febrile illness, and became ill herself at 7½ months gestation. Three days later she became extremely excited, scratching and biting; it required several people to restrain her. She had a bite on the leg and rabies was considered. She became comatose and died. She had a purulent meningitis from which both pneumococci and staphylococci were cultured.

Sheehan[271], among 360 women dying in pregnancy and puerperium, had 13 cases of meningitis – 8 pneumococcal, 3 tuberculous and 2 meningococcal. They usually developed during pregnancy, causing delirium, coma and seizures. Commandeur[445] also collected six cases of puerperal meningitis, of which three had fits, somnolence or coma, and three agitation or delirium, as in this example:

A *multipara* was admitted four hours after delivery. She had a rigor and fever (40°). In the night she was furiously delirious. The following day she had neck stiffness. She died three days later. Necropsy showed streptococcal meningitis.

Von Economo's Encephalitis

In Vienna, in the winter of 1916–1917, there was an epidemic of a new disease described by von Economo with the name *encephalitis lethargica*. The pathological lesions were mainly in the grey matter of the mesencephalon[446]. It spread to Paris in January 1918, and reached England later that year. The epidemic peaked in the autumn of 1919 and spring of 1920. The symptoms were headache, lethargy, eye palsies and fever, together with an overpowering desire to sleep. Parkinsonism was a sequel. Half the patients developed delirium or mania. Painless labour was reported in a number of cases[447]. This case had onset just before delivery:

> A 28-year old was sweet, calm and well-behaved by nature. At 8½ months gestation, she complained of headache and somnolence. Three days later she suddenly became agitated, hit out, threw anything she got her hands on, and said she saw thousands of snails on the walls. All night long she talked coherently on many subjects, showing an astonishing memory. This motor and verbal excitation continued for several days and nights. During the day she was somnolent, but kept up a continual verbigeration. Her character changed and she became violent and vulgar. One day, when she was sleepily passing urine, the infant's head appeared at the vulva; she showed no sign of pain. When presented with her baby, she claimed it was her sister's; it was hard to convince her she had given birth. In the puerperium she was profoundly sleepy and had to be shaken in order to feed. She developed diplopia and strabismus. Somnolence lasted six months, after which she was apathetic and behaved like an infant, with terrible rages. She had lost all affection for her family and remained in hospital[448].

Roques[449] published 21 cases, and from the literature collected 149 cases with onset in pregnancy, 63 of whom died; he stated that 7 per cent of female cases were pregnant. If convulsions, myoclonus or choreiform movements were prominent, it could be mistaken for eclampsia or *chorea gravidarum*. Delirium or confusion was found in 6 of his series. Three developed parkinsonism after delivery, and 4 during a subsequent pregnancy. He had only one puerperal case in his personal series, but found 22 in the literature, of whom 9 died. Alpers and Palmer[450] reviewed 37 cases, of which 19 were fatal; they claimed that the death rate was higher when the disease appeared during pregnancy. They found two puerperal cases, without mental illness but with recurrences in the next pregnancy followed by parkinsonism. This is one of them:

> A 27-year old developed *encephalitis lethargica* in the 3rd month of pregnancy. She was semi-stuporous for four weeks. She improved after seven weeks, and made a full recovery after delivery. But when she conceived again nine months later she had a recurrence and spent the whole pregnancy in bed. Parturition was almost painless. After delivery she developed parkinsonism.

N-Methyl-D-Aspartate Receptor (NMDAR) Encephalitis

Recently a new form of encephalitis has been discovered, associated with antibodies to the NMDA receptor, and often with ovarian teratomas; five of this last group developed early in pregnancy[451,452] and these three cases after delivery[453–455]:

> A 29-year old *primipara*, with a family history of bipolar disorder, presented eleven weeks postpartum with 2–3 weeks insomnia, memory difficulties and *déjà vu*. She kept asking why she had lost her memory, and was unable to recall three words. Admitted to hospital, she developed catatonia and delusions. Three days after ECT she had a seizure, and was noted to have athetosis, facial dyskinesia and chorea. An MRI scan showed three small dense areas. An abdominal mass was removed and proved to be an ovarian teratoma. She recovered.

> A 25-year old gave birth to a son. Seven weeks later she developed rhinorrhoea and malaise, then bizarre behaviour and *status epilepticus*. She was hypoventilating and had to be intubated. The CSF contained 61 mg/100 ml protein and 111 lymphocytes/ml; the erythrocyte sedimentation rate was 75 mm in the 1st hour and the EEG showed diffuse slowing. Anti-NMDA-antibodies were present. She recovered.

> A 25-year old presented three months after childbirth with delusions that there were demons in her body, who would kill her. Treated with risperidone, she became confused, and, because of

cog-wheel rigidity and raised creatinine phosphokinase levels, was thought to have a neuroleptic malignant syndrome. She failed to respond to treatment and had a seizure. NMDAR antibodies were found in the CSF, and an MRI scan showed an ovarian teratoma. After it was removed she dramatically improved and remained well.

Puerperal Encephalitis

This is a controversial subject. Lieb[456] published this case of encephalitis developing after delivery:

> Ten days after childbirth, a 31-year old got up and suddenly vomited. She returned to bed, and felt well for two days. She then failed to recognize her husband. She lay in bed, apathetic, mute, and incontinent of urine. Her lochia were foul-smelling and she had a slight fever (38.6°). Admitted to hospital, she lay in bed without moving, not responding to questions, but following things with her eyes. She had catalepsy in both arms, and flaccid paresis of the legs. Her temperature rose to 39.5°. She died six days after the onset. Necropsy showed encephalitis.

Lieb found 11 cases in the literature, of which 4 had onset in pregnancy, and 7 in the puerperium. Feuillade[457] reported seven more cases, of whom six died, but without necropsy confirmation. A considerable number of other cases have been claimed[458–464]. Five had necropsy confirmation, all from France in the early 1930s[225,465,466], as in this example[465]:

> Four days after childbirth, a 31-year old became sleepless and anxious about her infant's safety, whether she would have enough milk and whether she would go mad or die. On day 6 she was admitted to hospital confused, violently agitated and speaking nonsense. She rolled on the floor, hit out, tore out her sutures, refused food, and was completely sleepless. Her temperature was 40.7°. Two weeks after delivery she died in coma. Necropsy showed encephalitis.

The strongest claim for the importance of this form of puerperal illness was made by Marchand[466]. In four years (1930–1934), 27/175 women with prepartum or postpartum psychosis, admitted to Henri-Rousselle hospital, had a diagnosis of acute delirium due to encephalitis; fifteen had necropsies. The clinical picture was always acute delirium, sometimes with symptoms of metritis. This may have been a localised epidemic, similar to v. Economo's encephalitis, but it is possible that some special interpretation was being placed on infective psychoses.

More recently this case, somewhat resembling *encephalitis lethargica*, was published at length from the Czech Republic[467]:

> A 37-year old became pregnant after years of infertility. Nine weeks postpartum she suddenly developed a fever of 40°. She became confused and disorientated, and twice jumped from a height, suffering multiple fractures. She recovered and was discharged, but became depressed, sleepy and sluggish. She developed visual impairment and could only see fingers at one metre. She had to be helped with feeding, drinking and excretion, misidentified people and had visual hallucinations. For several months she lay motionless and unresponsive even to painful stimuli, as if quietly sleeping, a state resembling catatonic stupor. Nine months after the birth she suddenly awoke, spoke clearly and answered questions. She did not know where she was, or the date. She remembered many details, and complained of invincible drowsiness. She relapsed into stupor, but in the next few days several times returned to consciousness for half-an-hour. A year after the birth she gradually recovered, with a partial recall of what had happened. She had CSF and EEG evidence of an inflammatory cerebral process.

Miscellaneous Causes

Kinzel[468] reported this case of ischaemic heart disease, presenting as an organic psychosis:

> A 35-year old became disorientated two days after a Caesarean section. She failed to recognize her husband or newborn child. She was so restless that it required four nurses to keep her in bed. She shouted and cried, failed to answer questions and seemed not to understand. Her consciousness was clouded and she lapsed into stupor. She became breathless and died a few days later. She had suffered a myocardial infarction.

De Smit and de Waart[469] reported a case of puerperal amentia with a low level of ascorbic acid, cured by vitamin C.

Banzhaf[470] reported three cases of puerperal psychosis associated with space-occupying lesions of the brain, including this one:

> A healthy young woman gave birth, and then complained of increasing anxiety and incapacity, making numerous mistakes. She was from time to time confused. She had seizures and bouts of unconsciousness. On admission she had a paranoid-hallucinatory psychosis, and later an amnestic and confusional state. She was found to have an inoperable occipito-parietal tumour. Necropsy showed that this was an astrocytoma.

This case of meningioma presented with confusion on day 1[346]:

> A woman with a history of Fallot's tetralogy (corrected surgically) developed absence seizures in the 3rd trimester of her second pregnancy. On the first day after a Caesarean section, she had a 30-minute episode of confusion with auditory hallucinations and *déja vu*. She had no memory of the episode. She then had a seizure. An MRI scan showed a meningioma near the sphenoid bone, which was removed surgically.

There is a single case of Pick's presenile dementia presenting with a postpartum psychosis[360]:

> A 37-year old developed hyperphagia, hypersexuality, disinhibition and impaired judgment, together with depression, after the birth of her 3rd child. She failed to respond to anti-depressants, and was found to have fronto-temporal dementia.

King[302] mentioned a number of other systemic and metabolic diseases that can occur in pregnancy and the puerperium – renal failure, diabetic and hypoglycaemic coma, acute yellow atrophy of the liver, and the side effects of drugs including general anaesthetics, thiopentone and sulphonamides. All are known causes of confusion and coma, but there are no detailed case reports mimicking puerperal psychosis.

Summary

There are about 20 distinct neuropsychiatric disorders with a specific link to childbearing that can present with psychosis in pregnancy or the postpartum period. These organic psychoses account for about one-third of the childbearing psychoses reported in the literature.

Many are rare, some with only a single case description. Even those that used to be common (infective delirium and eclamptic psychosis) are now rare in high-income nations. But they may be prevalent in countries with high birth rates and high maternal morbidity. It is important to rescue and preserve knowledge of all the psychiatric complications of childbearing. Some of this knowledge has failed to cross language barriers, and some has been forgotten.

In many of these organic disorders, neurological or general medical symptoms predominate, with confusion or behaviour disturbances as a minor feature. But when psychiatric symptoms are prominent, this can lead to misdiagnosis.

The main forms of psychopathology seen are delirium and amnesic states. But severe, even fatal, organic disorders can present with a typical manic syndrome.

In addition to specific organic psychoses, there is a long list of infections and metabolic disorders that have occasionally caused sporadic complications in pregnancy or the puerperium.

References

1 Brockington IF. *Eileithyia's Mischief: the Organic Psychoses of Pregnancy, Parturition and the Puerperium*. Bredenbury: Eyry; 2006.

2 Hippocrates (5th Century BC). *Epidemics, books I and III*. Translated by WHS Jones, London, Heinemann; 1931.

3 Osiander FB. *Neue Denkwürdigkeiten für Ärzte und Geburtshelfer*. Volume 1. Göttingen: Rosenbusch; 1797. p. 52–89.

4 Brockington IF. *What Is Worth Knowing about 'Puerperal Psychosis'*. Bredenbury: Eyry; 2014.

5 Loudon I. *The Tragedy of Childbed Fever*. Oxford: Oxford University Press; 2000.

6 Burns J. *The principles of midwifery including the diseases of women and children*. London: Longman, Hurst, Rees, Orme & Brown; 1809. p. 275–279, 319–321.

7 Conolly J. Clinical lectures on the principal forms of insanity. Lecture 13. Description and treatment of puerperal insanity. *Lancet*. 1846;i:349–354.

8 Neumann KG. *Die Krankheiten des Vorstellungsvermögens*. Leipzig: Karl Knobloch; 1822. p. 152–175.

9 Leubuscher R. Über puerperalmanie. *Verhandlungen der Deutsche Gesellschaft für Geburtshilfe*. 1848;3:94–122.

10 Berndt. Bemerkungen über die Natur und die Behandlung der *Mania puerperalis*, und den Gebrauch des Kamphors in derselben, mit Beifügung einiger Krankheitsgeschichten. *Hufelands Journal der Practischen Heilkunde*. 1828;67:3–25.

11 Ritter Kiwisch v, Rotterau FA. *Die Krankheiten der Wöchnerinnen*. Part 2. Prague: JG Calve; 1841. p. 228–261.

12 Guislain J. *Leçons Orales sur les Phrénopathies ou Traité Théorique et Pratique des Maladies Mentales*. Paris: Baillière; 1852. p. 356.

13 Grant JA. Puerperal mania the result of metritic irritation from imperfectly developed scarlatinal exanthemata. *Canada Medical Journal*. 1865;1: 313–316.

14 Holm RA. Om Puerperalafsindighed. *Hospitals-Tidende*. 2nd series. 1874;15: 229–242, 245–250, 262–267 and 273–282.

15 Chaslin P. La confusion mentale primitive. *Annales Médico-psychologiques*. 7th series. 1892;16:225–273.

16 Bonhöffer K. *Die Symptomatische Psychosen*. Leipzig and Vienna: Deuticke; 1910.

17 Brockington IF. *Motherhood and mental health*. Oxford: Oxford University Press, p. 146; 1996.

18 Gooch R. *An account of some of the most important diseases peculiar to women*. London: Murray; 1829. p. 108–175.

19 Reid J. On the causes, symptoms and treatment of puerperal insanity. *Journal of Psychological Medicine*. 1848;1:128–151 and 284–294.

20 Campbell CA. Clinical illustrations of puerperal insanity. *Lancet*. 1883;ii 97–99, 180–181 and 277–279.

21 Clouston TS. Puerperal insanity, lactational insanity, the insanity of pregnancy. In *Clinical lectures in mental diseases*. Lecture XV. 4th ed. London: Churchill; 1896. p. 544–574.

22 Putnam S. Puerperal mania. *Transactions of the Vermont Medical Society*. 1878; 53–59.

23 Campbell CA. Aetiology, pathology and treatment of puerperal insanity. *Journal of Mental Science*. 1887;33:169–189, 372–379 and 487–496.

24 West RU. Fatal and other cases of puerperal mania. *Association Medical Journal*. 1854;79:716–720.

25 Meyer E. *Über puerperale Fieberpsychosen*. Inaugural-Dissertation, Strasbourg; 1888.

26 Bird F. No title. *London Medical Gazette.* 1845;36:1218–1219.

27 Warburg B. *Über die im Jahre 1909 in der Kieler psychiatrichen und Nervenklinik beobachteten Fälle von Generationspsychosen.* Inaugural-Dissertation, Kiel; 1915.

28 Arnold AB. Insanity occurring in the puerperal state. *Maryland Medical Journal.* 1880;7:73–76.

29 Drenk K. *Zur klinischen Einordnung und Prognose der Wochenbettpsychosen.* Inaugural-Dissertation, Köln; 1972.

30 Halim A, Utz B, Biswas A, Rahman F, van den Broek N. Cause of, and contributing factors, to maternal deaths: a cross-sectional study using verbal autopsy in four districts in Bangladesh. *British Journal of Obstetrics and Gynaecology.* 2014;121, supplement s4:86–94.

31 Guerrier G, Oluyide B, Keramarou M, Grais R. High maternal and neonatal mortality rates in northern Nigeria: an 8-month observational study. *International Journal of Women's Heath.* 2013;5: 495–499.

32 Vallely L, Ahmed Y, Murray SF. Postpartum maternal morbidity requiring hospital admission in Lusaka, Zambia – a descriptive study. *BMC Pregnancy Childbirth.* 2005;5:1–10.

33 Aranoff DM, Mulla ZD. Postpartum invasive group A streptococcal disease in the modern era. *Infectious Disease Obstetrics and Gynecology.* 2008. doi 10.1155/2008/796892.

34 Bauerschmitz GJ, Hellriegel M, Strauchmann J, Schäper J, Emons G. Fulminant postpartum sepsis caused by haemolytic group A streptococci and toxic shock syndrome – a case report and review of the literature. *Geburtshilfe und Frauenheilkunde.* 2014;74:764–767.

35 Karrosch M, Rodel F, Mühler N, Edel B, Sacher S, Schmidt KH, et al. Ovarian vein thrombosis following invasive group A streptococcus postpartum sepsis associated with expression of streptococcal pyrogenic exotoxin genes speC. *European Journal of Obstetrics & Gynecology and Reproductive Biology.* 2015;184:127–130.

36 Ghesquière L, Deruelle P, Charbonneau P, Puech F. Épidémiologie de la mortalité maternelle de cause infectieuse en France, période 2007–2009, à partir des données du rapport confidential de mortalité maternelle. *Journal de Gynécologie, Obstétrique et Biologie de la Réproduction.* 2014;44:1–9.

37 Turner CE, Dryden M, Holden MTG, Davies FJ, Lawrenson RA, Farzaneh L, et al. Molecular analysis of an outbreak of lethal postpartum sepsis caused by *Streptococcus pyogenes. Journal of Clinical Microbiology.* 2013;51:2089–2095.

38 Bilano VL, Ota E, Ganchimeg T, Mori R, Souza JP. Risk factors of pre-eclampsia/ eclampsia and its adverse outcomes in low- and middle-income countries: a WHO secondary analysis. *PLOS one.* 2014;9: 1–9 (e91198).

39 Merriman S. *A synopsis of the various kinds of difficult parturition, with practical remarks on the management of labours.* London: Callow, p. 129–142, 212–214, 267–277 and 299–301; 1920.

40 Lambert G, Brichant JF, Hartstein G, Bonhomme V, Dewandre PY. Preeclampsia: an update. *Acta Anaesthesiologica Belgica.* 2014;65:137–149.

41 Kleinknecht F. *Die posteklamptischen Psychosen.* Inaugural-Dissertation, Leipzig; 1914.

42 Cunningham FG, Twickler D. Cerebral edema complicating eclampsia. *American Journal of Obstetrics & Gynecology.* 2000;182:94–100.

43 Bathla S, Suneja A, Guleria K, Agarwal N. Dilantin as anticonvulsant in eclampsia. *Journal of the Indian Medical Association.* 2002;100:561–564.

44 Thapa K, Jha R. Magnesium sulphate: a life saving drug. *Journal of the Nepal Medical Association.* 2008; 47:104–108.

45 Obed JY, Dah T, Weerashinghe AS, Solomon EA. Hypoglycaemia: a major biochemical complication in eclampsia – its risk factors and prognostic value. *Journal of Obstetrics & Gynaecology.* 1997;17:535–539.

46 Pal A, Bhattacharyya R, Adhikary S , Roy A, Chakrabaty D, Ghosh P, et al.

Eclampsia-scenario in a hospital – a ten year study. *Bangladesh Medical Research Council Bulletin.* 2011;37:66–70.

47 Vega CEP, Kahhale S, Zugaib M. Maternal mortality due to arterial hypertension in São Paulo city (1995–1999). *Clinics.* 2007;62:679–684.

48 Mayi-Tsonga S, Ndombi I, Methogo M, Diallo T, Mendome G, Mounanga M. [Maternal mortality in Libreville, Gabon: assessment and challenges]. *Santé.* 2008;18:193–197.

49 Veloz-Martínez MG, Martínez-Rodríguez OA, Ahumada-Ramirez E, Puello-Tamara ER, Amezcua-Galindo FJ, Hernández-Valencia M. [Eclampsia, obstetric haemorrhage and heart disease as a cause of maternal mortality in 15 years of analysis]. *Ginecologia y Obstetrica Mexicana.* 2010;78:215–218.

50 Moodley J. Maternal deaths associated with eclampsia in South Africa: lessons to learn from the confidential enquiries into maternal deaths 2005–2007. *South African Medical Journal.* 2010;100: 717–719.

51 Hinchey J, Chaves C, Appignani B, Breen J, Pao L, Wang A, et al. A reversible posterior leukoencephalopathy syndrome. *New England Journal of Medicine.* 1996;334:494–500.

52 Page EW. The relation between hydatid moles, relative ischemia of the gravid uterus, and the placental origin of eclampsia. *American Journal of Obstetrics & Gynecology.* 1939;37:291–293.

53 Shembry MA, Noble AD. An instructive case of abdominal pregnancy. *Australian & New Zealand Journal of Obstetrics & Gynaecology.* 1995;35:220–221.

54 Roberts JM. Endothelial dysfunction in pre-eclampsia. *Seminars in Reproductive Endocrinology.* 1998;16:5–15.

55 Vatten LJ, Skjaerven R. Is pre-eclampsia more than one disease? *British Journal of Obstetrics & Gynaecology.* 2004;111: 298–302.

56 Roberts JM. Pathophysiology of ischaemic placental disease. *Seminars in Perinatology.* 2014;38:139–145.

57 Bourson Y. *Contribution à l'étude des psychoses puerpérales.* Thèse, Strasbourg; 1958.

58 Engelhard JLB. Über Generationspsychosen und den Einflus des Gestationsperiode auf schon bestehende psychische und neurologische Krankheiten. *Zeitschrift für Geburtshülfe und Gynäkologie.* 1912;70:727–812.

59 Hohmann A. *Über Puerperalpsychosen.* Inaugural-Dissertation, Königsberg; 1913.

60 Feldman M. Las psicosis puerperales. *Revista de Obstetricia y Ginecologia de Venezuela.* 1967;27:353–369.

61 Ndosi NK, Mtawali ML. The nature of puerperal psychosis at Muhimbili National Hospital: its physical co-morbidity, associated main obstetric and social factors. *African Journal of Reproductive Health.* 2002;6:41–49.

62 Anton G. Über Geistes- und Nervenkrankheiten in der Schwangerschaft, im Wochenbett und in der Säugungszeit. In Anton G, et al. editors, *Handbuch der Gynäkologie.* Wiesbaden: Bergmann; 1910. p. 1–41.

63 Sioli F. Eklamptische und post-eklamptische Psychosen. In Hinselmann H editor, *Die Eklampsie.* Bonn: Cohen; 1924. p. 597–524.

64 Guzman A. Trastornos psicóticos vinculados a la función reproductora de la mujer (las psicosis puerperales). *Revista de Obstetrica y Ginecologia de Venezuela.* 1986;46:7–18.

65 Wieger F. Recherches critiques sur l'éclampsie uroémique. Gazette Médicale de Strasbourg. 1854 ; 161–179, 288–303, 318–339, 362–378, 401–410, 443–469.

66 Bidon H. Note à propos d'un cas d'amnésie post-éclamptique. *Revue de Médecine.* 1891;11:961–970.

67 Olshausen R. Beitrag zu den puerperalen Psychosen, speciell den nach Eklampsie auftretenden. *Zeitschrift für Geburtshilfe und Gynäkologie.* 1891;21:371–385.

68 Atkin L. Post-partum macrocytic anaemia associated with confusional states. *Lancet.* 1938;i:434–435.

69 Joseph J. Puerperal cerebral venous thrombosis. *British Medical Journal* i.:1944;438–439.

70 Donkin AS. On the pathological relation between albuminuria and puerperal mania. *Edinburgh Medical Journal.* 1863;8:994–1004.

71 Case discussions from the University of Louisville Hospitals: eclampsia with postpartum psychosis. *Journal of the Kentucky Medical Association.* 1964;62:376–377.

72 Garcia Rijo M. *Contribution à l'étude de la folie puerpérale.* Thèse, Paris; 1879.

73 Buchmüller A. Ein Fall von geheilter Eclampsie mit darauf folgender mania puerperalis. *Allgemeine Wiener Medizinische Zeitung.* 1875;47:425, 467, 478–479.

74 Esquirol JED. Observations sur l'aliénation mentale à la suite de couches. *Journal Général de Médecine, de Chirurgie et de Pharmacie Françaises et Étrangères.* 1818;62:629–648.

75 Thaler H. Zur Klinik der Postpartum-Eklampsien. *Zentralblatt für Gynäkologie.* 1922;25:1019–1024.

76 Kutzinski A. Über eklamptische Psychosen. *Charité-Annalen.* 1909;33:216–260.

77 Lishman WA. Post-ictal disorders. In: *Organic Psychiatry: The Psychological Consequences of Cerebral Disorder.* Oxford: Blackwell; 1997. p. 257–258.

78 Herrmann E. *Die Eklampsie und ihre Prophylaxie.* Berlin and Vienna: Urban & Schwarzenberg; 1929. p. 150–159.

79 Fellner OO. Über Graviditätspsychosen. *Therapie der Gegenwart.* 1908;49:416–417.

80 Jahnel F. Ein Beitrag zur Kenntnis der geistigen Störungen bei der Eklampsie. *Archiv für Psychiatrie.* 1913;152:1095–1115.

81 Clauser F. Contributo allo studio delle psicosi puerperali. *Rivista Italiana di Ginecologia.* 1922;2:379–401.

82 Marzotko F. Seltene toxikosekomplikationen unter dem Bild einer Wochenbettspsychose. *Zentralblatt für Gynäkologie.* 1967;89:647–650.

83 Lértora A. En torno a una psicosis gravido-puerperal curada con cortone. *Obstetricia y Ginecologia Latino-Americanas.* 1955;13:20–30.

84 Franchini C. Contributo allo studio delle psicosi puerperali. *Sistema Nervoso.* 1955;7:81–101.

85 Smith T. Puerperal mania: recovery: frequent occurrence of twin pregnancy and placenta praevia in the same patient. *Lancet.* ii:1851;415–416.

86 Jenkins JF. Puerperal mania - has it any connection with toxaemia? *American Medical Monthly.* 1857;8:284–287.

87 Maynard JH. A case of puerperal mania, with convulsions. *Medical & Surgical Reporter.* 1872;27:216–217.

88 Rochaix P. *Contribution à l'étude des troubles mentaux d'origine puerpérale.* Thèse, Lyon; 1913.

89 Heidema ST. Puerperaalpsychosen. *Psychiatrische en Neurologische Bladen.* 1932;36:627–635.

90 Lauly MEE. *Dix cas de psychose post-puerpérale.* Thèse, Bordeaux; 1904.

91 Sélade E. Observation d'une grossesse compliquée d'éclampsie ayant nécessité l'accouchement forcé, et suivie de manie puerpérale. *Archives de Médecine Belge* 1847 and 1848; (April), 216–226.

92 Segeri DG. *Epilepsia gravidam eiusque embryonem per XXV hebdomadas infestante. Miscellanea Curiosa sive Ephemeridum Medico-Physicarum Germanicarum Academiae Naturae Curiosorum, decuriae* I: III, Observation 1672;160.

93 Jacquemier J. *Manuel des Accouchements et des Maladie des Femmes Grosses et Accouchées.* Paris: Baillière; 1846. p. 244.

94 Westphal A. Über seltenere Formen von traumatischen und Intoxikationspsychosen, insbesondere über aphasische, agnostische und apraktische Störungen bei denselben, zugleich ein Beitrag zur Pathologie des Gedächtnisses. *Archiv für Psychiatrie.* 1910;47:843–883.

95 Senlecq F. *Du délire post-éclamptique.* Thèse, Paris; 1896.

96 Jaffé M. *Beitrag zu den Puerperalpsychosen.* Inaugural-Dissertation, Rostock; 1905.

97 Hess M. *Über die sogenannten Puerperalpsychosen.* Inaugural-Dissertation, München; 1938.

98 Van Steenbergen-van der Noordaa MC. *Generatie-psychosen.* Academisch Proefschrift: Amsterdam; 1941.

99 Roberts JM, Redman CWG. Pre-eclampsia: more than pregnancy-induced hypertension. *Lancet.* 1993;i:1447–1451.

100 Granger JP, Alexander BT, Bennett WA, Khalil RA. Pathophysiology of pregnancy-induced hypertension. *American Journal of Hypertension.* 2001;14:178S–185S.

101 Roberts JM, Cooper DW. Pathogenesis and genetics of pre-eclampsia. *Lancet.* 2001;357:53–56.

102 Davison JM, Homuth V, Jeyabalan A, Conrad KP, Karumanchi SA, Quaggin S, et al. New aspects in the pathophysiology of pre-eclampsia. *Journal of the American Society of Nephrology.* 2004;15: 2440–2448.

103 Nader SK, Yemeni EA, Blann AD, Lip GYH. Thrombomodulin, von Willibrand factor and E-selectin as plasma markers of endothelial damage/dysfunction and activation in pregnancy-induced hypertension. *Thrombosis Research.* 2004;113:123–128.

104 Steinberg G, Khankin EV, Karumanchi SA. Angiogenic factors and preeclampsia. *Thrombosis Research.* 2009;123, supplement 2: S93–S99.

105 Masoura S, Kalogiannidis IA, Gitas G, Goutsioulis A, Kolou E, Athanasiadis A, et al. Biomarkers in pre-eclampsia: a novel approach to early detection of the disease. *Journal of Obstetrics & Gynaecology.* 2012;32:609–616.

106 Goel A, Rana S. Angiogenic factors in pre-eclampsia: potential for diagnosis and treatment. *Current Opinion in Nephrology & Hypertension.* 2013;22:643–650.

107 Griffin M, Shennan AH. Clinical applications of biomarkers in preeclampsia. *Biomarkers Medicine.* 2014;8:459–470.

108 Fairweather DVI. Nausea and vomiting in pregnancy. *American Journal of Obstetrics & Gynecology.* 1968;102:135–175.

109 Dubois P. L'avortement dans les cas de vomissements. *Bullétin de l'Académie Nationale de Médecine.* 1852;17:556–582.

110 Boulton P. Case of paraplegia occurring during pregnancy. *Transactions of the Obstetrical Society of London.* 1868;9: 12–15.

111 Madge HM. A case of paralysis during pregnancy. *British Medical Journal.* iv:1871;696–697.

112 Wernicke C. *Lehrbuch der Gehirnkrankheiten für Ärzte und Studirende.* Volume 2. Kassel and Berlin: Fischer; 1881. p. 229–242.

113 Korsakow SS. Über eine besondere Form psychischer Störung, combinirt mit multipler Neuritis. *Archiv für Psychiatrie und Nervenkrankheiten.* 1890;21:669–704.

114 Vinay C. Polynévrite consécutive à la grossesse et à l'accouchement – paralysie des quatres members – guérison. *Lyon Médical.* 1895;80:555–562.

115 Raimann E. Ein Fall von *cerebropathia psychica toxaemica* (Korsakoff) gastro-intestinalen Ursprunges. *Monatsschrift für Psychiatrie und Neurologie.* 1902;12: 330–339.

116 v. Hösslin R. Die Schwangerschaftslähmungen der Mütter. *Archiv für Psychiatrie.* 1904;38:730–861 and 40:446–576.

117 Victor M, Adams RD, Collins GH. *The Wernicke-Korsakoff syndrome.* Oxford: Blackwell; 1971.

118 Chiossi G, Neri I, Cavazzuti M, Basso G, Facchinetti F. Hyperemesis gravidarum complicated by Wernicke's encephalopathy: background, case report, and review of the literature. *Obstetric & Gynaecological Survey.* 2006;61:255–268.

119 Yoon CK, Chang MH, Lee DC. Wernicke-Korsakoff syndrome associated with hyperemesis gravidarum. *Korean Journal of Ophthalmology.* 2005;19:239–242.

120 Chitra S, Latha KVS. Jubilee, Professor Wernicke's encephalopathy with visual loss in a patient with hyperemesis gravidarum. *Journal of the Association of Physicians of India.* 2012;60:53–55.

121 Eijkman C. Eine Beriberiähnliche Krankheit der Hühner. *Archive für Pathologische Anatomie und Physiologie und für Klinische Medizin.* 1897;146: 523–532.

122 Funk C. On the chemical nature of the substance that cures polyneuritis in birds induced by a diet of polished rice. *Journal of Physiology.* 1911;43:395–400.

123 Hinze-Selch D, Weber MM, Zimmermann U, Pollmacher T. Thiamine treatment in psychiatry and neurology. *Fortschrift für Neurologie & Psychiatrie.* 2000;68:113–120.

124 Ironside R. Neuritis complicating pregnancy. *Proceedings of the Royal Society of Medicine.* 1939;32:588–595.

125 Purdon Martin J. No title. *Proceedings of the Royal Society of Medicine.* 1939;32:46.

126 Millson CE, Harding K, Hillson RM. Wernicke-Korsakoff syndrome due to hyperemesis gravidarum precipitated by thyrotoxicosis. *Postgraduate Medical Journal.* 1995;71:249–253.

127 Otsuka F, Tada K, Ogura T, Hayakawa N, Mimura Y, Yamauci T, et al. Gestational thyrotoxicosis manifesting as Wernicke encephalopathy: a case report. *Endocrine Journal.* 1997;44:447–452.

128 Ohmori N, Tushima T, Skine Y, Sato K, Shibagaki Y, Ijuchi S, et al. Gestational thyrotoxicosis with acute Wernicke encephalopathy: a case report. *Endocrine Journal.* 1996;46:787–793.

129 Sabourdy C, Baulon E, Tranchant C. Syndrome confusionnel au cours de la grossesse: encéphalopathy de Gayet Wernicke. *Revue Neurologique.* 2002;158:850–852.

130 Anaforoğlu I, Yildiz B, Inceçayir Ö, Algün E. A woman with thyrotoxicosis and hyperemesis gravidarum-associated Wernicke's encephalopathy. *Neuroendocrinology Letters.* 2012;33: 101–105.

131 Di Gangi S, Gizzo S, Patrelli TS, Saccardi C, D'Antona D, Nardelli GB. Wernicke's encephalopathy complicating hyperemesis gravidarum: from the background to the present. *Journal of Maternal–Fetal and Neonatal Medicine.* 2012;25:1499–1504.

132 Weill-Hallé B, Layani F. Polynévrite et syndrome de Korsakoff au cours de la gestation. *Bullétin et Mémoires de la Société Médicale des Hôpitaux de Paris,* 1927 February 4th; p. 145–148.

133 Duval RAE. *Les psychoses puerpérales.* Thèse, Lille; 1934.

134 Nayrac P, Gernez L, Duval R. Sur les psychoses gravidiques et puerpérales. *Gazette des Hôpitaux.* 1939;112:493–498.

135 Martin P. *Considérations sur la folie puerpérale.* Thèse, Paris; 1872.

136 Waindrach. (1889 or 1902). Ein Fall von polyuneuritische Psychose nach puerperale Parametritis. *Monatsschrift für Psychiatrie und Neurologie heft 4,* cited by Korsakoff and Serbski (1892, reference 144).

137 Williams RR, Cline JK. Synthesis of vitamin B_1. *Journal of the American Chemical Association.* 1936;58:1504–1505.

138 Séglas J, Sollier P. Folie puerpérale; amnésie; astasie et abasie. Idées délirantes communiqués. *Archives de Neurologie.* 1890;20:386–404.

139 Semon. Polyneuritis und Korsakoffsche Psychose bei Colipyelitis in der Gravidität. *Medizinische Klinik.* 1909;32:1185–1187.

140 Minski L. Non-alcoholic polyneuritis associated with Korsakow syndrome. *Journal of Neurology and Psychopathology.* 1936;16:219–224.

141 Maere M. Psychose de Korsakow avec polynévrite au cours d'une septicémie post-puerpérale. 1939:616–621.

142 Fischer R. Merkwürdiges Puerperalfieber, compliciert mit Encephalitis, Oophoritis, *Phlegmasia alba dolens* und geendigt mit einem Wechselfieber. *Medizinische Jahrbücher des Kaiserlichen und Königlichen Österreichischen Staates.* 1841;35:46–58.

143 Luzzatto A. Rilieve su taluni quadri neurologici e psicotici osservati durante il puerperio. *Rivista di Patologia Nervosa.* 1955;76:856–960.

144 Korsakow SS, Serbsky W. Ein Fall von polyneuritischer Psychose mit Autopsie. *Archiv für Psychiatrie und Nervenkrankheiten.* 1892;23:112–133.

145 Bayle LP. *Des névrites puerpérales (grossesse et puerpérium).* Thèse, Lyon; 1896.

146 Lapinsky M. Zur Casuistik der polyneuritischen Psychose. *Archiv für Psychiatrie.* 1908;43:1140–1174.

147 Dustin AP. La polynévrite gravidique. *Nouvelle Iconographie de la Salpêtrière.* 1909;4:349–367.

148 Anderodius J and Pery. Vomissements graves chez une femme enceinte: avortement provoqué; guérison des vomissements; psychose polynévritique consécutive. *Bullétin et Mémoires de la Société de Médecine et de Chirurgie de Bordeaux.* 1908; p. 446–451.

149 Anglade J. Psychose polynévritique d'origine puerpérale. *Bullétin et Mémoires de la Société de Médecine et de Chirurgie de Bordeaux.* 1908; p. 442–445.

150 Janssens G. Over Generatiepsychosen. *Nederlandsch Maandschrift voor Verlosk, Vrouwenziekten en voor Kindergeneesk.* 1918; 7:123–128 and 179–191.

151 Eulenberg. Über Puerperalwahnsinn. *Correspondenz-Blatt der Deutschen Gesellschaft für Psychiatrie und gerichtliche Psychologie.* 1856;3:121–122.

152 Kühne F. Beitrag zur Lehre von der Hyperemesis gravidarum. *Monatsschrift für Geburtshilfe und Gynäkologie.* 1899;10: 432–446.

153 Frigerio A. Psicosi polinevritica di Korsakow da gravidanza. *Rivista di Patologia Nervosa e Mentale.* 1917;22: 441–451.

154 Ely FA. Memory defect of Korsakoff type observed in multiple neuritis following toxaemia of pregnancy. *Journal of Nervous and Mental Disease.* 1922;56:115–125.

155 McGoogan LS. Toxic neuronitis of pregnancy. *Journal-Lancet.* 1933;52: 735–740.

156 Wagener HP, Weir JF. Ocular lesions associated with postoperative and gestational nutritional deficiency. *American Journal of Ophthalmology.* 1937;20: 253–259.

157 Schjøtt-Rivers E. Hyperemesis gravidarum: clinical and biochemical investigations. *Acta Obstetrica et Gynaecologica Scandinavica.* 1938;18: supplement 1.

158 Berkwitz NJ, Lufkin NH. Toxic neuronitis of pregnancy. *Surgery, Gynecology & Obstetrics.* 1932;54:743–757.

159 Lavin PJM, Smith D, Kori SH, Ellenberger C. Wernicke's encephalopathy: a predictable complication of hyperemesis gravidarum. *Obstetrics & Gynecology.* 1983;62: supplement 3:13–15.

160 Galloway PJ. Wernicke's encephalopathy and hyperemesis gravidarum. *British Medical Journal.* 1992;305:1096.

161 Ohkoshi N, Ishii A, Shoji S. Wernicke's encephalopathy induced by hyperemesis gravidarum, associated with bilateral caudate lesions on computed tomography and magnetic resonance imaging. *European Neurology.* 1994;34:177–180.

162 Marcé LV. *Traité de la Folie des Femmes Enceintes, des Nouvelles Accouchées et des Nourrices, et Considérations Médico-légales qui se rattachent à ce Sujet.* Paris: Baillière; 1858.

163 Faure E. *Contribution à l'étude de la folie chez les nouvelles accouchées.* Thèse, Lyon; 1890.

164 Devic E. Un cas de psychose polynévritique. *Province Médicale.* 1892;7:100–114.

165 Mader. Zur *polyneuritis peripherica puerperarum et gravidarum. Wiener Klinische Wochenschrift.* 1895;8: 537–559.

166 Turney HG. Polyneuritis in relation to gestation and the puerperium. *St Thomas' Hospital Reports.* 1897;25:1–47.

167 Perrin MNJ. *Des polynévrites.* Thèse, Nancy; 1901.

168 Lurà A. Della polinevrite in puerperio: la syndrome di Korsakow. *Bolletino delle Cliniche.* 1911;28:207–212.

169 Beck E. Zur Frage der Erbfaktors bei den symptomatischen Psychosen. *Monatsschrift für Psychiatrie.* 1930;77:38–70.

170 Byrne BM, Stronge JM. Wernicke's encephalopathy presenting in the puerperium. *Irish Medical Journal.* 1996;89:145–146.

171 Campbell ACP, Ritchie Russell W. Wernicke's encephalopathy: the clinical features and their probable relationship with vitamin B deficiency. *Quarterly Journal of Medicine. new series.* 1941; 37:41–51.

172 Olindo S, Smadja D, Cabre P, Mehdaoui H, Heinzlef O. Encéphalopathie de Gayet-Wernicke et myélinolyse centropontine induites par des vomissements gravides. *Revue Neurologique.* 1997;153:427–429.

173 Henderson DK. Korsakow's psychosis occurring during pregnancy. *Johns Hopkins Hospital Bulletin.* 1914;25:261–270.

174 Selitsky SA. *Cerebropathia et Psychopathia toxica gravidarum. Zentralblatt für Gynäkologie.* 1925;49:2070–2073.

175 Combemale P. À propos les psychoses gravidiques. *Écho Médicale du Nord,* April 29 1934; p. 616–620.

176 Biasci L. *Sulle psicosi in gravidanza. Archivi Italiani delle Malattie Nervosi e Rivista Sperimentale di Freniatria.* 1949;73: 507–520.

177 Tesfaye S, Achari V, Yang YC, Harding S, Bowden A, Vora JP. Pregnant, vomiting and going blind. *Lancet.* 1998;352:1594.

178 Lana-Peixoto MA, Claret dos Santos E, Pittella JEH. Coma and death in unrecognised Wernicke's encephalopathy. *Arquivio Neuro-Psiquiatrico.* 1992;50: 329–333.

179 Watanabe K, Tanaka K, Masuda J. Wernicke's encephalopathy in early pregnancy complicated by disseminated intravascular coagulation. *Virchows Archives.* 1983;400:213–218.

180 Sulaiman W, Othman A, Mohammad M, Salleh R, Mushahar L. Wernicke's encephalopathy associated with hyperemesis gravidarum – a case report. *Malaysian Journal of the Medical Sciences.* 2002;43–46.

181 Daaloul W, Jilli L, Ouerdiane N, Masmoudi A, Ben Hamouda S, Bouguerra B, et al. [Fatal complication of hyperemesis gravidarum: Wernicke's encephalopathy]. *Tunis Médical.* 2012;90:663.

182 Kantor S, Prakash S, Chandwani J, Gokhale A, Sarma K, Albahrani MJ. Wernicke's encephalopathy following hyperemesis gravidarum. *Indian Journal of Critical Care Medicine.* 2014;18:164–166.

183 Fraser D. Central pontine myelinolysis as a result of treatment of hyperemesis gravidarum: case report. *British Journal of Obstetrics and Gynaecology.* 1988;95: 621–623.

184 Biotti D, Osseby GV, Durand C, Lorcerie B, Couvreur S, Moreau T, et al. Wernicke's encephalopathy due to hyperemesis gravidarum . . . and fetal stroke: what relationship? *Clinical Neurology & Neurosurgery.* 2011;113:490–492.

185 Kumar D, Geller F, Wang L, Wagner B, Fitz-Gerald MJ, Schwendimann R. Wernicke's encephalopathy in a patient with hyperemesis gravidarum. *Psychosomatics.* 2012;53:172–174.

186 Zara G, Codemo V, Palmieri A, Schiff S, Cagnin AC, Citton V, et al. Neurological complications of hyperemesis gravidarum. *Neurological Sciences.* 2012;33:133–135.

187 Michel ME, Alanio E, Bois E, Gavillon N, Graesslin O. Wernicke's encephalopathy complicating hyperemesis gravidarum: a case report. *European Journal of Obstetrics & Gynecology & Reproductive Biology.* 2010;149:117–123.

188 Shalchian S, Maertens de Noordhout A, Fumal A, Tebache M. A rare complication of hyperemesis during pregnancy: Wernicke's encephalopathy. *Acta Neurologica Belgica.* 2010;110:2009–2011.

189 Palacios-Marquéz A, Delgado-García S, Martín-Bayón T, Martínez-Escoriza JC. Wernicke's encephalopathy induced by hyperemesis gravidarum. *BMJ Case Reports.* 2012. doi 10.1136/bcr-2012-006216.

190 Freo U, Rossi S, Ori C. Wernicke's encephalopathy complicating gestational hyperemesis. *European Journal of Obstetrics, Gynecology & Reproductive Biology.* 2014;180:204–205.

191 Chaturachinda K, McGregor EM. Wernicke's encephalopathy and pregnancy. *Journal of Obstetrics & Gynaecology of the British Commonwealth.* 1968;75: 969–971.

192 Scalzo SJ, Bowden SC, Ambrose ML, Whelan G, Cook MJ. Wernicke-Korsakoff syndrome not related to alcohol use: a systematic review. *Journal of Neurology, Neurosurgery & Psychiatry*. 2015. doi 10.1136/jnnp-s014-309598.

193 Sydenham T. *Praxis Medica Experimentalis, sive Opuscula Universa*. Leipzig: Fritsch; 1763. p. 661–662.

194 Pathania M, Upadhyaya S, Lali BS, Sharma A. Chorea gravidarum: a rarity in the West still haunts pregnant women in the East. *BMJ Case Reports*. 2013. doi 10.1136/bcr-2012-008096.

195 Harsch HH. Postpartum psychosis and systemic lupus erythematosus. *Psychiatric Medicine*. 1984;1:303–308.

196 Sanna G, Bertolaccini ML, Cuadrado MJ, Laing H, Khamashta MA, Mathieu A, et al. Neuropsychiatric manifestations in systemic lupus erythematosus: prevalence and association with antiphospholipid antibodies. *Journal of Rheumatology*. 2003;30:985–992.

197 Buist RC. Chorea gravidarum: a statistical review of the published cases. *Transactions of the Edinburgh Obstetric Society*. 1895;20: 134–153.

198 Willson P, Preece AA. Chorea gravidarum. *Archives of Internal Medicine*. 1932;49:471–553.

199 Gentin. *Contribution à l'étude des rapports de la chorée avec la menstruation et la puerpéralité*. Thèse, Paris; 1899.

200 Thiebaut F. Sydenham's chorea. In: Vinken PJ, Brauyn GW editors, *Handbook of Clinical Neurology*. Volume 6. *Diseases of the Basal Ganglia*. Amsterdam: North Holland, p. 409–434; 1968.

201 Cardioso F. Chorea gravidarum. *Archives of Neurology*. 2002;59:868–870.

202 Fam NP, Chisholm RJ. Chorea in a pregnant woman with rheumatic mitral stenosis. *Canadian Journal of Cardiology*. 2003;19:719–721.

203 Tekşut TK, Özcan H, Işik M, Karsli F. Konversiyon bozukluğu yanlış tanisi konan psikotik belirtilerin olduğu antifosfolipid sendromu ilişkili kore gravidarum: olgu sunumu. *Türk Psikiyatri Dergisi*. 2013;24:280–283.

204 Horstius. Quoted by Buist (1895, reference 197) ; 1661.

205 Breton A. *État mental dans la chorée*. Thèse, Paris; 1893.

206 Diefendorf AR. Mental symptoms of acute chorea. *Journal of Nervous and Mental Disease*. 1912;39:161–172.

207 Sandras CMS. and Bourgignon H. *Traité Pratique des Maladies Nerveuses*. Paris: Baillière; 1860.

208 Marcé LV. l'État mental dans la chorée. *Mémoires de l'Académie de Médecine*. 1860;24:30–38.

209 Maury A. Physiologie psychologique des hallucinations hypnagogiques, ou des erreurs des sens dans l'état intermédiaire entre la veille et le sommeil. *Annales Médico-psychologiques*. 1848;11: 26–40.

210 Vihvelin H. On the differentiation of some typical forms of hypnagogic hallucinations. *Acta Psychiatrica et Neurologica Scandinavica*. 1948;23: 360–389.

211 Schachter DL. The hypnagogic state: a critical review of the literature. *Psychological Bulletin*. 1976;83:452–481.

212 Frank JP. *Traité de Médecine-Pratique*. Paris: Baillière; 1842.

213 Arndt R. Chorea und Psychose. *Archiv für Psychiatrie*. 1868;1:510–544.

214 Lehmann F. *Casuistische Beiträge zur Kenntniss der im Verlaufe von Chorea auftretenden Psychosen*. Inaugural-Dissertation, Berlin; 1887.

215 Gatti FM and Rosenheim E. Sydenham's chorea associated with transient intellectual impairment. *American Journal of Disease in Childhood*. 1969;118:915–918.

216 Prichard JC. Remarks on the treatment of paralysis and some other diseases by issues and blisters. *London Medical Repository*. new series. 1824;1:3.

217 Vassitch MV. [*Mental derangement complicating chorea*]. Thèse, Paris; 1882.

218 Nicolauer. Chorea gravidarum mit Psychose. *Berliner Medizinische Wochenschrift.* 1912;49:670.

219 Léquyer M. *Contribution à l'étude de la chorée gravidique.* Thèse, Montpellier; 1904.

220 Royston GD. Chorea gravidarum. *Transactions of the American Association of Obstetricians & Gynecologists.* 1920;33: 303–317.

221 Reuter C. Geistesstörung während der Gravidität. *Ungarische Medizinische Presse.* 1903;3:47.

222 Jones R. A case of chorea and pregnancy with insanity. *Journal of Mental Science.* 1903;49:486–491.

223 Dupouy R. *Les psychoses puerpérales et les processus d'auto-intoxication.* Thèse, Paris; 1904.

224 Mühlbaum A. *Die Prognose bei Chorea gravidarum.* Inaugural-Dissertation, Wiesbaden; 1914.

225 Sivadon P. *Les psychoses puerpérales et leurs séquelles.* Thèse, Paris; 1933.

226 Beresford OD, Graham AM. Chorea gravidarum. *Journal of Obstetrics & Gynaecology of the British Empire.* 1950;57:616–625.

227 Barnes R. On chorea in pregnancy. *Transactions of the Obstetrical Society of London.* 1869;10:147–196.

228 Mundé PF. A case of puerperal chorea. *American Journal of Obstetrics.* 1882;15:187–190.

229 Peacock and Barnes' case, See Ruhemann (1889, reference 245)

230 Dakin. Seven cases of pregnancy complicated by chorea. *Practitioner.* 1897;59:571–584.

231 Sheill JS. 'Chorea gravidarum': a short monograph, with details of two recent cases. *Practitioner.* 1906;76:192–197.

232 Shaw WF. Chorea during pregnancy. *Journal of Obstetrics & Gynaecology of the British Empire.* 1907;11:289–304.

233 Runge W. Die Generationspsychosen des Weibes. *Archiv für Psychiatrie und Nervenkrankheiten.* 1911;48:545–690.

234 Strohmayer W. Künstliche Fehlgeburt und künstliche Unfruchtbarkeit vom Standpunkt der Psychiatrie. In Placzek et al., *Künstliche Fehlgeburt und künstliche Unfruchtbarkeit.* Leipzig: Thieme; 1918, p. 201–208.

235 Mackenzie S. Report on Inquiry no II, Chorea. *British Medical Journal.* 1887; i:425–436.

236 Festenberg. Ein Fall von schwerer Chorea während der Schwangerschaft mit Übergang in Manie. Heilung durch künstliche Fehlgeburt. *Deutsche Medizinische Wochenschrift.* 1897;23: 196–197.

237 Gundry R. Observations upon puerperal insanity. *American Journal of Insanity.* 1859; 294–320.

238 Treffers PE, Huidekoper BL, Weenink GH, Kloosterman GJ. Epidemiological observations of thrombo-embolic disease during pregnancy and in the puerperium, in 56,022 women. *International Journal of Gynaecology & Obstetrics.* 1983;21: 327–331.

239 Lloyd JH. *A System of Obstetrics.* Publisher unknown; 1888. p. 590–608.

240 Guinsbourg S. *Contribution à l'étude des psychoses puerpérales.* Thèse, Paris; 1912.

241 Thomas D, Byrne PD, Travers RL. Systemic lupus erythematosus presenting as post-partum chorea. *Australian & New Zealand Journal of Medicine.* 1979;9:568–570.

242 Pollock AJ. A case of acute chorea with pregnancy; induced premature labour; recovery. *Lancet.* 1886;i:686.

243 Hirst BC. A case of pregnancy complicated by anemia, chorea, insanity and pyelitis. *University Medical Magazine.* 1888;1: 151–152.

244 Routh A. In the discussion of the paper by Handfield-Jones on chorea in pregnancy. *Transactions of the Obstetrical Society of London.* 1889;31:243–251.

245 Ruhemann W. *Über Chorea gravidarum.* Inaugural-Dissertation, Berlin; 1889.

246 Piña FG. Corea gravídica: reporte de un caso. *Ginecologia y Obstetricia Mexicana.* 2009;77:156–159.

247 Mauriceau F. *Observations sur la Grossesse et l'Accouchement des Femmes et sur leurs Maladies, et celles des Enfans Nouveau-nés.* Paris: chez l'Auteur; 1694.

248 Morgagni JB. (1761), quoted by Huhn A. Die Hirnvenen- und Sinusthrombose. *Fortschritte der Neurologie, Psychiatrie und ihrer Grenzgebiete.* 1957;25:440–472.

249 Abercrombie. Quoted by Kalbag and Woolf (1967, reference 253); 1828.

250 Cruveiller. *Anatomie Pathologique du Corps Humain.* Paris: Baillière; 1829–1835.

251 Ducrest FM. De la phlébite cérébrale et méningée chez les femmes en couches. *Archives Générales de Médecine.* 4th series. 1847;15:1–39.

252 Hauser GA. In the discussion of a paper by Huggenberg HR and Kesselring F (1958) Postpartale cerebrale Komplikationen. *Gynaecologia.* 1958;146:312–317.

253 Kalbag RM, Woolf AL. *Cerebral Venous Thrombosis.* London: Oxford University Press; 1967.

254 Sheehan HL, Lynch JB. *Pathology of Toxaemia of Pregnancy.* Edinburgh and London: Churchill Livingstone; 1973.

255 Purdon Martin. Venous thrombosis in the central nervous system. *Proceedings of the Royal Society of Medicine.* 1944;37: 383–386.

256 Crouzon O, Foix C. Ramollissement hémorrhagique par phlébite des sinus et des veines encéphaliques: pseudo-syndrome de Weber. *Revue Neurologique.* 1913;25:341–344.

257 Lanska DJ, Kryscio RJ. Stroke and intracranial venous thrombosis during pregnancy and puerperium. *Neurology.* 1998;51:1622–1628.

258 Banerjee AK, Chopra JS, Sawhney BB. Postpartum cerebral venous thrombosis: study of autopsy material. *Neurology India.* 1973;21:19–24.

259 Bansal BC, Gupta RR, Prakash C. Stroke during pregnancy and puerperium in young females below the age of 40 years as a result of cerebral venous/venous sinus thrombosis. *Japanese Heart Journal.* 1980;21:171–183.

260 Chopra JS, Prabhakar S. Clinical features and risk factors in stroke in young. *Acta Neurologica Scandinavica.* 1979;60: 289–300.

261 Srinavasan K. Cerebral venous and arterial thrombosis in pregnancy and the puerperium: a study of 135 patients. *Angiology.* 1983;34:731–746.

262 Srinavasan K. Ischemic cerebrovascular disease in the young: two common causes in India. *Stroke.* 1984;15: 733–735.

263 Srinavasan K. Puerperal cerebral venous and arterial thrombosis. *Seminars in Neurology.* 1988;8:222–225.

264 Prasad A. *Puerperal cerebral venous thrombosis: a follow up study.* DM Thesis, Bangalore; 1991.

265 Estanol B, Rodriguez A, Conte G, Aleman JM, Loyo M, Pizzuto J. Intracranial venous thrombosis in young women. *Stroke.* 1979;10:680–684.

266 Purdon Martin J. Thrombosis in the superior longitudinal sinus following childbirth. *British Medical Journal.* 1941; ii:537–540.

267 Huhn A. Die Hirnvenen- und Sinusthrombosen in Schwangerschaft und Wochenbett. In: Bürger-Prinz H, Fischer PA editors, *Psychiatrie und Neurologie der Schwangerschaft.* Stuttgart: Enke; 1968. p. 181–194.

268 Kendall D. Thrombosis of the intracranial veins. *Brain.* 1948;71:386–402.

269 Garcin R, Pestel M. *Thrombo-phlébites Cérébrales.* Paris: Masson; 1949.

270 Dubois J. Les thrombo-phlébites cérébrales du post-partum. *Gynécologie et Obstétrique.* 1956;55:472–493.

271 Sheehan HL. Neurological complications of pregnancy. *Proceedings of the Royal Society of Medicine.* 1939;32:585–588.

272 Motet A. Manie puerpérale. *Moniteur des Sciences Médicales et Pharmaceutiques.* 1859;1:52–52.

273 Bauman KH, Brouwer B. Delirium acutum and primary sinus thrombosis. *Journal of Nervous & Mental Disease.* 1922;55: 273–293.

274 Hilpert P. Zur Symptomatologie der nichteitrigen Sinusthrombosen. *Klinische Wochenschrift.* 1929;8:496–500.

275 Skottowe I. Mental Disorders in Pregnancy and the Puerperium. *Practitioner.* 1942;148:157–163.

276 Scheid. See Noetzel H, Jerusalem F (1965) Die Hirnvenen- und Sinusthrombosen. In *Monographien aus dem Gesamtgebiete der Neurologie und Psychiatrie.* Berlin: Springer; 1961.

277 Goldman JA, Eckerling B, Gans B. Intracranial venous sinus thrombosis in pregnancy and the puerperium. *Journal of Obstetrics & Gynaecology of the British Commonwealth.* 1964;71:791–796.

278 Grünes JU. Zu einigen neurologisch-psychiatrischen Problemen von Schwangerschaft und Wochenbett. *Zeitschrift für Ärztliche Fortbildung.* 1973;67:614–617.

279 Aresin L. *Psychopathologische, Psychiatrische und Neurologische Aspekte der Schwangerschaft.* Leipzig: Thieme; 1976.

280 Visscher GRA. *Generatie-psychoses en hersenstam. Een katamenstisch onderzoek.* Thesis, Groningen; 1949.

281 Combs JD. Psychoses associated with childbearing. *Diseases of the Nervous System.* 1956;17:166–169.

282 Koek HC, Schreuder JTR. Intracranial venous thrombosis. *Acta Psychiatrica et Neurologica Scandinavica.* 1951;26: 353–357.

283 Stertz G. Katatonische Psychose als symptomatisches Bild bei Sinusthrombose. *Berliner Klinische Wochenschrift.* 1909;46:685–688.

284 Schröder P. Anatomische Befunde bei einigen Fällen von akuten Psychosen. *Allgemeine Zeitschrift für Psychiatrie.* 1909;66.

285 Corazza L. Thrombose des *sinus longitudinalis superior* mit subarachnoidealem Bluterguss. *Schmidts Jahrbücher.* 1866;131:324–327.

286 Vorpahl F. Über Sinusthrombose und ihre Beziehung zu Gehirn- und Piablutungen. *Ziegler's Beiträge zur Pathologischen Anatomie und zur Allgemeinen Pathologie.* 1913;55:323–344.

287 Zangmeister W. Sinusthrombose im Wochenbett unter einem der Eklampsie ähnlichen Bild. *Zentralblatt für Gynäkologie.* 1925;49:225–227.

288 Lindeman J, Beyer-Boon ME. Een patiënt met een hemolytisch-uremisch syndroom post partum. *Nederlander Tijdschrift voor Geneeskunde.* 1972;116:841–842.

289 Morin P, Guilly P, Badin J, Choukroun J. Étiologie de certaines psychoses puerpérales. *Bullétin de la Féderale Société de Gynécologie et Obstétrique Française.* 1952;4:600–602.

290 Saintfort R, Stern TA. Cross-cultural and neuropsychiatric aspects of a postpartum delusional state. *Harvard Review of Psychiatry.* 2000;8:141–147.

291 Hunt JR. Thrombosis of the cerebral sinuses and veins as complication of the puerperium. *Bulletin of the Lying-in Hospital of the City of New York.* 1917;11:73–80.

292 Constantinescu I, Constantinescu S, Constantinescu D. Thrombo-phlébite des sinus cérébraux dans une confusion mentale post-partum. *Bullétin de la Société de Psychiatrie de Bucarest.* 1937;2:68–73.

293 Ashkenazy HM, Kosary IZ, Braham J. Thrombosis of the longitudinal sinus: diagnosis by carotid angiography. *Neurology.* 1962;12:288–292.

294 Dhasmana DJ, Brockington IF, Roberts A. Postpartum transverse sinus thrombosis presenting as acute psychosis. *Archives of Women's Mental Health.* 2010;13:365–368.

295 Jennett WB, Cross JN. Influence of pregnancy and oral contraception on the incidence of strokes in women of childbearing age. *Lancet.* 1967;i:1019–1023.

296 Cross JN, Castro PO, Jennett WB. Cerebral strokes associated with pregnancy and the puerperium. *British Medical Journal.* 1968; iii:214–218.

297 Kittner SJ, Stern BJ, Feeser BR, Hebel JR, Nagey DA, Buchholz DW, et al. Pregnancy and the risk of stroke. *New England Journal of Medicine.* 1996;335:768–774.

298 Finola GC. Cerebral vascular accidents in pregnancy. *American Journal of Obstetrics & Gynecology.* 1957;74:1342–1352.

299 Resnik R, Swartz WH, Plumer MH, Benirschke K, Stratthaus ME. Amniotic fluid embolism with survival. *Obstetrics & Gynecology.* 1976;47:295–298.

300 Steiner PE, Lushbaugh CC. Maternal pulmonary embolism by amniotic fluid. *Journal of the American Medical Association.* 1941;117:1245–1254.

301 Peterson EP, Taylor HB. Amniotic fluid embolism. An analysis of 40 cases. *Obstetrics & Gynecology.* 1970;35:787–793.

302 King A. Neurological conditions occurring as complications of pregnancy. *Archives of Neurology and Psychiatry.* 1950;63: 471–499 and 611–644.

303 Churchill F. On paralysis occurring during gestation and childbed. *Dublin Quarterly Journal of Medical Science.* 1854;17:276–294.

304 Rangell L. Cerebral air embolism. *Journal of Nervous and Mental Disease.* 1942;96:542–555.

305 Rascol. See Janssens (1995, reference 306); 1979.

306 Janssens E, Mommel M, Mounier-Vehier F, Leclerc X, Guerin du Masgenet B. Postpartum cerebral angiopathy possibly due to bromocriptine therapy. *Stroke.* 1995;26:128–130.

307 De Carle. See Finola (1957, reference 298); 1949.

308 Amias AG. Cerebral vascular disease in pregnancy:1. Haemorrhage. *Journal of Obstetrics & Gynaecology of the British Commonwealth.* 1970;77:100–120.

309 Delattre JY, Pertuiset BF, Poisson M, Mashaly R, Grosskopf D, Buge A. [Hypoglycorrhachia and postpartum aseptic cerebral thrombophlebitis with meningeal haemorrhage]. *Revue Neurologique.* 1985;141:58–60.

310 Hansen T. *Om forholdet mellem puerperal Sindssygdom og puerperal Infection.* Thesis, Kopenhaagen; 1888.

311 Jack TM. Post-partum intracranial subdural haematoma. *Anaesthesia.* 1979;34:176–180.

312 Miyazaki S, Fukushima H, Kamata K, Ishii S. Chronic subdural hematoma after lumbar-subarachnoid analgesia for a Caesarean Section. *Surgical Neurology.* 1983;19:459–460.

313 Campbell DA, Varma TRK. Chronic subdural haematoma following epidural anaesthesia, presenting as puerperal psychosis. *British Journal of Obstetrics & Gynaecology.* 1993;100:782–784.

314 Mercieri M, Mercieri A, Paolini S, Arcioni R, Lupoi D, Passarelli F, et al. Postpartum cerebral ischaemia after accidental dural puncture and epidural blood patch. *British Journal of Anaesthesia.* 2002;90: 98–100.

315 Logsdale SJ, Toone BK. Post-ictal psychoses: a clinical and phenomenological description. *British Journal of Psychiatry.* 1988;152:246–252.

316 Dongier S. Statistical study of clinical and electroencephalographic manifestations of 536 psychotic episodes occurring in 516 epileptics between clinical seizures. *Epilepsia.* 1959;1:117–142.

317 Wells CE. Transient ictal psychosis. *Archives of General Psychiatry.* 1975;32:1201–1203.

318 Richard P, Brenner RP. Absence status. *Case reports and a review of the literature. Encéphale.* 1980;6:385–392.

319 Béraud R. Grossesse et épilepsie. *Encéphale.* 1984;4:320–325.

320 Mattson RH, Cramer JA. Epilepsy, sex hormones and anti-epileptic drugs. *Epilepsia.* 1985;26, supplement 1: S40–S41.

321 Clemmesen C. Epilepsie und Schwangerschaft. *Zeitschrift für die gesamte Neurologie und Psychiatrie.* 1927;110: 793–795.

322 Hoppe H. Symptomatologie und Prognose der im Wochenbett entstehenden Geistesstörungen (zugleich ein Beitrag zur Lehre von der acuten hallucinatorischen Verwirrtheit). *Archiv für Psychiatrie und Nervenkrankheiten.* 1893;25:137–210.

323 Cruchet R, Rivière M. Sur deux cas de psychose puerpérale. *Bullétin de la Société d'Obstétrique et de Gynécologie de Paris.* 1923;22:232–237.

324 Guder. Über den Einfluss der Schwangerschaft auf Epilepsie und epileptische Geistesstörung. *Irrenfreund.* 1886;28:1–11.

325 Elfes K. *Katatonie mit besonderer Berücksichtigung des Verlaufs in der Gravidität.* Inaugural-Dissertation, Kiel; 1912.

326 Jolly P. Beitrag zur Statistik und Klinik der Puerperalpsychosen. *Archiv für Psychiatrie und Nervenkrankheiten.* 1911;48:792–823.

327 Stouffs L. Psychose et accouchement. *Bullétin de la Société Belge de Gynécologie et d'Obstétrique.* 1902;13:69–71.

328 Solomons B. Insanity and its relation to the parturient state. *Journal of Mental Science.* 1931;77:701–707.

329 Mori L, Mingozzi M. L'elettroshock in gravidanza. *Annali dell'Ospedale Psichiatrico di Perugia.* 1944;1:1–20.

330 McSwiney SM. Report of a case in midwifery practice. *Dublin Journal of Medical Science.* 1875;59:462–469.

331 Quensel F. Psychosen und Generationsvorgänge beim Weibe. *Medizinische Klinik.* 1907;50: 1509–1515.

332 Mayer CEL. *Die Beziehungen der krankhaften Zustände und Vorgänge in den Sexual-Organen des Weibes.* Berlin: Hirschwald; 1869.

333 Sullivan WC. A note on the influence of maternal inebriety on the offspring. *Journal of Mental Science.* 1899;45:489–503.

334 Lienau A. Über künstliche Unterbrechung der Schwangerschaft bei Psychosen in psychiatrische, rechtliche und sittliche Beleuchtung. *Archiv für Psychiatrie und Nervenkrankheiten.* 1914;53:915–942.

335 Kaestner G. *Über Psychose und Schwangerschaft und Berücksichtigung der einschlägigen Fälle aus der Erlanger Universitätsklinik.* Inaugural-Dissertation, Erlangen; 1919.

336 Jacobs B. Aetiological factors and reaction types in psychoses following childbirth. *Journal of Mental Science.* 1943;89: 242–250.

337 Gregory MS. Mental diseases associated with childbearing. *American Journal of Obstetrics & Gynecology.* 1924;8: 420–430.

338 Chartrou JMM. *Contribution à l'étude de la psychose post-eclamptique.* Thèse, Bordeaux; 1899.

339 Meissner F. *Zwei Fälle von Psychosen im Wochenbett.* Inaugural-Dissertation, Greifswald; 1899.

340 Bretonville P. *Contributions à l'étude des psychopathies puerpérales.* Thèse, Paris; 1901.

341 Masieri N. Contributo allo studio della patogenesi delle psicosi puerperali. *Rivista Italiana di Ginecologia.* 4:163–183.

342 Lemoine P, Harousseau H, Borteyru JP, Menuet JC. Les enfants de parents alcooliques: anomalies observées. *Ouest Médical.* 1968;25:476–482.

343 Schaefer O. Alcohol withdrawal syndrome in a newborn infant of a Yukon Indian mother. *Canadian Medical Association Journal.* 1962;87:1333–1334.

344 Gill JL. Haematemesis – post-partum haemorrhage – puerperal mania. *Medical Circular.* 1858;13:146.

345 Lemeland. Aperçu général sur les psychoses puerpérales. *Archives Internes de Neurologie.* 21st series. 1892;October/November:140–144.

346 Khong SY, Leach J, Greenwood C. Meningioma mimicking puerperal psychosis. *Obstetrics & Gynecology.* 2007;109:515–516.

347 Ballantine EP. Psychosis occurring during pregnancy and the puerperium. *New York State Journal of Medicine.* 1909;9:460–464.

348 Karnosh LJ, Hope JM. Puerperal psychoses and their sequelae. *American Journal of Psychiatry.* 1937;94:537–550.

349 Herlihy CE. The management of postoperative and postpartum acute psychiatric emergencies. *Alabama Journal of the Medical Sciences.* 1965;2:259–263.

350 Herzer G. Beitrag zur Klinik der Puerperalpsychosen (Generationpsychosen). *Allgemeine Zeitschrift für Psychiatrie.* 1906;63:244–274.

351 Schmidt M. Beitrage zur Kentniss der Puerperalpsychosen. *Archiv für Psychiatrie und Nervenkrankheiten.* 1881;11:75–95.

352 de Gorsky Z. *Considérations sur la folie puerpérale.* Thèse, Paris; 1888.

353 Ballet G. Les psychoses puerpérales. *Médecine Moderne.* 1892;3:661–665 and 677–682.

354 Castin P. *Des psychoses puerpérales dans leur rapports avec la dégénerescence mentale.* Thèse, Paris; 1899.

355 Privat de Fortunié J. *Étude sur le délire post-partum.* Thèse, Paris; 1904.

356 Nichols MM. Acute alcohol withdrawal syndrome in a newborn. *American Journal of Diseases of Childhood.* 1967;113: 714–715.

357 Hill NM. Four cases of puerperal insanity. *Transactions of the Iowa State Medical Society.* 1891;9:132–134.

358 Baker AA. *Psychiatric Disorders in Obstetrics.* Oxford: Blackwell; 1967.

359 Simpson AR. 1883, cited by Sheehan (1939, reference 271)

360 Dell DL, Halford JJ. Dementia presenting as postpartum depression. *Obstetrics & Gynecology.* 2002;99:925–928.

361 Glinski LK. Anatomische Veränderungen der Hypophyse. *Deutsche Medizinische Wochenschrift.* 1913;39:473 (German summary).

362 Simmonds M. Über Hypophysisschwund mit tödlichem Ausgang. *Deutsche Medizinische Wochenschrift.* 1914;40: 322–323.

363 Sheehan HL. Post-partum necrosis of the anterior pituitary. *Journal of Pathology & Bacteriology.* 1937;45:189–214.

364 Sheehan HL, Somers VK. The syndrome of hypopituitarism. *Quarterly Journal of Medicine.* new series. 1949;72:319–362.

365 Sheehan HL, Davis JC. *Post-partum Hypopituitarism.* Springfield: Charles C Thomas; 1982.

366 Bunch TJ, Dunn WF, Basu A, Gosman RI. Hyponatraemia and hypoglycaemia in acute Sheehan's syndrome. *Gynecological Endocrinology.* 2002;16:419–423.

367 Özkan Y, Colak R. Sheehan syndrome: clinical and laboratory evaluation of 20 cases. *Neuroendocrinology Letters.* 2005;26:257–260.

368 Diri H, Tanriverdi F, Karaca Z, Senol S, Unluhizarci K, Durak AC, et al. Extensive investigation of 114 patients with Sheehan's syndrome: a continuing disorder. *European Journal of Endocrinology.* 2014;171:311–318.

369 Tanriverdi F, Dokmetas HS, Kebapci N, Kilicli F, Atmaca H, Yarman S, et al. Etiology of hypopituitarism in tertiary case institutions in Turkish population: analysis of 773 patients from pituitary study group database. *Endocrine.* 2014;47:198–205.

370 Hughes RR, Summers VK. Changes in the electro-encephalogram associated with hypopituitarism due to post-partum necrosis. *EEG & Clinical Neurophysiology.* 1956;8:87–96.

371 Bethune JE, Nelson DH. Hyponatraemia in hypopituitarism. *New England Journal of Medicine.* 1965;272:771–776.

372 Clarke EC, Franklin M, Sahs AL. Postpartum necrosis of the adenohypophysis with hypoglycaemic convulsions. *Archives of Neurology & Psychiatry.* 1951;65:724–731.

373 Oelbaum MH. The variability of endocrine dysfunction in post-partum hypopituitarism. *British Medical Journal.* 1952;ii:110–113.

374 Staehelin B. Die psychopathologie des Sheehan-syndroms. *Acta Endocrinologica.* 1953;14:145–152.

375 Blau JN, Hinton JM. Hypopituitary coma and psychosis. *Lancet.* 1960;i:408–409.

376 Bourgeois M. Syndrome de Sheehan et troubles neuro-psychiatriques. *Annales Médico-psychologiques.* 1967;125:796–800.

377 Parker RR, Isaacs AD, McKerron CG. Recoverable organic psychosis after hypopituitary coma. *British Medical Journal.* 1976;i:132–133.

378 Bahemuka M, Rees PH. Sheehan's syndrome presenting with psychosis. *East African Medical Journal.* 1981;58: 324–329.

379 Sidorov J, Mitnick P. Postpartum hyponatremia. *American Journal of Medicine.* 1987;83:183–184.

380 Boulanger E, Pagniez D, Roueff S, Binaut R, Valaat AS, Provost N, et al. Sheehan syndrome presenting as early post-partum hyponatraemia. *Nephrology, Dialysis & Transplantation.* 1999;14:2714–1715.

381 Munz W, Seufert R, Knapstein PG, Pollow K. Early postpartum hyponatraemia in a patient with transient Sheehan's syndrome. *Experimental & Clinical Endocrinology & Diabetes.* 2004;112:278–280.

382 Anfuso S, Patrelli S, Soncini E, Chiodera P, Fadda GM, Nardelli GB. A case report of Sheehan's syndrome with acute onset, hyponatraemia and severe anemia. *Acta Biomedica.* 2009;80:73–76.

383 Zuker N, Bissessor M, Korber M, Conrads M, Margolis J, Massel P, et al. Acute hypoglycaemic coma – a rare, potentially lethal form of early onset Sheehan syndrome. *Australian & New Zealand Journal of Obstetrics & Gynaecology.* 1995;35:318–320.

384 Verga P. Contributo allo studio dell'infarto della ipofisi. *Pathologica.* 1930;22:4–15.

385 Putterman C, Almog Y, Caraco Y, Gross DJ, Ben-Chetrit E. Inappropriate secretion of antidiuretic hormone in Sheehan's syndrome: a rare cause of postpartum hyponatraemia. *American Journal of Obstetrics & Gynecology.* 1991;165: 1330–1333.

386 Kale K, Nihalani N, Karnik N, Shah N. Postpartum psychosis in a case of Sheehan's syndrome. *Indian Journal of Psychiatry.* 1999;41:70–72.

387 Dwivedi A, Dwivedi S. Acute post-partum pituitary necrosis presenting as bradycardia. *Journal of the Indian Academy of Clinical Medicine.* 2002;4:63–65.

388 Shoib S, Dar MM, Arif T, Bashir H, Bhat MH, Ahmed J. Sheehan's syndrome presenting as psychosis: a rare clinical presentation. *Medical Journal of the Republic of Iran.* 2013;27:35–37.

389 Guiraud P, Nodet C. Les psychoses puerpérales et leur traitement (action de la vitamine E). *Paris Médicale.* 1936;ii: 194–199.

390 Rowntree LG. The effects on mammals of the administration of excessive quantities of water. *Journal of Pharmacology & Experimental Therapeutics.* 1926;29: 135–159.

391 Liggins GC. The treatment of missed abortion by high dosage syntocinon intravenous infusion. *Journal of Obstetrics & Gynaecology of the British Commonwealth.* 1962;69:277–281.

392 Ahmad AJ, Clark EH, Jacobs HS. Water intoxication associated with oxytocin infusion. *Postgraduate Medical Journal.* 1975;51:249–252.

393 Lilien AA. Oxytocin-induced water intoxication: a report of a maternal death. *Obstetrics & Gynecology.* 1968;32:171–173.

394 Gupta DR, Cohen NH. Oxytocin, 'salting out' and water intoxication. *Journal of the American Medical Association.* 1972;220; 681–683.

395 Lauerson NH, Birnbaum SJ. Water intoxication associated with oxytocin administration during saline-induced abortion. *American Journal of Obstetrics & Gynecology.* 1975;121:2–6.

396 Whalley PJ, Prichard JA. Oxytocin and water intoxication. *Journal of the American Medical Association.* 1963;186:601–603.

397 Graham K, Palmer J. Severe hyponatraemia as a result of primary polydipsia in labour. *Australian & New Zealand Journal of Obstetrics & Gynaecology.* 2004;44:586–587.

398 Enns GM, O'Brien WE, Kobayashi K, Shinzawa H, Pellegrino JE. Postpartum 'psychosis' in mild arginosuccinate synthetase deficiency. *Obstetrics & Gynecology.* 2005;105:1244–1246.

399 Yamada N, Fukui M, Ishii K, Shibata H, Okabe H, Ohomiya H, et al. [Adult hypercitrullinaemia with consciousness disturbance and marked hypertransaminasemia after delivery]. *Nihon Shokakibyo Gakkai Zasshi.* 1980;77:1655–1660.

400 Kurasawa G, Shiotsuka S, Nakajo J, Nagao M, Ohisi M, Aida T, et al. A case report of citrullinemia induced by pregnancy. *Nippon Sanka Fujinka Gakkai Kantorengo Chihobukai Kaiho.* 1998;35:3–7.

401 Ito S. Mastitis and puerperal psychosis. *Japanese Journal of Obstetrics*. 1934;17: 373–377.

402 Häberle J, Vilaseca MA, Meli C, Rigoldi M, Jara F, Vecchio I, et al. First manifestation of citrullinemia type 1 as differential diagnosis to postpartum psychosis in the puerperal period. *European Journal of Obstetrics & Gynecology and Reproductive Biology*. 2010;149:225–231.

403 Russell A, Levin B, Oberholzer VG, Sinclair L. Hyperammonaemia: a new instance of an inborn enzymatic defect of the biosynthesis of urea. *Lancet*. 1962;ii: 699–700.

404 Maestri NE, Lord C, Glynn M, Bale A, Brusilow SW. The phenotype of ostensibly healthy women who are carriers for ornithine transcarbamylase deficiency. *Medicine (Baltimore)*. 1998;77:389–397.

405 Legras A, Labarthe F, Maillot F, Garrigue MA, Kouatchet A, Ogier D. Late diagnosis of ornithine transcarbamylase defect in three related female patients: polymorphic presentations. *Critical Care Medicine*. 2002;30:241–244.

406 Cordero DR, Baker J, Dorinzi D, Toffle R. Ornithine transcarbamylase deficiency in pregnancy. *Journal of Inherited Metabolic Disorders*. 2005;28:237–240.

407 Arn PH, Hauser ER, Thomas GH, Herman G, Hess D, Brusilow SW. Hyperammonaemia in women with a mutation at the ornithine carbamoyltransferase locus. *New England Journal of Medicine*. 1990;322:1652–1655.

408 Peterson DE. Acute postpartum mental status change and coma caused by previously undiagnosed ornithine transcarbamylase deficiency. *Obstetrics & Gynecology*. 2003;102:1212–1215.

409 Wong LJC, Craigen WJ, O'Brien WE. Postpartum coma and death due to carbamoyl-phosphate synthetase I deficiency. *Annals of Internal Medicine*. 1994;120:216–217.

410 Grody WW, Chang RJ, Panagiotis NM, Matz D, Cederbaum SD. Menstrual cycle and gonadal steroid effects on symptomatic hyperammonaemia of urea-cycle-based and idiopathic aetiologies. *Journal of Inherited Metabolic Disease*. 1994;17: 566–574.

411 Wakutani Y, Nakayasu H, Takeshima T, Mori N, Kobayashi K, Endo F, et al. [A case of late-onset carbamoyl phosphate synthetase 1 deficiency, presenting periodic psychotic episodes coinciding with menstrual periods]. *Rinsho Shinkeigaku*. 2001;41:780–785.

412 Frankl-Hochwart L. Über Psychosen bei Tetanie. *Jährbücher für Psychiatry*. 1890;9:128–136.

413 Greene JA, Swanson LW. Psychosis in hypoparathyroidism, with a report of five cases. *Annals of Internal Medicine*. 1941;14:1233–1236.

414 Anderson GW, Musselman L. The treatment of tetany in pregnancy. *American Journal of Obstetrics & Gynecology*. 1942;43:547–567.

415 v. Frankl-Hochwart L. Die Prognose der Tetanie der Erwachsenen. *Neurologisches Centralblatt*. 1906;25:642–651 and 694–704.

416 Allen TE, Agus B. Hyperventilation leading to hallucinations. *American Journal of Psychiatry*. 1968;125:632–637.

417 Lum LC. Hallucinations during hyperventilation. Personal communication; 1985.

418 Magarian GJ, Olney RK. Absence spells: Hyperventilation syndrome as a previously unrecognised cause. *American Journal of Medicine*. 1984;76:905–909.

419 Engel GL, Ferris EB, Logan M. Hyperventilation: analysis of clinical symptomatology. *Annals of Internal Medicine*. 1947;27:683–704.

420 Patil NJ, Yadav SS, Gokhale YA, Padwa N. Primary hypoparathyroidism: psychosis in the postpartum period. *Journal of the Association of Physicians of India*. 2010;58:506–508.

421 Birnbach DJ, Bourlier RA, Choi R, Thys DM. Anaesthetic management of Caesarean section in a patient with recurrent genital herpes and AIDS-related

dementia. *British Journal of Anaesthesia.* 1995;75:639–641.

422 Weiskorn J. *Transitorische Geistesstörung beim Geburtsakt und im Wochenbett.* Inaugural-dissertation, Bonn; 1897.

423 Friedrich E. *Über Psychosen bei secundärer puerperaler Anämie.* Inaugural-Dissertation, Münster; 1941.

424 Shulman R. Psychiatric aspects of pernicious anaemia: a prospective controlled investigation. *British Medical Journal.* 1967;ii:266–270.

425 Zucker DK, Livinston RL, Nakra R, Clayton PJ. B$_{12}$ deficiency and psychiatric disorders: case report and literature review. *Biological Psychiatry.* 1981;16: 196–105.

426 Evans DL, Edelsohn GA, Golden RN. Organic psychosis without anemia or spinal cord symptoms in patients with vitamin B$_{12}$ deficiency. *American Journal of Psychiatry.* 1983;140:218–221.

427 Payinda G, Hansen T. Vitamin B$_{12}$ deficiency manifested as psychosis without anemia. *American Journal of Psychiatry.* 2000;157:660–661.

428 Durand C, Mary S, Brazo P, Dollfus S. [Psychiatric manifestations of vitamin B$_{12}$ deficiency: a case report] *Encéphale.* 2003;29:560–565.

429 Thornton WE. Folate deficiency in puerperal psychosis. *American Journal of Obstetrics & Gynecology.* 1977;129: 222–223.

430 Van Schoot H. Katalepsie bij eene zwangere en haar jonggeboren kind. *Nederlands Tijdschrift voor Geneeskunde.* 1887;23: 110–113.

431 Schultze E. Über pathologische Schlafzustände und deren Beziehung zur Narkolepsie. *Zeitschrift für Psychiatrie.* 1895;52:724–740.

432 Perritti J. Über die Beeinflussung der Geistesstoerung durch Schwangerschaft. *Archiv für Psychiatrie.* 1885;16:442–463.

433 Menzies WF. Puerperal insanity. *American Journal of Insanity.* 1893;50:147–185.

434 Aschaffenburg G. Über die klinischen Formen der Wochenbettpsychosen.

Allgemeine Zeitschrift für Psychiatrie. 1901;58:337–355.

435 Rolland JA. *Contribution à l'étude des rapports de la grossesse et de l'aliénation mentale recherches statistiques faites a l'asile de Bailleul (Nord) 1870–1910.* Thèse, Lille; 1910.

436 Cristiani A. Demenza paralitica di origine puerperale. *Riforma Medicina.* 1894;3: 772–775.

437 Joseph S, Rabau E. Akute Meningoencephalitis im Wochenbett unter dem Bilde der Eklampsie. *Zentralblatt für Gynäkologie.* 1926;50:525–529.

438 Bernard MPC. *Contribution à l'étude des psychoses puerpérales, de leur étiologie en particulier.* Thèse, Nancy; 1922.

439 Colin H, Robin G. Paralysie générale à invasion foudroyante et puerpéralité. *Annales Médico-psychologiques.* 1923;81:463–468.

440 Kohler CG, Pickholtz J, Ballas C. Neurosyphilis presenting as a schizophrenia-like psychosis. *Neuropsychiatry, Neuropsychology & Behavioural Neurology.* 2000;13:297–302.

441 Anonymous. A case of mania. *Medical Repository.* 1816;6:377–378.

442 Harrar JA. Puerperal hysteria, pregnancy toxaemia or acute poliomyelitis. *New York Lying-in Hospital Bulletin.* 1917;11: 123–124.

443 Krupp S. Klinischer Beitrag zur Kenntnis der Schwangerschaftsmyelitis und Schwangerschaftsencephalitis. *Zentralblatt für Gynäkologie.* 1919;43:915–922.

444 Lôo P, Saba S, Sauvage J, Lôo H, Pouzols Y. Une démence puerpérale? *Annales Médico-psychologiques.* 1971;129:592–600.

445 Commandeur F. Des meningitis cérébrales et cérébro-spinales suppurées au cours de la puerpéralité. *Obstétrique.* 1908;13:289–315.

446 Couvelaire A, Trillat P. Un cas d'encéphalite léthargique au cours de la puerpéralité. *Gynécologie et Obstétrique.* 1920;1:63–70.

447 Haultain WFT, Thornton GO. Labour in a case of encephalitis lethargica. *British Medical Journal.* 1921;i:382.

448 Klippel and Baruk. Encéphalitie léthargique et grossesse: état du nouveau-né. *Revue Neurologique.* 1923;i:381–386.

449 Roques F. Epidemic encephalitis in association with pregnancy, labour and the puerperium – a review and report of twenty-one cases. *Journal of Obstetrics & Gynaecology of the British Empire.* 1928;35:1–113.

450 Alpers BJ, Palmer HD. The cerebral and spinal complications occurring during pregnancy and the puerperium. *Journal of Nervous and Mental Disease.* 1929;70: 465–484 and 606–621.

451 Ito Y, Abe T, Tomioka R, Komori T, Araki N. [Anti-NMDA receptor encephalitis during pregnancy] *Rinsho Shinkeigaku.* 2010;50:103–107.

452 Kumar M, Jain A, Dechant VE, Saito T, Rafael T, Aizawa H, et al. Anti-N-methyl-D–aspartate receptor encephalitis during pregnancy. *Archives of Neurology.* 2010;67:884–887.

453 Yu AYX, Moore FGA. Paraneoplastic encephalitis presenting as postpartum psychosis. *Psychosomatics.* 2011;52: 568–580.

454 Shaaban HS, Choo HF, Sensakovic JW. Anti-NMDA-receptor encephalitis presenting as postpartum psychosis in a young woman, treated with rituximab. *Annals of Saudi Medicine.* 2012;32:421–423.

455 Koksal A, Baybas S, Mutluay B, Altunkaynak Y, Keskek A. A case of NMDAR encephalitis misdiagnosed as postpartum psychosis and neuroleptic malignant syndrome. *Neuroscience Letters.* 2014. doi 10.1007/s10072-014-1966-3.

456 Lieb H. Ein Fall von Encephalitis im Puerperium als Beitrag zur Frage der Schwangerschaftstoxikosen. *Schweizerische Medizinische Wochenschrift.* 1924;54: 550–551.

457 Feuillade M. Sept cas d'encéphalites psychosiques aigues post-puerpérales mortelles. *Lyon Médicale.* 1938;161: 53–58.

458 Delay J. Encéphalite azotémique post-puerpérale et pénicillinothérapie. *Presse Médicale.* 1946;54:506.

459 Delay J, Corteel A, Lainé B. Sur une observation de psychose puerpérale guérie après curettage. *Annales d'Endocrinologie.* 1949;10:566–569.

460 Coumel H, Paraire J, Hosotte P. Un cas d'encéphalite psychosique aigue asotémique du 'post-partum', guéri par la pénicilline et la convulsivo-thérapie. *Búllétin et Mémoires de la Société des Hôpitaux de Paris.* 1948;64:681–683.

461 Yaskin JC. Nonsuppurative nonepidemic encephalitis following labor and in the puerperium *Archives of Neurology & Psychiatry.* 1931;26:371–391.

462 Smith BC. The psychoses associated with pregnancy. *Journal of the Kansas Medical Society.* 1934;35:203–209.

463 Steinmann I. Die Verursachung der Wochenbettpsychosen. *Archiv für Psychiatrie und Nervenkrankheiten.* 1935;103:552–579.

464 Morrant JCA. A catatonic syndrome resulting in death. *Canadian Journal of Psychiatry.* 1984;29:147–150.

465 Toulouse E, Marchand L, Courtois A. Deux cas d'encéphalites psychosiques aigues post-puerpérales. *Annales Méd-psychologiques.* 12th series. 1930;2:316–325.

466 Marchand L, Courtois A. Deux cas de psychose post-puerpérale: encéphalite hémorrhagique. *Annales Médico-psycholiques.* 1932;90:55–65.

467 Dobiás J, Skaličková O, Macek Z, Riegerová H, Kubelka V. Porucha vědomí s katatonickými symptomy při encefalitidě v poporodní době. *Československá Psychiatrie.* 1958;2: 122–128.

468 Kinzel U. Organische Psychose bei Herzinfarkt im Wochenbett. *Psychiatrische Praxis.* 2000;27:414.

469 De Smit DNW, de Waart C. Relatie tussen amentiële psychose in het puerperium en het ascorbinezuur-gehalte in het plasma. *Nederlaande Tijdschift voor Geneeskunde.* 1962;106:159–162.

470 Banzhaf E, Endler S, Besel R, Genzel U. Raumfordernde intrakranielle Prozesse im Wochenbett. *Zentralblatt für Gynäkologie.* 1979;19:1262–1263.

The Psychopathology of Parturition

10

Introduction

Little has been written about the mental disorders that occur during the birth of a child. For that reason this chapter, which is an abridgement and revision of chapter 3 of *Eileithyia's Mischief*[1], will cover some states of mind that do not fall under the rubric of 'psychoses'. It does not, however, cover the most important complication – neonaticide; that literature, with more than 2,000 publications, demands a monograph of its own.

Remarkable Circumstances

There are many strange things about childbirth. It may be feigned – as occurs in obstetric factitious disorder: some women who strongly desire the end of the pregnancy have simulated premature rupture of membranes and the contractions of labour[2–5]. It may be false – as occurs in delusions of pregnancy and pseudocyesis: in Bivin and Klinger's monograph on pseudocyesis[6], which analysed 333 cases, labour pains were experienced by 138 women. It may be concealed, as is common in the literature on neonaticide. It can be painless, not only in women who have neurological lesions affecting the lower body[7–9], but in women with normal sensation; there are at least 30 detailed reports of painless labour, with an estimated frequency of 1/10,000 births[10]; this can be familial[9] and recurrent[11] and can result in unexpected births during normal activities[12,13]. It can occur during sleep[11,12,14–19]; one mother fell into a state of somnolence and complete insensibility each time the uterus contracted, and woke at the end of the contraction[13]. It can be incomplete: in about 1/20,000 pregnancies, the uterus is unable to expel the foetus (usually in the abdomen), which is walled off, remaining in the body as a lithopaedion ('stone child'). Most remarkable is the birth of infants after death: this is not post-mortem Caesarean section, but the expulsion of the foetal corpse through the vaginal canal after the burial of the mother (*Sarggeburt*, coffin birth), probably under the pressure of gas in the abdomen[20].

Three Settings for Childbirth

Throughout history, childbirth, for pain and terror, has ranked with torture as one of the most severe human ordeals. Tyler Smith[21,22] wrote that no human suffering could surpass the piercing agony of childbirth. These are statements made by obstetricians, writing before the discovery of effective anaesthesia[23,24]:

> Labour pains torment a woman so much that her whole body trembles with fear. She can reach the point where she no longer knows what she is doing, and speaks and acts like a mad woman. One moment she turns on the midwife, then the obstetrician, bombarding them with demands for help – to get the babe out dead or alive, and release her from this agonizing pain. If these importunate demands are refused, she swears at them and covers them with bitter reproaches, curses her situation and above all her child, throws herself about the bed or jumps out in a futile attempt to find relief. As the infant

reaches the vulva, she tries to get a grip on the head and pull it out herself. No matter if she is injured or the infant dies, she will perish if her torture is not brought to an end.

Each pain begins with an almost convulsive trembling of the limbs. The face burns, the whole body is covered with sweat, the eye is fixed and haggard, the features decompose. The unfortunate woman cries out, calls for death, prays that someone kill her to put an immediate end to her suffering.

(Cazeau cited by Degaud[24])

It is not surprising that, although women spend, at the most, a few days in labour – brief episodes in a lifetime – it is, for many, an extreme experience and has severe psychiatric complications.

The discovery of anaesthetics has ameliorated this ordeal. Mesmer developed 'animal magnetism' about 1775, but hypnotism was not used in surgery until 1845[25] and in obstetrics until 1860[7,12]. Davy discovered the effects of nitrous oxide in 1795, but it was not used for tooth extraction until 1844, and in obstetrics until 1881. Ether was introduced in 1842. On 9 January 1847 it was used, by Simpson in Edinburgh, in obstetric patients; on 8 November he used chloroform. Cocaine, the first local anaesthetic, was introduced into eye surgery in 1884[25]; eventually spinal and epidural anaesthesia followed.

Even under optimal circumstances – when pregnancy occurs in the context of a stable relationship, and is completed by planned parturition supervised by obstetricians or midwives – parturition is often a stressful experience. In the first description of puerperal post-traumatic stress disorder (PTSD), Bydlowsky and Raoul-Duval[26] wrote,

Parturition – especially the first – can, by its obligatory violence, and by its confrontation with an imminent and lonely death, put the mother under extreme stress.

Since then, more than 50 papers have been published on this topic, including 8 quantitative studies showing frequencies of PTSD up to 5.6 per cent[27]. Querulant (complaining) disorders also complicate stressful childbirth[28].

These reports have come from nations with advanced obstetrics, but many women in the third world have to endure labour without professional help. AbouZahr and Wardlaw[29] summarized figures from WHO and UNICEF databases on the percentage of deliveries attended by skilled attendants (doctors, nurses or midwives): in sub-Saharan Africa it was 37 per cent and in South Asia 29 per cent. By 2014, in Bangladesh, it was still only 40 per cent[30]. Maternal death rates run in parallel. Estimates made in 1990–2013[31] show that 26 European nations (plus Australia, Israel, Japan, New Zealand, Qatar, Singapore and the United Arab Emirates) have death rates below $10/10^5$ live births; but 15 African nations have rates above $500/10^5$ – approximately 100 times as high, with Sierra Leone highest at $1,100/10^5$. The conditions under which many or most babies are born are comparable with those of the early nineteenth century in Europe and North America.

There is a third, totally different, setting – clandestine delivery. When a child is brought into the world hugger-mugger after a concealed pregnancy, there is no analgesia, no support from mother or friends, and no professional advice on complications. In addition, there is a nightmare of despair, shame, dread of humiliation and denunciation (or even, in some cultures, the spectre of 'honour murder'), and in many cases anger about exploitation or desertion. These deliveries are primaeval. There is almost no information about the mental states of these women, but the severity and frequency of psychopathology are certainly much higher[8]. Clandestine delivery still occurs in high-income nations, and will be more frequent in parts of the world that forbid termination of pregnancy and punish childbirth out of wedlock.

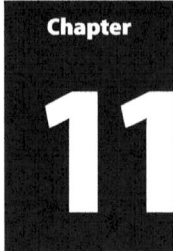

Chapter

11

Delirium during Labour

Definition

In the eighteenth century it was realized that women could become confused during severe labour. Parturient delirium can be defined as follows:

1. An acute (usually sudden) clouding of consciousness, lasting minutes or hours, with full recovery. Onset is usually towards the end of labour, and recovery after the birth.
2. Any of the following may be observed – incoherent speech, misidentification of persons or situation, visual hallucinations, inappropriate behaviour such as singing, or memory loss for the episode.

Description

The first account was by Kirkland[32]:

> A young married lady, of an healthful and vigorous constitution but naturally irritable habit, was seized with regular pains as the birth advanced. She became restless, and when the child's head began to pass the cervix, delirious during each pain; but instantly became sensible again, upon the pain going off. When the head was so very low, that it was expected every pain would bring matters to a crisis, but they were insufficient to bring the head any farther, she grew more restless, and the delirium was of longer continuance. The forceps were applied with perfect success. Her spirits were afterward very good, and she seemed to be tolerably well. But she died on the 9th day of puerperal fever.

Not long afterwards, Osiander[33] described this case:

> A small weak and irritable woman, veteran of many pregnancies, was in obstructed labour. With severe pains she spoke in a crazy way. She complained ceaselessly, writhed about in the bed, sprang up and tried to jump out of the window. When the doctor arrived she was completely delirious, and could hardly be restrained by two strong men from repeated attempts to throw herself out of the window. While she was being held down, the doctor extracted one child, and found a twin, which he extracted by the foot. After delivery she returned to her senses.

More than 30 years later, an Irishman, Montgomery[14], wrote about 'incoherence during natural labour', in an article[a] that many have cited as the original description. When the infant's head stretched the cervix, it caused extreme pain that was, in so many cases, accompanied by sudden incoherence or temporary delirium that this no longer surprised him.

---

[a] I found this famous article in the library of the British Medical Association; 164 years after its publication, I borrowed a knife to cut the pages.

Well into the nineteenth century the literature was full of descriptions of delirium during labour. Its importance was underlined by Reid[34], who proposed an early classification recognizing the distinction between transitory delirium and puerperal insanity:

> There are two forms of delirium, occurring during labour and after it, which some authors have included under puerperal insanity.

More than 50 cases have been published – 12 British, 19 German, 7 French, 5 Dutch, 5 American, 4 Hungarian[35] and one Italian[36]. Because this phenomenon has been so completely forgotten, and because of its medico-legal importance, I will summarize a number of cases. These are two of Montgomery's[14]:

> A 25-year old was in her first labour. When the membranes had been ruptured for ½ hour and the cervix was fully stretched, she turned to Dr Montgomery and said she would not go down to the drawing-room; for what would visitors think if they saw her sitting there, and she in labour? And I need say no more on the subject, for she would not do it, but she would have no objection to step into the coach and start off for Ballybay. She dozed a little and gave birth to a very large boy an hour later.

> A 40-year old was in her 9th labour. When the pains were quick and forcing, she turned to Dr Montgomery and said she thought it would be time for her to get up and see the children dressed and sent to school, otherwise they would be late. Then she expressed surprise at what could be preventing her mother from coming to town, to be with her during her confinement. (Her mother was holding her hand.) When the head descended fully into the pelvis, the incoherence ceased, after lasting about five minutes.

These are two German cases[37,39]:

> A 20-year old was in her first labour. After the waters broke, the pains became so strong that she screamed and bellowed like an animal, became cyanotic, threw herself about and pleaded for medicine to kill her. Suddenly she looked about her with staring eyes and no longer knew where she was – did not know she was in labour and did not recognize the doctor. She must go home – her mother was calling her. She swore over the presence of strangers in her house. After a dose of morphine, she lost consciousness. Immediately after delivery, she woke and asked what was crying, and why her belly had become so small. She would not believe her baby had been born because she had felt nothing. Gradually she came to her senses, realised that she was in the delivery room, and recognized the doctor. She had absolutely no knowledge of the birth.

> A 21-year old was in labour with her first child. After four hours she seemed dazed. She complained of headache and soon began to say weird things. She believed herself to be at work, where she was sewing ties. She cursed her boss, blaming him for some defect in the cloth. Then she praised her craft and showed her beautiful red and yellow pieces of silk. She could not see for darkness and asked her friend to turn on the light. With the pains, she gripped her body and asked what was pressing on her. She denied being pregnant or in labour. After two hours she gave birth, and shortly afterwards these phenomena disappeared.

In this French example, delirium continued after delivery[40]:

> A 32-year old was in her 4th labour. After seven hours, at the moment when dilatation of the cervix was almost complete, she failed to recognize her husband and the doctor, looked round vaguely, forgot she was pregnant, and hurled coarse insults. This state continued beyond her delivery two hours later; for another hour she still failed to recognise people, would not believe she had given birth and refused to see the infant. She gradually recovered, but it was not until the following day that she remembered the pregnancy. She had no memory for events during her period of confusion.

This is one of Engelhard's[10] Dutch cases, with a recurrence after the next birth, which continued afterwards:

> A 26-year old developed a similar state in both of her two deliveries. Her 2nd labour lasted 17 hours, the pains being neither very strong nor very painful. As the head began to appear, she became delirious, and reacted neither to questions nor contractions; she lay apparently unconscious. Twenty minutes after the birth she opened her eyes; she was still disorientated, and had auditory hallucinations. After recovery she had severe headache for an hour, and complete amnesia for the birth (case 30).

The interest of the next (American) case is that it was reported recently, with a diagnosis of 'brief reactive psychosis'[41]:

> A 20-year old Hispanic woman, with a history of childhood epilepsy, had auditory and visual hallucinations during her 1st labour, confirmed by her husband. During her 2nd labour she was again responding to visual hallucinations. She scanned the ceiling in a frightened and suspicious manner, and saw unfamiliar faces above her bed. She heard male and female voices instructing her to remove her intravenous catheter. She got the date wrong by two months. At this point she had not received any medication. After delivery the hallucinations ceased.

In the British literature this phenomenon was last mentioned in 1891[42], in the American 1921[43], in the French 1928[44], in the German 1930[45] and in the Dutch 1937[46]. It then disappeared from the literature, except for occasional cases without reference to earlier literature, and garbled accounts, like Chinese whispers, that linked the cause to the toxic effects of drugs, not pain[47].

Features of the Disorder

Loss of memory was often mentioned. In this patient of Kutzinski[48] there was an element of retrograde amnesia, recalling Snoeck's patient[49] (see later discussion), who was unconscious during delivery:

> A 26-year old developed a clouded state lasting several hours during her 2nd delivery. She was restless and mute, with a tense expression and closed eyes. She reacted with irritation to pin prick. She spoke spontaneously ¼ hour after the birth, but remained disorientated for 1½ hours. She had no memory of the birth – the last thing she could remember was having her supper some hours before the attack. She had received no medication.

The duration has varied from a few minutes to three, four, five and eight hours. Continuation into the puerperium was noted in five fully described cases[10,36,40,48,50]. Two[8,14] had phases of delirium and clarity. Two[10,41] had recurrences in different deliveries, and the following case of Lüning[51] four episodes:

> A 32-year old 'hysterical' woman was delirious during her 4th labour, which was rapid with strong contractions, aided by forceps. She had no memory of the event. The midwife said that she had been unconscious during each of her three earlier deliveries.

The possible role of drugs, such as nitrous oxide[52], is important, but many cases were described before the discovery of ether and chloroform.

There is one investigation that might be relevant to aetiology. Degaud[24] published data on hyperventilation: paroxysms of pain corresponded to the maximum respiratory rate; some women in labour have respiratory rates of 68/minute. Hyperventilation causes constriction of the cerebral arteries. It can lead to slowing of the electro-encephalogram and impaired consciousness (as mentioned in Section 2). This can, however, hardly explain retrograde amnesia or continuation after the birth.

Frequency

This form of delirium was one of the first childbirth psychoses to be recognized; that is perhaps an indication of its frequency in the dark ages of childbirth without analgesia. Certain German authors in the early nineteenth century made extravagant claims. Platner[53] wrote that loss of consciousness of some degree almost always occurred during the agitation accompanying birth. Nägele[54] stated that mothers' behaviour in the 3rd and 4th stages of labour often resembled a true episode of *Wahnsinn* [insanity], in which they lost all control and ceased to be master of their senses. Henke[55] made the extreme claim that

> *Verwirrung der Sinne* [delirium] occurs in more or less every delivery. The daily experience of obstetricians and midwives establishes the occurrence of brief confusion in married women. It is certain that the delirium induced by the mere process of childbirth can be prolonged. Numbing and fading of the senses in various nuances, for a shorter or longer time, is a daily occurrence in women giving birth.

K. G. Neumann of Berlin[56] wrote,

> It is not so rare for women to be formally insane during the whole of labour and not to have the slightest recollection of the birth. With astonishment they see the baby lying nearby and realise that they have been freed from their burden.

In America, Macdonald[57] observed incoherence and temporary delirium in so many instances that he ceased to regard it as a matter for surprise. As late as 1896, Andriezen[58] stated that 4 or 5 of 120 women he had attended in labour had well-marked mental symptoms.

Almost all other and later accounts have given much more cautious estimates of the frequency. Mende (writing in 1826)[59], while acknowledging that delirium occurred, said he had never seen a case in hundreds of deliveries. Another Neumann (of Aachen)[60] wrote in 1832 that *Raserei* [frenzy] during birth was a very rare event – he had seen only three cases. Kremling's case[61] of unconscious delivery was the only one encountered in 42 years of practice. Worthington[62] wrote in 1861:

> All obstetrical authors describe the agitation and anxiety of the moment when the head of the child is passing through the uterine neck, and it is not wonderful that an acute attack of mania should occasionally supervene. But temporary insanity at the moment of delivery, in consequence of the accompanying physical suffering, rarely occurs.

Barker[63] wrote in 1872,

> Most who have been in long practice have occasionally met such cases. Since the use of anaesthetics in midwifery, these cases must be very rare. I have seen but one case in the past 24 years.

Some quantitative studies, all published after 1890, are summarized in Table 11.1.

Sarrat[66] questioned obstetricians in Lyon: one said there was no such thing as transitory madness of delivery, but another stated that quite frequently, at the moment of dilatation, the woman was in a state of almost absolute unconsciousness, recognizing no-one not even her husband, biting, crying and pinching. Engelhard's[10] 11-year quantitative study in Utrecht stands out: among 19,910 deliveries, there were 5 transitory

Table 11.1 Frequency of delirium during parturition

First author		Number of cases	Number of births
Debus (1896)[38]		1	7,360
Degaud (1904)[24]		1	12,215
Bischoff (1908)[64]		Nil	1,700
Englehard (1912)[10]		5	19,910
Fehling	Cited by Becker	Nil	30,000
Fellner	(1926)[65]	Nil	40,000
Sarwey		1	10,000
Pollák (1929)[35]		4	20,000

mental disturbances and one loss of consciousness during the birth; this is about 1/4,000 deliveries. Willer[67] circulated university obstetric units in Germany, Austria and Switzerland asking for details during the decade 1915–1925 – a retrospective postal enquiry among state-of-the-art obstetric units. He received 16 replies: most obstetricians denied seeing cases that could not be explained by eclampsia or other organic lesions; only two matched the transitory delirium reported previously; idiopathic delirium had disappeared from university clinics. As for psychiatrists, Weiskorn[39] collected 4 cases in a year (1896) at Bonn. Bourson[68] in Strasbourg 1945–1957 (13 years), found only one case among 48,000 deliveries. Although the methodology differed among these several quantifications, they agree that, in supervised deliveries and after the introduction of anaesthetics, delirium had become rare. But it was probably common in the early nineteenth century, and may still be common in parts of the world where childbirth is unsupervised.

Chapter

12

Unconscious Delivery

Drugs

In the seventeenth century there was the *cause celèbre* of the Countess of St Géran ('medico-legal landmark')[69] (See Clinical Gem 12.1).

The content of the sedative draft was not stated in the original report; at the time only the hyoscine-containing plants (mandragora, henbane) and opium were available. This was not a medical document, and we do not have to accept Gayot de Pitaval's version. It was either the first recorded case of unconscious delivery, or a unique case of pseudocyesis followed by a delusion of maternity.

Women can give birth without knowing it, not only when anaesthetised, but also when profoundly drunk. Dorfmüller[70] wrote:

> I would like to say something about the way childbirth is handled in our neck of the woods. On the whole it is very dangerous and ineffective. I have often observed these procedures with astonishment and sadness. When a woman goes into labour, liberal use of the beloved spirit bottle gives her Dutch courage, and enables her to forget the pain. To my certain knowledge, some women were so drunk they did not feel a thing.

Others have supported this, but there are only two clear descriptions of parturition in alcoholic coma:

> A miner's wife was in early labour with her 6th child. The doctor left instructions that she should take a little tea, but (knowing her irregular habits) nothing stronger. When he returned, he found her insensible – there was no rousing her. The head was just emerging. She remained unconscious for six hours. On his insistent enquiries, the women attending admitted they had 'fetched a bottle of gin'. At the time they thought they would each get a share, but she drank the whole pint[71].

> A prostitute was admitted to hospital in Amiens in alcoholic coma. She gave birth in this state, and her sleep lasted a little longer. She was surprised to have been delivered, and delighted to have made such a useful discovery, which she could exploit next time[16].

Eclampsia

This is the most common cause of unconscious delivery. Henke[55] summarised a case of *Schlafsucht* [pathological somnolence] published by Platner[53] in another famous 'medico-legal landmark' (see Clinical Gem 12.2).

This was a typical case of eclampsia, and the mention of 'sleep' in a comatose patient betrays the ignorance of physicians and medico-legal experts at the time. Most of the early cases collected by Behrens[72] and Freyer[8] were eclamptic, and similar early cases were reported by Kirkland[32], Ulrich[73] and Spiegelthal[74].

Clinical Gem 12.1   Medico-Legal Landmark: Drugged Delivery

The Count of Saint-Géran was a wealthy widower with one son, Claude de la Guiche. On 17 February 1619, the Count and his son (then aged 18) had a double wedding to a widow and her daughter – Susanne de Longaunay. Despite many a pious pilgrimage, Susanne remained childless, and the family fortune was destined for Claude's sister, the Marquise de Bouillé. A ne'er-do-well, the Marquis de Saint-Maixent, already accused of magic, incest and strangling one wife to marry another, parked himself on the family. He started a liaison with the Marquise de Bouillé, who secretly agreed to marry him after the death of her aged husband. The Count died, and Claude succeeded him. At this point, Susanne conceived and the birth of the new heir was eagerly awaited. The Marquis de Saint-Maixent and Marquise de Bouillé ('the conspirators') corrupted the butler (Beaulieu), bribed two chamber-maids (the sisters Quinet) and engaged a midwife, Louise Goillard, called by Dumas, who recounted this case in his *Crimes Celèbres, une faiseuse d'anges* [an angel-maker]. On 16 August 1641, Susanne went into labour. The conspirators cleared the room and the midwife gave Susanne a *breuvage* [beverage], which sent her into a deep sleep ('the perfect image of death') until the next day. That night she gave birth to a boy, whom the midwife attempted to crush to death. For unexplained reasons her hands were torn away, though his skull ever after bore the marks of her murderous assault. Beaulieu spirited the babe away, and took it on horseback many leagues, stopping only to engage temporary wet-nurses. One refused to foster the babe, because he would not name the parents. But another, Marie Pigoreau, who had recently lost a son, took him for a sum of money. He was baptized Bernard, with fictitious parents and hired godparents. Meanwhile Susanne awoke, bleeding heavily. She demanded the baby. At first she was told she had not yet given birth, then that she had never been pregnant. With the help of religion she eventually accepted her disappointment. But two years later, Pigoreau, who had exhausted the money, returned the child to Beaulieu. Not knowing what to do, he persuaded Claude and Susanne to take the toddler ('his nephew') into their own household. Susanne became attached to him – a fair-haired, blue-eyed child about the same age as the one she thought she never had. Beaulieu, troubled in his conscience, began to express remorse. The Marquise de Bouillé had him poisoned. When the boy was seven years old, he was made a page. Rumours began to circulate. Susanne caught the Marquise de Bouillé in consultation with the midwife. Goillard was arrested and interrogated. First she said the baby had been stillborn, then that it had never been delivered, then that it was a mole pregnancy. Twice, under torture, she admitted that it had been stolen. But she never named the conspirators. The boy (now Bernard de la Guiche, Compte de la Palice) was introduced to the King. All the conspirators and their accomplices died (none confessing), but Susanne (now a widow) was determined to prove she was the boy's mother. Pigoreau (financed by rival heirs to the St Géran fortune) also claimed to be the mother, and a protracted legal tussle ensued. One of Susanne's difficulties was that unconscious delivery was considered impossible because of Genesis 3:16 – 'In sorrow thou shalt bring forth children'. She declared that if the court did not decide in her favour, she would marry the boy to ensure his inheritance. She won (1659), and Pigoreau was sentenced to death. Since she had made good her emigration, she was hanged in effigy. The young Count married and had a daughter who became a nun, extinguishing an illustrious family.

Clinical Gem 12.2 Medico-Legal Landmark: Eclampsia Not Neonaticide

An 18-year old domestic servant (Mielerin), normally good humoured and of good character, complained of colic, and was sent to bed by her mistress, who thought she had caught cold walking barefoot in January. When she failed to appear the next morning, her sister sought her out, and beheld a frightful sight. Mielerin was lying on the straw half-dressed. Bed linen and clothing were strewn about the room. The placenta lay on the floor in a mass of blood. The infant was found nearby, covered in a little straw, but not enough to look like deliberate concealment. The umbilical cord was torn. While all this was going on, the girl lay in the deepest 'sleep', gripped by strong convulsions, almost like epilepsy, especially in the face and arms. Her face was glowing red, her appearance wild and contorted. Shaking and shouting failed to awaken her. Putting the child on her arm, in order to stimulate maternal feelings, made as little impression as the midwife's vaginal examination. She opened her eyes momentarily when the doctor arrived, but promptly 'fell asleep' again. She was not weak and faint, because she resisted an attempt to clothe her, and move her to the bedroom. The following day, when taken to prison on a charge of infanticide, she was blind, deaf, completely insensitive and without consciousness, and took no notice of these events. Her capacity to reason was destroyed. On the 3rd day she gave a deep sigh and made a meaningless noise, as if she had been shaken out of slumber. But her memory and consciousness had not fully returned. She was able to give some answers, but the sense was disturbed by dreams and nonsense. She knew nothing of the birth or the events before and after it. Full consciousness gradually returned, and a month later she could be interrogated. She did not deny the birth, but claimed with the greatest certainty that she knew nothing of the time and place of the event, nor the fate of the baby. She insisted that neither on that day nor afterwards had she any consciousness. She accepted that she had been pregnant, but knew nothing about it until the onset of labour. She never had regular periods, and had only once been with a man (whom she named). The judge counted against her that she had torn or cut the umbilical cord, and covered the infant in straw. The case was heard in Leipzig, where the famous Dr Platner gave evidence with his customary clarity. He diagnosed epilepsy or somnambulism, and gave his opinion that birth in a sleep-like state or with *betäubung* [a dazed state], could occur naturally or artificially, without consciousness or memory of the birth. It was rare but by no means unheard of, as reliable observations had shown.

Other Lesions

Unconscious childbirth can follow trauma, or any other medical condition that leads to coma. Reported cases have been due to head injury, antepartum haemorrhage, apoplexy and the terminal stages of tuberculosis. Poppel[75] described a unique case of birth during hypothermia:

> A naïve 19-year old, so ignorant that she believed babies were delivered through the abdominal wall, denied her pregnancy. When she went into labour, notwithstanding the severe wintry conditions, she rushed home to her mother – a 3-hour journey in an open sleigh at a temperature of −17°. She lost consciousness. The baby was born and fell into the snow, where it was found alive.

In several cases, loss of consciousness was probably due to syncope. If the fall in peripheral resistance is severe enough, a patient who has fainted can remain unconscious even when lying down[76].

> An 18-year old obstinately denied the possibility of pregnancy. Her lover, a doctor, had talked her into believing that their intimacies could not lead to pregnancy. When examined on the morning of her confinement, the foetal head could be felt distinctly; nonetheless she maintained her denial. At noon she complained of pain and went to the lavatory, from where a scream was heard. She had passed out, and had to be dragged into the room. The doctor found her in a state of complete unconsciousness. The foetal head was already in the birth canal and was extracted without difficulty, during which she made no sound. When the shoulders were passing the perineum she groaned and cried out. She recovered half an hour later. It was hard to convince her of what had happened.

Unexplained Stupor or Coma

Not all cases of unconscious delivery are due to drugs, trauma, syncope, eclampsia or other medical disorders. These are some unexplained cases:

> A delicate 20-year old twice gave birth in a state of complete unconsciousness. On the second occasion, she became speechless and unconscious as soon as labour began. Her face was pale, her lips blue and her eyes closed. Her breathing was unnoticeable except when interrupted by deep sighs. In spite of smelling salts and other stimulants, she remained in this state throughout her two-hour delivery. As soon as the child passed the perineum, she came to, without any memory for what had happened[77].

> A woman in labour suddenly lapsed into a death-like state. A surgeon from the neighbourhood set about opening her abdomen with a pair of scissors. But before he could open the uterus, the infant was delivered. The mother recovered in two months[12].

> A healthy labourer's wife, in the 9th month of pregnancy, suddenly developed chills and fever, and was somnolent for a while. For two days she remained well. Towards evening on the third day she groaned and fell into a state of *Scheintod* [suspended animation]. Her extremities were ice cold, her sphincters paralysed, her pulse, heart-beat and breathing not discernable, and her body insensitive to the strongest stimulus. Apart from foetal movements there were no signs of life. After ¾ hour and using all possible means to rouse her, the doctor decided to rescue the child by Caesarean section, and departed to get the necessary instruments. On his return half an hour later, he was intercepted by her husband with the news that his moribund wife had woken with a sigh. Fully conscious, she gave birth to a healthy child[78].

> A delicate, 'hysterical' married woman during her first labour made a great deal of noise with every pain, and was highly restless and disturbed. But during the delivery of the infant's head, she lay still for five minutes, showing no reaction, in a state of complete abolition of consciousness. She had not the slightest memory of the birth[61].

A woman went into labour with her second child. After eight hours, when all was going well but slowly, she became agitated and confused. When the waters broke and the pains became continuous, she lost consciousness and became unresponsive to speech and stimulation. A live but asphyxiated child was delivered by forceps. During this operation, she sighed but did not cry out. Immediately after delivery she regained consciousness. She had only a vague notion of what had happened[49].

A 28-year old felt her first labour pains in the evening. The midwife advised rest and she fell asleep. At 1 am, her husband was awakened by a sigh. He called his wife, then shook her, but there was no response. The midwife was unable to wake her, and called the doctor. Physical examination was normal. Her pupils reacted to light. A cold wet towel and smelling salts had no effect. A hot iron and needle prick produced only a slight movement of the arm. Labour progressed without any sign of pain. The infant was born at 7 am, with no change in her condition. She remained 'asleep' for three days, without eating, or passing water or stool, then woke up. It was difficult to convince her she had been a mother for so long. She had no memories since the onset of labour, and had even forgotten a visit to a neighbour that afternoon. Her second birth was normal[49].

A 20-year old of low intelligence had an 8-hour 1st delivery. She screamed with every contraction. But in the last hour, with equally strong contractions, she lay still and silent, with closed eyes, reacting neither to speech nor the infant's passage through the vulva, which was badly torn. As the perineum was being sewn, 45 minutes later, she opened her eyes, but said nothing and showed no sign of pain[10].

An unmarried girl became completely mute, shut into herself and stuporose during the expulsive stage. Within three hours of delivery this passed off[36].

Two patients have shown catatonic features[76], as in this example[79]:

A 26-year old was in labour for the second time. Shortly after the waters broke, she laid both hands on her head and drew her knees high up, maintaining this position motionless for the last half hour of the birth. She gave no answer to questions. Her eyes were staring, fixed on a point, and she blinked only when her cornea was touched. Her breathing was slow and deep. The birth seemed to cause no pain whatsoever. Immediately afterwards, she suddenly threw herself on her back, pushed her head back on the pillow and for two minutes maintained an *arc-de-circle*. She seemed completely unconscious, and reacted neither to questions nor pin-prick. Ten minutes later she did the same again, then lay still. With the delivery of the placenta she let out a small cry, as if in pain. An hour after the birth she suddenly awoke and looked around bewildered, seeming not to understand where she was, although she recognized the doctor and nurse. When told she was the mother of a healthy boy, she looked incredulous and said, "How can that be?" Given her baby, she said, "God! Doctor! What a strange thing to happen! I knew nothing about it". The last thing she remembered was hearing that the waters had broken.

In two of the cases described[59,79] stupor continued into the puerperium. But Snoek's[49] second patient is in a class of her own, continuing for three days after the birth and followed by retrograde amnesia. Schmidt's patient[77] had a recurrence during another delivery. There is controversy over the possible role of dissociation, which is not unconsciousness, but distraction to the point that the person feels no pain and is unaware of events; the paradigm is hypnosis, and hysteria is a related phenomenon. Occasional cases of unconscious delivery might have been due to hysterical dissociation, but the diagnosis of hysteria is a matter of great difficulty. There is no electro-encephalographic evidence to resolve the dispute. It seems likely that most of these states of stupor and coma are a more severe and prolonged manifestation of the cerebral disturbance leading to delirium. Indeed, Snoek's first patient[49] progressed from delirium to coma.

Chapter

Acts of Desperation

13

Parturient Rage

Nineteenth century obstetricians and medico-legal experts recognized pathological anger (*Wut der Gebärenden, colère d'accouchées*) as a consequence of the pains of childbirth. This phenomenon is important in the understanding of some cases of neonaticide. Wigand[80] wrote,

> I have known several worthy, educated and pious women who, in the anger and rage of the last strong pains, for hours after delivery have refused to see their dearly beloved husband or their ardently desired child.

Luther[81] wrote that in 40 years of obstetric experience he had often seen women driven to anger by pain, fear and despair in the third and fourth stages of labour; he remembered several occasions when four strong men had to hold down a raging woman, in order to complete the delivery. Mende[59] wrote,

> Anger, against the husband who was responsible for putting her in her present predicament, and against the foetus, who caused her such pain . . . could lead to hitting its head against the floor, without knowing what she was doing.

Flemming[82] mentioned a married woman, a mother of several children, who suddenly became disturbed at the end of labour and had to be forcibly prevented from killing her child; afterwards she had no memory of these events. Jörg[23] described women who hit and kicked the midwives, scratched and bit anyone within reach. He and JF Osiander[83] said they not infrequently had to protect the nose or hair of the husband. Scanzoni[84] wrote:

> At the crucial moment of childbirth, the parturient, covered in sweat, moaning and wailing in despair, suddenly escapes control, gathers herself up and demands to be released from her torture, never mind the child. Her eyes are rolling, her carotids pulsating and her face suffused. Gnashing her teeth and with menace, she hits out with balled fist. Neither soothing words, nor strict commands can quell the storm. When a foetal part emerges, out of her mind with pain, she often reaches down with both hands to seize it and haul it out. This is a moment of peril. Sometimes the paroxysm ends with the expulsion of the child. It usually lasts a little longer, though not more than half an hour, leaving no trace. She sinks back exhausted, sometimes breaking into tears and begging forgiveness, and lavishes tender kisses and devotion on the child.

He saw 4 cases in about 10,000 deliveries, during unusually painful or prolonged labours. Morris[85] gave evidence in a case of infanticide:

He had seen quite a number of cases in which women have attempted to strangle their offspring at the time of birth, owing to a temporary insanity occasioned by extreme suffering. This brief insanity, which does not last more than 5–10 minutes, occurs just at the moment when the head is expelled and the body is still *in utero*. Driven wild by the last agonizing pain, the mother attempts to grasp the cause of her suffering and effect its destruction. Being prevented, she turns savagely on the attendants. Every medical man who has a large experience in midwifery must have witnessed this exhibition of uncontrollable impulse.

Many other authors refer to this phenomenon[21,86,87], most recently a Brazilian review[88]. Von Krafft-Ebing[89] included *mania transitoria*, mostly rage followed by amnesia, among his five categories of mental disorder during parturition. Anton[90] stated that aggression against the child was typical, and there were cases in the literature involving married women who have thrown, strangled or throttled the child; one (no citation) took her much desired infant by the feet and struck it on the wall. The following incident led to the death of the child in the presence of a midwife[91]:

A 40-year old nervous woman experienced such stormy pains during her first delivery that each contraction caused her whole body to tremble. This increased with every pain until, as the head was passing through the vulva, she hit out, kicked the midwife out of the way, grabbed hold of the head, tore the baby out of the birth canal, and smashed it against the bedpost, killing it instantly.

Albert[91] linked this behaviour to veterinary observations, citing a cow which calved seven times: as soon as she saw or heard the calf, she flew into a rage and tried to kill it, and anyone else nearby. The first time, giving birth in the field, she mutilated the calf. Thereafter she was firmly tethered, and the calf removed from her presence. This state lasted no more than three days, after which she tended her calf with care.

Though it was widely recognized in the nineteenth century, there are few detailed accounts. Clinical Gem 13.1 is a marvel of description[92]. These are some other cases:

A woman in labour was raving at the moment of birth and for ¼ hour afterwards. She sprang out of bed, hitting out, demanded a knife to cut herself open, and bit the arms of bystanders trying to restrain her[93].

A young woman with gentle disposition, from the onset of labour, began to rave, scream, bite and rage until she was delivered. After the birth she quietened down and asked for her child. She gripped it so fiercely, with such a blistering look in her eye, that she would have murdered it, but for the caution of the attendants. After hours of raging she slept for 16 hours. On waking she had no memory of what had gone before, was delighted the delivery was over, and shed a flood of tears over the absence of her baby, which she looked after with tender care[94].

A 40-year old was in her 6th labour. Just as the head was passing the outlet, she raised herself up and, uttering a terrible imprecation, grasped the infant's head and tried to strangle it. The doctor rescued the baby but not without her husband's help. As soon as the delivery was completed she fell into a deep sleep that lasted several hours. When she awoke she was entirely oblivious of what had happened[97].

A 32-year old mother of six was exhausted after three days in labour. The doctor put on the forceps. As he began to exert gentle traction, a sudden change came over her. She looked wildly round the room with an expression of astonishment. When he started to pull again, she took hold of his arms and hurled a torrent of abuse at her husband, the nurse and himself. She shrieked, fought and struggled frantically. With the aid of all the women in the house, and under a stream of

Clinical Gem 13.1 Parturient Rage

A 24-year old single woman was admitted at the end of the 9th month of pregnancy to the Berlin Obstetric Institute. She was a robust farm girl, and throughout pregnancy maintained her customary good health. This continued during her month-long stay in the Institute, where she worked diligently and gained a reputation as a quiet, modest, friendly and good-natured young lady. But this behaviour suddenly changed when she went into labour. From the first contraction she disobeyed every ordinance of obstetric care, tried to escape from the delivery room, insulted those trying to help her, kicked the young doctor (examining her) on the head, and made a thoroughly nasty impression. However disconcerting this behaviour, no-one suspected she was out of her mind, because there was no change in her pulse or temperature, no inconsistency in her verbal utterances, no disorientation in time, place or situation, and no apparent clouding of her sensorium. It was supposed that labour pains revealed her true character, up till then concealed. The birth canal, contractions and foetal position were normal, but labour was slow because she tried to suppress the contractions. The foetal head remained for hours at the pelvic exit, and her pulse rate and jerking limbs gave cause for concern. It was decided to complete the delivery with forceps. While her child was being extracted, she showed the same behaviour as before, making insulting remarks and kicking the doctor in the chest, so that she had to be restrained by his students. Hardly was the infant born than she tried to grab it, in order (so she said) to tear off its head. She was rebuked for her atrocious behaviour and kept under close observation, while the infant was placed in the care of another mother. She lay quietly in bed, awake but mute, for four hours. When an attendant chanced to pass by, she asked in a tone of amazement how it happened that she was in the ward for newly delivered mothers. The attendant, likewise amazed, gave her the appropriate answer. Verifying her delivery by feeling her body, she asked for her child. The attendant refused, telling her the doctor had forbidden it, because she had tried to harm it, and went on to give an uncensored account of all that had happened. This caused such dismay that the midwife sent for the doctor. He found her in a state of inconsolable remorse. She begged for her child. To calm her, he allowed it to be brought, and witnessed a moving scene of maternal tenderness and pleading for forgiveness. Neither at this time, nor later, had she any memory of her 18-hour labour and the first four hours postpartum; between the preliminary examination at the onset of labour and the attendant passing her bed, she had complete amnesia. Miss Schultz became, as before, modest, friendly and good-hearted. She looked after her baby with great care and left the hospital in perfect health five weeks later.

foul language, blows and kicks, he delivered a healthy boy. She immediately fell back exhausted and slept. When she woke she said, "Papa, why don't you send for the doctor. I will die if this lasts much longer". She partly remembered some of the things she had said, and asked for forgiveness. It all seemed like a dream[98].

I personally encountered this case:

A patient went into labour for the second time. She asked for her (deceased) mother 4–5 times, and refused to give birth until she came. During her ordeal, she hit her husband several times.

These cases, described by medical men in attendance on married women having the full benefits of obstetric care, give an insight into what may be happening during clandestine deliveries. In some neonaticides, the infant is decapitated, or stabbed many times, or its head smashed. The relationship to delirium is important. Anger or violence was a feature in at least 6 of the well-described cases of delirium[10,14,39,40,60,99]. Of 10 detailed cases of parturient rage, 4[92,96–98] had amnesia for the episode. Amnesia claimed by a person accused of homicide must be viewed with scepticism, but these were all clinical observations, none resulting in criminal charges. In a clandestine delivery, it would be impossible to know whether or not rage was part of a wider cognitive disturbance.

Auto-Caesarean Section

With Szabo[100] I reviewed more than 20 cases. The first record of a mother performing the operation on herself occurred in Jamaica; it was published in two separate reports, one by Cawley[101] and the other by Moseley[102], of which the 'historical curiosity' described in Clinical Gem 13.2 is a synthesis.

We divided the cases into three groups, according to the apparent motivation for the act. In a few cases, details were insufficient to assess the mother's psychological state[103–105].

Destruction of an Unwanted Child

In four cases, the pregnant woman probably acted to get rid of an unwanted child at an advanced stage of gestation, without risking a charge of infanticide (which is usually defined as murder of a child that has lived outside the body). Other mothers have murdered the infant at an even later stage – during the birth process itself – first reported by Hoffmann[106].

In 1822, in Nassau, Rensselaer County, New York State, a 14-year old quadroon, pregnant with twins and in active labour, performed a Caesarean section on herself lying in a snow bank 200 yards from the house. Her employer found her covering the first child with snow. She ran to the house, with some intestines hanging out of the wound. She put away the razor and a large needle she had brought with her. A doctor came and removed the 2nd child and placenta. Dr McClellen arrived and noted that there was a double incision, one at right angles to the other, with a total length of four inches. The abdomen was full of blood. He sewed up the wound. He deduced that she had delivered the first child by the natural route. She recovered in a few weeks and was alive six years later[107].

A 23-year old unmarried peasant woman from Viterbo (Italy), under interrogation by her family about her increasing girth, opened her abdomen with a kitchen knife. The wound measured five inches, directed obliquely outward and downwards. She opened the uterus, cut off an arm and the infant's head, and removed the placenta. She bound her abdomen, hid the foetus and returned to work. In a nearby city she showed her sister a blood-stained cloth as evidence of menstrual

Clinical Gem 13.2   Historical Curiosity

Auto-Caesarean Section

In the year 1769, a black woman belonging to Mrs Bland, a midwife, at Mr Campbell's grass plantation at the Ferry, between Kingston and Spanish Town, being in labour, performed the Caesarean operation on herself, and took her child out of the left side of her abdomen, by cutting boldly through the uterus. She performed this operation with a broken butcher's knife. The position of the child was natural; the cut was near the linea alba, on her left side, about three lines deep, and two inches and a half long; it cut into the child's right thigh. The child came out by its own struggling. A lay midwife cut the umbilical cord, freed the child, returned some intestines, and stitched the abdomen. A few hours later the surgeon who attended the plantation[§] was called. He found her in a dirty situation, with dirt in wound. He cut open the stitches, extracted the placenta, carefully washed the wound, and stitched it up again. On the third day, she had recovered from her sunken state, but developed a fever, which was treated by antiphlogistics and bark. The wound was fomented and dressed, and soon cured. In six weeks she was well, and able to return to work. The child came into the world healthy and strong, but died on the sixth day, with the jaw-falling [*trismus neonatorum*]. The woman remained well, menstruated regularly, and was pregnant again a year or two afterwards. She attempted the same operation again, but was watched and prevented, and had a regular and proper labour. She had borne three children before this affair, all natural and easy births. She was an impatient and turbulent woman, whose violence of temper was the only cause assigned to her conduct.

[§] In Cawley's account this was a 'horse doctor'. That report stated that the child died on the second day and the mother herself died from dysentery on the 9th day. But there is no doubt that this was the same case, because the woman was enslaved to the same woman – Mrs Bland.

bleeding. Walking home (a five-hour journey on foot), she fainted and doctors were called: 13 hours after the extraction, most of the intestines protruded. She recovered[108,109].

A 19-year old had concealed her pregnancy. She felt suicidal and, before the onset of labour, decided to put an end to her life. She opened her abdomen with a 20 cm incision and cut open the uterus. Intestine was protruding from the wound. Her mother came in and called a doctor. She was admitted to hospital with an abdominal wound, severely anaemic. Signs of pregnancy were found, and the uterus and abdomen sutured. The following morning, her father found the baby and placenta in a bucket, partly submerged in water. There were cuts in the placenta and the child's back. She was accused of infanticide. She had a raging fever for six weeks, but recovered. Later she was married and gave birth after a normal delivery[110,111].

In Sošice (Croatia), a 26-year old farmer's wife became pregnant while her husband was working in America. In the second trimester she cut open her abdomen from the navel to the left hip, and removed a foetus, which she threw into a bush. She sewed up her abdomen but not her uterus. She made her way home half an hour away, and lay in bed for ten days, after which she was admitted to Karlovac hospital (Croatia), but died some days later. Necropsy showed the placenta *in situ*, and widespread sepsis[104].

In another case, auto-Caesarean Section was attempted, but the baby was born vaginally, and then killed.

In Hokkaido a 40-year old unmarried woman presented with an abdominal wound, which she said had been inflicted by a street gang. But one of her relatives found a dead baby in the washing machine. She said she had tried to cut her abdomen when the pains were severe. The baby was born by the natural route. Five other infant corpses were found in plastic bags. She was convicted of infanticide[112].

In this sixth case, the circumstances were shameful, but the mother did not destroy the child.

In Malo Pornaveno (Russia), a 40-year old soldier's wife was pregnant for the 6th time. Conception was extra-marital, in the absence of her husband. When he heard about it, he said, "What will the world say!" At the end of the pregnancy she cut herself open with an axe, making a 14 cm wound in the abdomen and 11 cm in the uterus. Her daughter heard her cry out, and found her covered with blood with a baby in her arms. She made her confession to a priest and died the same day. The baby seemed well, but died on the 9th day[113].

Psychiatric Illness

In three cases, there was no clear reason for the action that was taken by mentally ill mothers. There is a huge literature on self-mutilation, which can take many forms. At the extreme, both eyes have been enucleated (oedipism). It is not surprising that it may involve the uterus.

In this transitory delusional disorder, the operation was performed with the intention of delivering a snake, although the child had already been born:

A 28-year old had spent only 14 days with her bridegroom before he was transferred to another locality. When she became pregnant she formed the delusion that she had been impregnated with immature sperm, and had a snake in her belly. She could not be persuaded that she had a child within. She gave birth to a live infant, but would not acknowledge it. On day 2, when left alone, she seized a bread knife, which she had hidden, and stuck it up to the hilt in her abdomen. A handful of intestine emerged, which she said was the snake. She pulled out a piece of omentum. She recovered from her wound and from insanity, and lived to be the mother of children[114].

This Turkish mother had a chronic delusional state:

> A 32-year old had a 9-year history of psychiatric symptoms: she was suspicious and complained of people gossiping about her; she believed she had given birth to 36 children, and that 30 of them had been stolen by her husband's relatives. She cut open her abdomen and uterus with a razor blade and removed the baby and placenta. The incision curved round the umbilicus on the left side. Her son, aged 11, called the police. She was admitted to hospital in shock and transfused with six pints of blood. Mother and infant survived[115].[a]

The third mother had an unspecified chronic disorder:

> In County Clare, a 34-year old had already given birth to six children and 'had not been of sound mind' for 4–5 years. She laid open her abdomen with a razor, and plucked out a live child, together with the placenta. Unfortunately the neighbours, frightened by the awful sight, ran away, and the child was dead by the time the doctor arrived three hours later. The wound extended from an inch above the umbilicus straight down for five inches. Intestine protruded, but the uterus was firmly contracted and there was little bleeding. The infant had a two-inch wound on the buttock. The wound was cleansed and sewn, but the woman died from peritonitis on the 2nd day[116].

Obstructed Labour

In the other eight cases, the mother resorted to desperate remedies in prolonged labour. Two believed they were on the point of death[117,118]; in others, the unendurable ordeal of labour was the only evident factor. One has been summarized previously (Clinical gem 13.2). These are the others:

> A Lancashire woman, mother of four, after being in labour for 36 hours, on being abused by her husband, made a 5-inch incision on the left side of her abdomen with a weaver's knife. When the doctor arrived she was drenched in blood and moribund. A dead child was removed from the abdomen and the wound dressed, but she died two days later[119].

> In 1879, a peasant woman in Priština (then in Turkey, now Kosovo) who had been in labour for three days with unbearable pains, cut open her abdomen and uterus with her husband's razor. Holding the wound edges with her hands, she asked a neighbour to stitch them, providing her with needle and silk thread. Mother and child survived[120].[a]

> In Biela (Bohemia) a 37-year old, mother of six, went into labour in the 8th month. After three days in labour she had convulsions, and believed she was going to die. Using a razor, she made repeated cuts 9 cm long, extracted the infant and placenta and cut the umbilical cord. She said foetal movements had already ceased. A physician found her in a miserable house, on a dirty bed, exhausted, bloodless and only able to respond with signs, with a dead child between her knees. A large coil of intestine protruded through the wound. The womb was firmly contracted. He dealt with the wound and she made a full recovery[117].

> In 1901 the 42-year old wife of a Turkish farmer, suffering from pulmonary tuberculosis and osteomalacia, was at full term in her 16th pregnancy. Believing she was at death's door, she opened her abdomen with a rusty jagged knife, which she had hidden for three days. The child fell out and she lost consciousness. When she came round, she awoke her 13-year old daughter, who removed the placenta, and sewed up her wound with a rusty needle and thread, and dressed the wound with moss. Dr Löffler arrived two days later. Mother and child recovered[118].

---

[a] Papaloucas[121] briefly summarized a case in a woman from Radovo (now in Macedonia) using almost exactly the same words – perhaps the same case.

A 38-year old Viennese metal-worker's wife had a slow labour. The midwife went home at midnight. At 4.15 am, the husband found her sitting on the bed, with blood on the floor. She had made a 10 cm cut in her abdomen, from which omentum escaped. She said she had been in severe pain, so used a pocket-knife, seeking relief. Several hours later, a Caesarean section was completed in hospital. The child was dead. There were four small wounds in the uterus, six in the child and one in the placenta. The mother died from sepsis[110].

A woman from the Kitosh tribe in Kenya was in labour with her 10th child. She could not stand the pains of labour and cut open her abdomen with a safety razor, making an 8-inch incision, with three separate cuts. She was driven to the hospital 45 miles away in a 3-ton lorry. On arrival, most of the intestines had prolapsed. The child was alive, but both buttocks had been amputated by the incisions, and it died on the 3rd day. The mother was anaemic and developed a uterine infection. She recovered and was discharged well ten weeks later[122].

A 40-year old Mexican woman, living in a village without water, electricity or sanitation, who lost her 8th child through obstructed labour two years before, went into labour and was again obstructed. Using her skills in slaughtering animals, she drank three glasses of spirits, and sliced open her abdomen with a kitchen knife. On the third attempt, she was able to cut the uterus longitudinally and deliver a live infant. She asked one of her children to call a nurse before she lost consciousness. The nurse replaced her bowels and sutured the skin, then transferred her to hospital by car, eight hours distant. The abdomen was reopened, her tubes tied and the uterine and abdominal walls sutured in layers. She had to have a second laparotomy to release a twisted colon. She recovered[123].

This phenomenon may be less rare in countries that lack modern obstetric services – nations whose contributions to literature are at present light. If there is no other means of delivery, and the nearest hospital many hours away, and reachable for example by 'mammy wagon' or canoe, such desperate measures are only to be expected. According to Näcke[124], Ploss-Bartels asserted that such events occurred occasionally in the East, and in Africa. AbouZahr and Wardlaw's[29] data on the low percentage of deliveries attended by skilled personnel in sub-Saharan Africa and South Asia outline the circumstances in which courageous mothers in obstructed labour may take a knife to themselves.

Only five of these women are known to have died from the operation[104,110,113,116,119]. If we include Barker's[119] second case and Rosenzweig's Montenegran woman[104], the survival rate was 15/21 (71 per cent). This agrees with the findings of Harris[125], who collected 12 cases of pregnant women gored by cattle: 9 survived. Three women in our series had at least one further child[102,111,114]. The survival rate for the infants was lower, because five were deliberately killed, and probably two more[107]. Three died in the neonatal period[102,113,122]. Five are known to have survived[114,115,118,120,123].

Auto-Episiotomy

The literature contains an instance of this obstetric procedure, self-performed[126]:

Perrin de la Touche performed an autopsy on a new-born child, a suspected victim of infanticide. It had lived, but there were no signs of violence and only three small sub-pleural ecchymoses. The mother was a poor 21-year old seamstress, small, sickly and hunch-backed. She did not hide her pregnancy, and warned the neighbours. She summoned them when she went into labour, but they had gone out for a walk. Delivery was obstructed at the pelvic floor, so she took a pair of scissors, introduced them as deeply as she could, one blade between the vulva and the infant head (protected by a finger to avoid wounding it), and closed them sharply. At that moment she lost consciousness. The baby died accidentally from asphyxia between the thighs of its mother. The police took no further action.

Suicide

The literature consists of 12 cases of attempted suicide during labour[18,33,127–132,134–136,138–143].
Most unsuccessful attempts had all the hallmarks of psychological determination – three
threw themselves out of a window[18,133,140]. This mother tried to hang herself[135]:

> A mother of five developed oedema and albuminuria in her next pregnancy. Before the birth
> she said, "Strike me dead before I suffer such pain". Two days after the onset of labour, and
> 16 hours after the waters broke, she was found in deep coma. She had hanged herself from the
> door jam. She was revived by artificial respiration. She was delivered of a very large child, with
> a face presentation. When she came to, she was struggling, hitting out and biting; it was ten
> hours before she calmed down. She remembered the suicide attempt, which she carried out in a
> state of frightful fear: she thought no-one would help her and the doctors would tear her apart.
> She did not know she had given birth. She developed a postpartum fever, but recovered after 30
> days.

These are eight accounts of completed suicide:

> A woman denied her pregnancy. One night she left her bed and disappeared. Her body was found
> by a fisherman near the mill where she worked. Necropsy showed she was in labour when she
> died[144].

> A young lady was seized by labour pains in the middle of the night. She got up, dressed, walked
> 250 yards and drowned herself in the river. When she was found two hours later, the baby's
> head had traversed the vulva[145].

> The doctor saw his patient, known to be melancholic, falling past the window as he was climbing
> the stairs. Mother and child died[146].

> A 20-year old jumped out of a 3rd floor window and died from multiple fractures – skull,
> pelvis, spine, and many other bones. The child had a fractured skull[147].

> A woman drowned herself during labour[148].

> A patient committed suicide by jumping out of the window, because she could not stand the pains
> of birth[24].

> A fully clothed woman was buried as a suicide. On the rumour that she was pregnant, and had
> been murdered, she was exhumed 18 days later: a new born baby was found among her clothes,
> and the placenta was in the vulva[149]. (The alternative diagnosis is post-mortem birth.)

> A 22-year old was not known to be pregnant. She went shopping and was last seen alive by a shop
> assistant. Shortly afterwards she was found in a pool of blood at the bottom of a ventilation shaft,
> having jumped from the second floor. She was in early labour, and the uterus had ruptured in the
> fall[150].

> A mother was in labour when she gassed herself and her two children[151].

Chapter
14
Other Parturient Psychoses, Organic and Non-Organic

Parturient delirium, and birth in stupor or coma, are by no means the only organic disorders observed during parturition. Five eclamptic psychoses and one Donkin psychosis began during labour, as did four epileptic psychoses and six infective psychoses.

There are also 15 non-organic psychoses, which differ from parturient delirium in their long duration (at least two weeks and usually more than two months), and psychopathology of mania rather than delirium. They were first described by an American[57]:

> A 28-year old complained of headache and depression during the last month of her 4th pregnancy. Towards the end she became sleepless and excited about religious subjects and in great anxiety about her confinement [prodromal symptoms, but insufficient evidence of prepartum psychosis]. In the 1st stage of labour, her mind was wandering; she talked incoherently on religious subjects, imitating the Quaker tone of preaching. As labour failed to progress, she became more and more delirious. A putrefied infant was born. She slept for a time, and awoke in a wild state of mind, and attempted to jump out of the window. She became so violent that it was necessary to fasten her to the bed. On day 6 she was raving uninterruptedly and incoherently, repeatedly using indecent words. By day 7 she had less than six hours sleep since the birth. She improved, but 17 days after the birth relapsed and was removed to an asylum (case 3).

This is another example[152]:

> A 20-year old mother of four had a mentally ill sister. Two days before term in her 5th pregnancy she became anxious, fearing she would not survive. During labour she spoke in a confused way, disputing the fact that a child was about to be born. After an easy delivery, restlessness increased from day to day. She prayed, laughed, sang, spoke nonsense, tore her bedding, was incontinent and hardly slept. Admitted to hospital after three weeks she lay still and took no interest in her surroundings, then wandered about, started singing and said she would be murdered by ghosts and saw her husband and children in the next bed. She spoke little and in a confused way, misidentified the doctor as the Kaiser and kept talking about not having murdered children. Two months after the birth she recovered.

Allowing one day for parturition, the frequency is 1,274 published cases/trimester, which is lower than that of day 1 and early postpartum onset, but higher than any other onset group (see Section 4 page 199). Three had a relapsing pattern, three had previous psychotic episodes and two had other postpartum episodes. Four mothers in my series had parturient onsets. This is one:

> A woman was reared by a paranoid mother in a noisy and chaotic home. At the age of 24 she had the first of two cycloid episodes. At 27 she gave birth to her only child @ 42 weeks gestation. During her 36-hour labour, she misidentified a student midwife as an acquaintance from a religious cult. She could feel insanity coming on. "I got very paranoid, thinking that staff were saying negative things about me". Within hours she was 'dipping in and out of psychosis'. After the

birth she became confused and frightened. By day 3 she was staring blankly, not speaking, refusing food, drink and medication, and incontinent of urine. By day 8 she improved, as if awaking from a bad dream. A week later she relapsed, but with six ECT again recovered within two weeks. In the course of 24 years she had five unrelated episodes, with a variety of diagnoses including hypomanic, paranoid and schizophreniform episodes.

With the reservation that there is much diagnostic uncertainty in this group of patients, I consider that, on the balance of probability, a trigger of bipolar-cycloid episodes is already active during labour.

Chapter

15

Postpartum Delirium and Stupor Immediately after the Birth

Introduction

As soon as the infant is born, there is a dramatic change, physically and psychologically. There is little or no pain, but there is a risk of infection and anaemia, and a slide in blood levels of several hormones. The mental disorders found in the immediate aftermath of parturition include exhaustion, fainting and shock, confusion and stupor.

Exhaustion and Fainting

The ordeal of labour, including the exertion and pain, and in some cases lack of sleep and emotional turmoil, can be followed by extreme weakness and inertia[153,154]. Mende[59] wrote:

> A state of numbness can follow, rendering the mother incapable of making the smallest effort to look after the newborn.

The exhausted mother submits passively and drowsily to any procedures. Döffler[94] included *Erschöpfungszustände* [exhaustion states] as one of his categories of mental illness – so well known to midwives and obstetricians that there was no need to provide examples. Its forensic importance, in clandestine deliveries, was recognized at an early stage[55]. The infant often needs stimulation to breathe and can die from suffocation by mucus. Exhaustion alone, without fainting or delirium, can prevent a mother from succouring a moribund infant.

Fainting is due to brain anaemia, usually with prodromal signs such as yawning, dizziness, noises in the ears and visual effects. It was mentioned by many other authorities, but especially Freyer[8], who wrote a comprehensive monograph, *Die Ohnmacht bei der Geburt* [fainting in childbirth]. He conducted two contemporary enquiries.

(1) He sent a questionnaire to 517 doctors in Prussia and the rest of Germany, receiving 290 answers. Only three cases of fainting not due to other causes of loss of consciousness were reported. Systematically searching two major journals, he came across this example, reported by a physician from his own household[155]:

> In the night, there were cries for help from the kitchen. The cook, known to be pregnant, was on her knees in a lake of blood. A newborn infant was lying on the ground, its head cradled by the woman's left hand. She suddenly lost consciousness and fell on the child. It required a lot of effort to lift her up, and the baby would have been crushed if no help was at hand. Dr Kamnitzer cut the cord, removed the placenta, and got the mother into bed. She was roused by cold water and friction, not less than 15 minutes after she fell. She had two other fainting attacks during the day. The child lived. If it had died, and he had not been there to observe the mother's condition, no-one would have believed she had fainted, and she would have been convicted of infanticide.

(2) He conducted a unique investigation into clandestine delivery. Everyone believed that complications were much more common in these cases, but without confirmatory data. He considered the legal reports on 195 clandestine deliveries that came to court in 1879–1885. A large minority claimed to have lost consciousness – 34 during the birth and 28 afterwards (32 per cent). He critically examined the evidence, and accepted 20 cases:

- In five, witnesses arrived in time to observe the mother in a collapsed state.

A woman gave birth on the toilet: the child cried and people came running; she then, before their eyes, lost consciousness (case 121).

- In ten, the mother described fainting or loss of consciousness during the birth, but this formed no part of her defence, because she confessed to killing the child at a time when she was fully conscious.

A woman gave birth standing and then fainted. She recovered half an hour later, and went to wake up the householders. She returned to find the child still living and hit it with a piece of wood (case 25).

- In five, she claimed to have lost consciousness during or immediately after the lethal act, but nevertheless confessed to infanticide.

A woman was disturbed and fearful that she could be discovered at any minute. She immediately suffocated the babe with a vest and stuffed it in a cupboard. She then fainted (case 130).

These 20 cases made up 1/10 of the series of 195 clandestine deliveries associated with neonaticide. This compares with 1/4,000 for all such complications on academic obstetric units[10]. He concluded that fainting in clandestine delivery was less common than claimed, but much more common than in supervised deliveries.

Debus[38] conducted an extensive review, trawling the textbooks. The rarity of fainting suggested that hospital delivery, with births in a horizontal position, a tranquilizing and comforting ambience, and restriction of blood loss, prevented their occurrence. Clandestine deliveries were usually first deliveries, often in upright, crouching or sitting position, sometimes with *Sturzgeburt* [precipitate delivery], as well as emotional crises, postpartum haemorrhage, and perineal or cervical tears; all these factors increased the risk. Collet's thesis[9] on *accouchement spontané rapide* [rapid births] is a mine of information – detailed and well documented, logical and concise; he discussed whether rapid delivery (as opposed to haemorrhage) could itself lead to fainting, which was a matter of dispute between obstetricians and forensic experts: each case had to be considered on its merits after a detailed and sceptical analysis of the circumstances. Montel[156] collected evidence in a thesis on 'nervous shock'. He claimed that a state of collapse could occur in the postpartum period without uterine haemorrhage, rupture or inversion, collecting four cases. There seems, therefore, to be sufficient evidence that fainting can occur without haemorrhage or uterine catastrophes. Döffler[94] claimed that one of its features, in contrast to exhaustion, was amnesia. But this depends on loss of consciousness, which does not occur in all cases, but only in those sitting upright, or with sufficiently severe hypotension.

Postpartum Delirium

In the section on parturient delirium, it was mentioned that some episodes continued into the puerperium for a few hours. Delirium can also start after delivery. The first description was associated with pain during the delivery of the placenta[157]:

A 24-year old married woman, pregnant for the first time, gave birth to a healthy boy after a 13-hour labour. Ten minutes later, the placenta was delivered, immediately followed by strong after-pains returning every 4–8 minutes. She began to rave and rage. She recognized none of those present (not even her husband), hit out violently, tried to get out of bed and could only be held down by several attendants. She said she was being threatened by murderers and thieves and shouted for help. She kicked out at the child when it was brought to calm her. She cursed her husband, with whom she lived in harmony. The uterus felt as hard as a stone. The doctor prescribed opium and castor oil. She gradually became quieter, and fell asleep. After a few hours, she woke completely restored, and had no memory for these events.

In other cases postpartum delirium has occurred without pain. There are 20 in the literature[10,39,68,157–170]. Several were associated with violence[39,161,162,164,167], as in this example[162]:

A 28-year old was delivered of her 2nd infant after a 3-hour painful labour. Immediately after the birth she started to rave, sprang out of bed, hit out, scratched and bit everyone in sight. She hit the midwife on the head with a water jug, and required four people to restrain her. After 4½ hours she sank into a state of exhaustion for 15 minutes, then slept for 10 hours. When the doctor returned, she had no knowledge of his earlier attendance. All she remembered was the midwife saying, "It's a girl!"

Two mothers had recurrent episodes involving two pregnancies[160,171]. A third had a single episode after one birth and a phasic disturbance after another[163]:

Immediately after her 5th child was born, a 30-year old suffered a *délire* with cries and agitation; this settled down after two hours. Her 6th pregnancy was complicated by frequent vomiting. She went into labour a month overdue. It was severe and prolonged and she became agitated. After delivery she had a postpartum haemorrhage. She was given some ergot and the uterus contracted. Suddenly she was seized by *délire*, with agitation and incessant movements. The memory of a deceased relative came to her mind, and she spoke as if this person was present. She was exasperated by the efforts made by the doctor, the nurse and her husband to restrain her, and became violent. She cried out, wept and demanded why she was not allowed to visit this dead person. This lasted 4–5 minutes, after which she seemed to wake, and take note of where she was. But, after a pause, it all started again with the same manifestations, but was this time more violent and persistent. She had nine more attacks in two hours. The penultimate attack occurred four hours after the birth, and then she fell asleep. She awoke with no memory for these events. Eleven hours after delivery she had another attack lasting 30 minutes. She slept for seven hours and remained well.

Amnesia was mentioned in nine cases. An alternative cause was present in six cases – severe blood loss[39], Donkin psychosis[10], and in four cases anaesthetics or other drugs[68,166,169,170]. As for frequency, Kirchberg[50], citing Neubürger, stated that his was the only case of the kind in 3,160 births, and Engelhard[10] had one possible case in nearly 20,000 deliveries. Thus, it is less common than parturient confusion.

Postpartum Stupor

Kelso[172] described two cases of 'nervous exhaustion' seen in his own practice of 1,000 deliveries, one of which was recurrent. By this he meant labour followed by a protracted state of insensibility. The eyes remained partly open and fixed, or the lids drooped languidly showing some portion of the eyeballs. Respiration was imperceptible, the heart regular but weak. The countenance was wan and expressionless, the skin pallid and cold. The limbs were feeble and lifeless, but retained for a short time the position in which they were placed. All consciousness was suspended. From this state of alarming prostration, the patient could be aroused, with difficulty and only temporarily, by pinching, bellowing in the ears, volatile salts, burning feathers applied to the nostrils or cold water. The total span was 3–4 hours, but this was divisible into paroxysmal attacks, diminishing in severity and duration, with each recovery more complete. During remissions the mother could give slow and hesitant answers. When fully recovered, she was 'affrighted and wondered what in all the world could have occasioned such an assemblage of anxious relatives and friends.' She had only a feeble recollection of what occurred since her delivery. This is not like syncope, which rarely persisted for more than five minutes. Each of his patients received an oral dose of laudanum after delivery.

> His first case followed a second labour, lasting 18 hours. She had headache, a sense of praecordial oppression, slight giddiness and pallor. Ten minutes later she lapsed into complete insensibility with periods of remission, with total length nearly 3½ hours.

> His second case followed the 7th delivery of a 38-year old, lasting 20 hours. After delivery of the placenta she complained of headache and a crushing sensation in the lower chest. Ten minutes later she was speechless and apparently dying. She was in profound stupor. After half an hour she briefly rallied, then relapsed. A series of episodes continued until she recovered after four hours. Another obstetrician who attended two previous confinements said she had similar attacks on each occasion.

Under the name of *melancholia attonita*, Tott[173] described three cases:

> A 20-year old, whose sister suffered from puerperal melancholia, gave birth to her first child. Immediately after delivery she lay motionless as if struck by lightning. Her eyes were open and she appeared to be lost in amazed contemplation, as if unable to grasp the immensity of the extraordinary event that had happened to her. Entreaty, shouting and shaking had no effect. With open eyes she seemed to see nothing, hear nothing and feel nothing. She took something to drink without a murmur. There was no catalepsy. She recovered in 24 hours.

> Another woman, immediately after the difficult delivery of her 8th child, became somnolent. Speech and shaking had no effect. She woke after 24 hours, but remained stuporose, like the first case, but more mildly. This lasted two days and disappeared without trace.

> A farmer's wife, immediately after a severe delivery, lay with her eyes open, seeing, hearing and feeling nothing. She could not be stimulated to move, speak or take anything to drink. Her pulse was small and slow and she breathed gently. She seemed sunk in endless spaces of contemplation, as if struck by something her intellect could not grasp. An emetic was introduced into her mouth, which she swallowed, and then recovered her faculties.

It is extraordinary that no other cases of this well-defined disorder, somewhat similar to catatonia, have appeared in the literature since the graphic reports published 160 years ago. The most likely reason is that these papers have hardly ever been read; each has been cited only once.

Other Transitory Disturbances Occurring in the First 10 Postpartum Days

Sieche and Giedke[171] described a unique recurrent and familial delirium that may have been due to an inherited metabolic disorder:

> A 26-year old suddenly became agitated and aggressive four days after her first delivery. She had uncontrolled movements, did not recognize familiar people, was disorientated and could only

repeat single words in a stereotyped way. This lasted for 24 hours, with amnesia for the episode. Four years later she gave birth to her 2nd child. On day 1 she felt anxious and complained of nausea. In the evening of day 2 she was making uncontrolled movements of her mouth and arms. She talked in a bewildered way, was disorientated in time, place and situation, did not recognize her husband and confused the names of her daughters. She became agitated and hit people. She recovered the next morning, with partial amnesia for the episode. The EEG showed generalized slowing with delta waves. Her twin sister developed the same complication after her 2nd child was born: on day 3 she became confused, disorientated, agitated and aggressive. On day 4 she had seizures and lapsed into coma. The EEG showed generalized slowing. A CAT scan showed cerebral oedema. On day 5 she died and necropsy showed necrosis of the pituitary and ischaemic lesions especially in the hippocampus.

There are several other transitory disorders occurring some days after parturition that it is convenient to mention here. Although they occur in the same time and space as early onset puerperal mania, their course and psychopathology are different. Steinberger[174] published a case of stupor that started on day 7, lasting less than 24 hours:

A 22-year old gave birth to her 1st child. On day 6 she imprudently stood on the cold floor (in February) with bare feet; she started shivering. On day 7 she became melancholic and still, staring in front of her and looking confused. She answered no questions. The doctor arrived to find her standing upright, stiff, staring at her hands. She responded to questions by a melancholic gaze. She began to improve after 12 hours, and recovered the next day.

Two similar cases have been reported[165,175]:

A 17-year old gave birth to her 1st child. On day 4 she suddenly became confused and tried to throw the child out of the window, because it had a white head. From that moment she sat quite still, stared in front of her all day and took no notice of her surroundings. She was admitted to hospital, and it was not possible to get a word out of her. Three days later she recovered and could not understand how she came to try to jettison her child. She remained well thereafter.

A 36-year old was *sans conscience* two days after a difficult delivery, and responded to questions with a vague gesture. She had stereotypic movements. In hospital she became excited at times, shouted and recited the Lord's prayer at the top of her voice, saw devils, and heard the voice of her dead mother. After two days she recovered but 24 hours later had another brief period of excitement. There was no follow-up.

A London mother consulted me because she felt aggrieved about her obstetric and psychiatric management. She had two similar episodes on days 4 and 9 (see Clinical Gem 15.1). She had an infection, but the clinical picture was unlike an infective psychosis.

There are several other brief (sometimes recurrent) disturbances, closely related to the birth[35,176-181], which differ in clinical picture and duration from puerperal bipolar disorder and organic psychoses. Their cause is unknown. They may belong with the transient delirium known to occur during labour and shortly afterwards, which is also of unknown cause. It is notable that most of these cases date from the mid-nineteenth century, when parturition was an even more severe ordeal. My London patient had a severe labour.

Clinical Gem 15.1   Recurrent Early Postpartum Stupor

A strong and determined, thoughtful and caring, well-educated 35-year old, holding down a responsible job, became pregnant for the 1st and only time. The 20-week scan showed foetal hydronephrosis, but otherwise the pregnancy was uncomplicated. At 42 weeks gestation, after a 10-hour labour, she was delivered by emergency forceps (for foetal distress), of a baby weighing 8 lb 8 oz. In spite of epidural anaesthesia, the pain was 'insane' and continuous. She required blood transfusions, and suffered from perineal discomfort due to an infected episiotomy wound, but without fever. She had no post-traumatic symptoms, but, on a noisy postnatal ward, slept little. On day 3 (75 hours after the birth), she felt 'quite creative'. "I had all these ideas for paintings. I started drawing, and writing ideas on the back of a paper towel". Later that morning she entered a dream-like state. "There was a wall of ice between me and the world. I felt paralysed, and could only move my arms". She could hear people talking but was unable to answer. She could not understand why she was unable to move or speak, and had a sense of doom. "The main thing I felt was complete fear. I thought I had died, and maybe this is what death is like – an in-between world". The blanket felt itchy and uncomfortable, due to skin hypersensitivity, "as if someone had put a chemical on my skin, or iron filings, anything caustic that would irritate". Her husband described her as 'stiff and statuesque, on a frieze, eyes open but not talking, somewhere else'. She was incontinent of urine, and disorientated in time and space. As a mark of the severity of her disorder, the obstetric team ordered a brain scan, which she refused. On the next day she awoke perfectly well, and remembered the experience as a bad dream. She was transferred to the psychiatric hospital. By this time she had a painful perineal suture, haemoglobin 7.6 g/100 ml and leucocyte cell count 16.3/mm^3 with 87 per cent neutrophils. Six days later she had a second episode: she lapsed into a trance, as if she had smoked 'dope', and became 'paranoid'. "I thought they would section my husband and were poisoning me. I was in a floating state, unable to get up off the bed". All that night she could not move, lying rigid. She was incontinent of urine. In the morning, she returned to normal. A community midwife diagnosed the perineal infection (now accompanied by fever), and alerted the obstetric team. She was transferred to the women's hospital and recovered after treatment with intravenous antibiotics.

Summary

Childbirth is often stressful even when it occurs under optimal circumstances. But, in some parts of the world, infants are born without analgesia and without skilled assistance. Clandestine births are an even more extreme ordeal.

The psychiatric complications of parturition include delirium, coma, rage and acts of desperation. They are important in the understanding of neonaticide.

Parturient delirium is now hardly ever mentioned, but more than 50 cases have been described, many of them in the pre-analgesic era. There are various causes of unconscious delivery, but in 9 published cases there was no apparent cause, and this may be a severe variant of the same phenomenon.

Rage was a recognized reaction to severe labour in the nineteenth century.

Acts of desperation include more than 20 cases of auto-caesarean section and 10 of suicide.

Several organic psychoses have begun during labour. It is probable that puerperal bipolar disorder can also start at this time.

The birth of the child may be followed by exhaustion or shock. There are more than 20 detailed reports of postpartum delirium or stupor. Transient delirium or stupor may also occur later in the first 10 days.

References

1   Brockington IF. *Eileithyia's Mischief: the Organic Psychoses of Pregnancy, Parturition and the Puerperium.* Bredenbury: Eyry; 2006.

2   Lee CY, Lau, MPH. Manipulation of external tachodynamometer by the patient: case report. *Henry Ford Hospital Medical Journal.* 1983;31:170–172.

3   Goodlin RC. Pregnant women with Munchausen syndrome. *American Journal of Obstetrics & Gynecology.* 1985;153: 207–210.

4   Pickford E, Buchanan N, McLaughlin S. Munchausen syndrome by proxy: a family anthology. *Medical Journal of Australia.* 1988;148:646–650.

5   Jureidini J. Obstetric factitious disorder and Munchausen syndrome by proxy. *Journal of Nervous & Mental Disease.* 1992;181:135–137.

6   Bivin GD, Klinger MP. *Pseudocyesis.* Bloomington: Principia; 1937.

7   Kiproff I. *Contribution à l'étude des accouchements par surprise.* Thèse, Paris; 1903.

8   Freyer M. *Die Ohnmacht bei der Geburt vom gerichtsärztlichen Standpunkt.* Berlin: Springer; 1887.

9   Collet MJ. *l'Accouchement spontané rapide.* Thèse, Paris; 1904.

10 Engelhard JLB. Über Generationspsychosen und den Einflus des Gestationsperiode auf schon bestehende psychische und neurologische Krankheiten. *Zeitschrift für Geburtshülfe und Gynäkologie.* 1912;70:727–812.

11 Tarnier S, Chantreuil G. *Traité de l'Art des Accouchements.* Volume 1. Paris : Lauwereyns; 1882. p. 590.

12 Coliez. *Accouchements inconscients et sans douleur.* Thèse, Paris; 1898–1899.

13 Depaul. Accouchements sans douleur. *Journal d'Accouchements.* 1907;28:73–74.

14 Montgomery WF. On the occasional occurrence of mental incoherence during natural labour. *Dublin Journal of Medical and Chemical Science.* 1834;5:52–69.

15 Case MW. Labour during sleep. *American Journal of the Medical Sciences.* 1868;279–280.

16 Panis A. *Une femme peut-elle accoucher sans en avoir conscience?* Thèse, Paris; 1861.

17 Palfrey J. Twin labour in which uterine action commenced and progressed to the second stage during sleep. *Lancet.* 1864;i :36.

18 Tardieu A. *Étude Médico-Légale sur l'Infanticide.* Paris : Baillière; 1868.

19 Wescott W. A remarkable case. *Lancet.* 1897;i:607.

20 Taylor AS. Death from rupture of the uterus: inversion of the uterus and expulsion of the child by gaseous putrefaction. *Guy's Hospital Reports.* 3rd series. 1864;10:253–260.

21 Tyler Smith W. A course of lectures on the theory and practice of obstetrics: lecture 39: puerperal mania. *Lancet.* 1856;ii:423–425.

22 Tyler Smith W. *A Manual of Midwifery.* London: Churchill; 1858. p. 489–498.

23 Jörg JCG. *Die Zurechnungsfähigkeit der Schwangern und Gebärenden.* Leipzig: Weygand; 1837.

24 Degaud. *Douleurs exagérées pendant le travail.* Thèse, Lyon; 1904.

25 Editorial. Hypnosis. *New Scientist.* August 6, 2005;35–36.

26 Bydlowski M, Raoul-Duval A. Un avatar psychique méconnu de la puerpéralité: la névrose traumatique post-obstétricale. *Perspectives Psychiatriques.* 1978;4:321–328.

27 Brockington, IF. Postpartum psychiatric disorders. *Lancet.* 2004;363:303–309.

28 Brockington IF. *Motherhood and Mental Health*. Oxford: Oxford University Press; 1996. p. 154–156.

29 AbouZahr C, Wardlaw T. Maternal mortality at the end of the decade. *Bulletin of the World Health Organization*. 2001;79:561–573.

30 Halim A, Utz B, Biswas A, Rahman F, van den Broek N. Cause of and contributing factors to maternal deaths: a cross-sectional study using verbal autopsy in four districts in Bangladesh. *British Journal of Obstetrics & Gynaecology*. 121, supplement 2014;4:86–94.

31 World Health Organization. *Trends in maternal mortality 1990 to 2013*. Geneva: WHO; 2014.

32 Kirkland T. *A Treatise on Childbed Fevers and on the Methods of Preventing Them*. London: Baldwin & Dawson; 1774. p. 56–63, 72–73 and 92–95.

33 Osiander FB. Wahnsinn von Geburtsschmerzen, und Wendung eines Zwillingspaares. In: *Neue Denkwürdigkeiten für Ärzte und Geburtshelfer*. Volume 1. Göttingen: Rosenbusch; 1797. p. 134–140.

34 Reid J. On the causes, symptoms and treatment of puerperal insanity. *Journal of Psychological Medicine*. 1848;1:128–151 and 284–294.

35 Pollák J. Psychosisok a terhesség, szülés és gyermekágy alatt. *Orvosi Hetilap*. 1929;44:1100–1104.

36 Ciulla U. Disturbi psichici e psicosi nello stato puerperale. *Monitore Ostetrico-Ginecologico*. 1940;12:577–626.

37 Sarwey O. see Debus (1896, reference 38).

38 Debus H. *Über Bewusstlosigkeit während der Geburt*. Inaugural-Dissertation, Tübingen; 1896.

39 Weiskorn J. *Transitorische Geistesstörung beim Geburtsakt und im Wochenbett*. Inaugural-Dissertation, Bonn; 1897.

40 Évrot JB. *Essai de classification pathogénetique des délires liés à la puerpéralité*. Thèse, Lyon; 1894.

41 Ticknor CB, Vogtsberger KN. Development of psychosis during premature labour. *Hospital and Community Psychiatry*. 1987;38:406–407.

42 Finlayson J. *Clinical Manual for the Study of Medical Cases*. 3rd ed. London: Smith, Elder; 1891. p. 320–321.

43 Bear J. Associated nervous manifestations and psychoses in obstetrics. *Virginia Medical Monthly*. 1921;48:151–154.

44 Lemeland. Aperçu générale sur les psychoses puerpérales. *Pratique Médicale Francaise*. 1928;9:315–334.

45 Pappenheim. Neurosen und Psychosen der Weiblichen Generationsphasen. *Bücher der ärztlicher Praxis*. 1930;26.

46 Carp EADE. *Psychosen op Exogenen Grondslag en Geestelijke Defect Toestand*. Amsterdam: Scheltema & Holkeme; 1937.

47 Cohen LH. Psychiatric aspects of childbearing. *Yale Journal of Biology and Medicine*. 1943;16:77–92.

48 Kutzinski A. Ungewöhnlicher Verlauf eklamptischer Delirien. *Allgemeine Zeitschrift für Psychiatrie*. 1813;70: 313–317.

49 Snoeck J. Psychoses survenant pendant l'accouchement. *Bullétin de la Société Medical de Gand*. 1902;69:56–62.

50 Kirchberg P. Psychische Störungen während der Geburt. *Archiv für Psychiatrie*. 1913;52:1153–1163.

51 Luning see Freyer (1887, reference 8).

52 Bergström H, Bernstein K. Psychic reactions after analgesia with nitrous oxide for Caesarean section. *Lancet*. 1968; ii:541–542.

53 Platner. Geschichte eines schlafwachenden Zustandes bei Gebärenden, in Bezug auf den Verdacht des Kindmordes erzählt. In: E Hedrich's translation of *Untersuchungen über einige Hauptcapitel der gerichtlichen Arznei-Wissenschaft*. Leipzig: Kummer; 1820. p. 403–415.

54 Nägele FC. *Erfahrungen und Abhandlungen aus dem Gebiethe der Krankheiten des weiblichen Geschlechtes*. Mannheim: Löffler; 1812. p. 114–115.

55 Henke A. Über die zweifelhaften psychischen Zustände bei Gebärenden. *Abhandlung aus dem Gebiete der Gerichtlichen Medicin*. 1820;4:197–232.

56 Neumann KG. *Die Krankheiten des Vorstellungsvermögens*. Leipzig: Karl Knobloch; 1822. p. 152–175.

57 Macdonald J. Puerperal insanity. *American Journal of Insanity*. 1847;4:113–163.

58 Andriezen. In the discussion of a paper by Savage, in Crichton-Browne, chairman. Prevention and treatment of insanity of pregnancy and the puerperal period. *Lancet*. 1896;i:164–165.

59 Mende LJC. *Ausführliches Handbuch der gerichtlichen Medizin für Gesetzgeber, Rechtsgelehrte, Ärzte und Wundärzte*. Volume 2. Leipzig: Duk'schen Buchhandlung; 1826. p. 615–627.

60 Neumann CG. Der Einfluss der Schwangerschaft und des Wochenbetts auf das Gemüth der Frauen. *Journal für Geburtshülfe, Frauenzimmer- und Kinderkrankheiten* 1832;11:234–273 and 437–479.

61 Kremling-Walsrode. see Freyer (1887, reference 8).

62 Worthington JH. On puerperal insanity. *American Journal of Insanity*. 1861;18:42–60.

63 Barker F. Puerperal mania. *New York Medical Journal*. 1872;16:449–472.

64 Bischoff E. Der Geisteszustand der Schwangeren und Gebärenden. *Archiv für Kriminalanthropologie und Kriminalistik*. 1908;29:109–165.

65 Becker FT. *Über transitorischen Dämmerzustand bei der Geburt*. Inaugural-Dissertation, Frankfurt; 1926.

66 Sarrat J. *De l'infanticide dans ses rapports avec les psychoses transitoires des femmes en couches*. Thèse, Lyon; 1911.

67 Willer H. Transitorische Störungen unter der Geburt und ihre forensische Bedeutung. *Deutsche Zeitschrift für die Gesamte Gerichtlichen Medizin*. 1929;15:47–58.

68 Bourson Y. *Contribution à l'étude des psychoses puerpérales*. Thèse, Strasbourg; 1958.

69 Gayot de Pitaval F. Enfant réclamé par deux mères. In: *Causes Célèbres et Intéressantes avec les Jugements qui ont Décidées*. Volume 1. The Hague, Neaulm; 1775.

70 Dorfmüller. Beytrag zur Behandlung des Wahnsinns oder Raserey der Kindbetterinnen (*mania puerperarum*). *Neues Archiv für der Geburtshilfe*. 1804;3:58–74.

71 Clay C. On the prevalence of almost unconscious parturition in manufacturing districts. *Lancet*. 1841;404–407.

72 Behrens JBH. *De partu mirabili foetus vivi in somno matris profundo*. Inaugural-Dissertation, Helmstedt; 1751.

73 Ulrich of Halle. Entbindung ohne Bewusstseyn Gebärenden. *Rusts Magazin für die gesamte Heilkunde*. 1823;14:379.

74 Spiegelthal of Paderborn. Entbindung ohne Bewusstseyn der Gebärenden. *Rusts Magazin für die gesamte Heilkunde*. 1825;20:183–184.

75 Poppel J. Über einen Fall con durch Kälte bewirktem, bewusstlosem Zustande während und nach der Geburt. *Monatsschrift für Geburtskunde und Frauenkrankheiten*. 1865;25:387–392.

76 Schreyer. Gutachten über eine verheimlichte Schwangerschaft und Geburt, ein Beitrag zu Beurtheilung der Zurechnungsfähigkeit der Schwangern und Gebärenden. *Henke's Zeitschrift für der Staatsarzneikunde, Ergänzungsheft*. 1837;24:194–214.

77 Schmidt WJ. Übersicht der Vorfallenheiten an dem klinischen Entbindungs-Institute der K.K. medicinisch-chirurgischen Josephs-Akademie zu Wien vom 1 Nov. 1810 bis lezten Oct. 1812. *Medicinisch-Chirurgische Zeitung*. 1813;1:97–98.

78 Outrepond. 1843 See Döffler (1893, reference 94).

79 Van Rooy. Een geval van bewusteloosheid tijdens de baring. Verslag van het behandelde in de Vergarderomgem vam Januari to Mei 1908, der Nederlansche Gynaecologische Vereeniging te Amsterdam door Dr. Catharine van Tussenbroek. *Nederlander Tijdschrift voor Verloskunde en Gynaecologie*. 1908;18:284–287.

80 Wigand JH. In: Nägele FC editor, *Die Geburt des Menschen*. Berlin: Nicolai; 1820. p. 80–81.

81 Luther H. Etwas über Zurechnungsfähigkeit bei gesetzwidrigen Handlungen in Beziehung auf die neuern Grundsätze in der gerichtlichen Arznei-Wissenschaft. *Hufelands Journal für die Praktische Heilkunde*. supplement, 1826;136–183.

82 Flemming, of Schwerin. Erörterungen über die Frage der Zurechnungsfähigkeit bei zweifelhaften Gemüthszuständen. *Archiv für Medizinische Erfahrung*. July/August 1830;604–653.

83 Osiander JF. *Die Ursachen und Hülfsanzeigen der unregelmässigen und schweren Geburten*. 2nd ed. Tübingen: Osiander; 1833, p. 55–59 and 61–70.

84 Scanzoni FW. *Franz A Kiwisch Ritter von Rotterau's Klinische Vorträge über specielle Pathologie und Therapie der Krankheiten des Weiblichen Geschlechtes*. Prag, Calve; 1855. p. 520.

85 Morris J. Insanity during parturition. *Maryland Medical Journal*. 1894;32:248–251.

86 Winslow. On puerperal insanity. *Journal of Psychological Medicine*. 1859;12:9–38.

87 Hirsch W. Puerperal insanity. *Medical Record*. 1900;57:10–14.

88 Garcia JA. Psicoses no ciclo gravido-puerperal. *Anais Brasileiros de Ginecologia*. 1953;35:305–317.

89 v. Krafft-Ebing R. *Die transitorischen Störungen des Selbstbewusstseins. Ein Beitrag zur Lehre vom transitorischen Irresein in klinisch-forensischer Hinsicht, für Ärzte, Richter, Staatsanwälte und Vertheidiger*. Erlangen: Enke; 1868.

90 Anton G. Über Geistes- und Nervenkrankheiten in der Schwangerschaft, im Wochenbett und in der Säugungszeit. In: Anton G. et al. editors, *Handbuch der Gynäkologie*. Wiesbaden: Bergmann; 1910. p. 1–41.

91 Albert of Euerdorf. Wut der Gebärenden und Wöchnerinnen. *Medizinisches Correspondenz-Blatt Bayerische Ärzte*. 1850;11:737–738.

92 Kluge. *Mania parturientium transitoria*. *Medizinische Zeitung*. 1833;2:97–98.

93 Runge W. Die Generationspsychosen des Weibes. *Archiv für Psychiatrie und Nervenkrankheiten*. 1911;48:545–690.

94 Dörffler H. Der Geisteszustand der Gebärenden. *Friedreich's Blätter für Gerichtliche Medizin und Sanitätspolizei*. 1892;44:269–294.

95 Neumann CG. see Eulenberg (1856, reference 96); 1844.

96 Eulenberg. Über Puerperalwahnsinn. *Correspondenz-Blatt der Deutschen Gesellschaft für Psychiatrie und Gerichtliche Psychologie*. 1856;3:121–122.

97 Arnold AB. Insanity occurring in the puerperal state. *Maryland Medical Journal*. 1880;7:73–76.

98 Zinke G. Three cases of puerperal insanity with remarks upon the history, causes, pathology and treatment of the disease. *Transactions of the Obstetrical Society of Cincinnati*. 1884;2:352–364.

99 Busch. *Mania parturientium transitoria*. *Neue Zeitschrift für Geburtskunde*. 1837;5:129–130.

100 Szabo A, Brockington IF. Auto-Caesarean section: a review of 22 cases. *Archives of Women's Mental Health*. 2014;17:79–81.

101 Cawley. No title. *London Medical Journal*. 1785;6:372–373.

102 Moseley B. *A Treatise on Tropical Diseases and on the Climate of the West Indies*. London: Cadell; 1787. p. 62–63.

103 Young JH. *Caesarean Section: The History and Development of the Operation from Earliest Times*. London: Lewis; 1944. p. 12–21.

104 Rosenzweig E. *Auto-sectio caesarea*. *Zentralblatt für Gynäkologie*. 1960;46: 1787–1790.

105 Granier C. *La Femme Criminelle (1906)*. Reprinted by Nabu Press ; 2012. p. 86–87.

106 Hoffmann F. *Infanticidio subparta ex raptu furioso patrato*. In: *Medicinae Rationalis Systematicae*. Dec. V, casus II, Venice: Coltei; 1721. p. 318–327.

107 McClellen S. Case of self-performed Caesarean section. *New York Medical & Physical Journal.* 1823;2:40–42.

108 Baliva R. Una strana e nuova laparo isterotomia. *Raccogliatore Medica.* 5th series. 1886;1:340–341.

109 Serpieri A. Ulteriori notizie sulla ormai celebre Nazzarena de Alexandris di Viterbo. *Raccogliatore Medica.* 5th series. 1886;1:367–368.

110 v. Sury K. Selbstverletzung durch Bauchschnitt während der Schwangerschaft und der Geburt. *Korrespondenzblatt für Schweizer Ärzte.* 1910;4:100–103.

111 Patek R. Ein Beitrag zur Widerstandskraft des Peritoneums und der Uterusnaht nach *sectio caesarea* (von der Patientin selbst ausgeführt). *Zentralblatt für Gynäkologie.* 1913;37:1105–1109.

112 Funayama M, Ikeda T, Tabata N, Azumi JI, Morita M. Case report: repeated neonaticides in Hokkaido. *Forensic Science International.* 1994;64:147–150.

113 Aisenstadt. Opération Césarienne pratiquée avec une hache par la malade elle-même (French summary of a Russian paper). *Répertorium Universitaire d'Obstétrique et Gynécologie.* 1887;150.

114 Osiander JF. Einige Bemerkungen und Beobachtungen über Puerperal-Manie. *Annalen für die Gesamte Heilkunde.* 1843;3:297.

115 Yoldas Z, Iscan A, Yoldas T, Ermete L, Akyürek C. A woman who did her own Caesarean section. *Lancet.* 1996;348:135.

116 Madigan B. Death from injuries inflicted while under delusion. *Lancet.* 1884;i:146.

117 v. Guggenberg O. Entbindung durch Laparotomie, von der Gebärenden selbst ausgeführt. *Prager Medizinische Wochenschrift.* 1885;10:3–4.

118 Löffler R. Ein Fall von *auto-sectio caesarea*. *Wiener Medicinische Wochenschrift.* 1901;10:472–473.

119 Barker L. The history of a case of self-performed Caesarean operation. *New York Medical Journal.* 1930;1:381–383.

120 Gjorgjevic V. No title. *Wiener Medizinische Wochenschrift.* 1880;13:360.

121 Papaloucas C. Autosurgery in women. *Journal of the Royal Society of Medicine.* 2005;98:337–338.

122 Sandford AR. Self-inflicted Caesarean section. *East African Medical Journal.* 1951;28:254.

123 Molina-Sosa A, Galvan-Espinosa H, Gabriel-Guzman J, Valle RF. Self-inflicted Caesarean section with maternal and fetal survival. *International Journal of Gynecology & Obstetrics.* 2004;84:287–290.

124 Näcke P. Ausführung des Kaiserschnitts an sich Selbst. *Archiv für Kriminalanthropologie und Kriminalistik.* 1910;38:158.

125 Harris RP. Cattle-horn lacerations of the abdomen and uterus in pregnant women. *American Journal of Obstetrics and Diseases of Women & Children.* 1887;20:673–685.

126 Perrin de la Touche of Rennes. Cause exceptionelle de syncope au moment de l'accouchement (auto-épisiotomie). *Bullétin de la Société de Médecine Légale de France.* 1899;16:43–46.

127 Anonymous. Wahnsinn von Geburtsschmerzen und Wendung eines Zwillingspaars. *Hartenkeils Medicinisch-Chirurgische Zeitung.* 1798;2:41–42 (probably a summary of Osiander's case, reference 33).

128 Jeffery JD. Case of puerperal mania, with remarks. *London Medical Gazette. new series.* 1839;2:114–116.

129 Blot. 1848. see Tardieu (1868, reference 18).

130 Simpson JY. Lectures on puerperal mania (lecture 35). In: *Works: Diseases of Women.* Edinburgh: Adam & Charles Black; 1872.

131 v. Winckel F. Die Eklampsie der Wöchnerinnen. In: *Die Pathologie und Therapie des Wochenbetts.* 3rd ed. Berlin: Hirschwald; 1878. p. 485–497.

132 Kraepelin E. see Hoppe (1893, reference 133).

133 Hoppe H. Symptomatologie und Prognose der im Wochenbett entstehenden Geistesstörungen (zugleich ein Beitrag zur Lehre von der acuten hallucinatorischen

Verwirrtheit). *Archiv für Psychiatrie und Nervenkrankheiten.* 1893;25:137–210.

134 Hucklenbroich. see Sigwart (1907, reference 135).

135 Sigwart W. Selbstmordversuch während der Geburt. *Archiv für Psychiatrie.* 1907;42:249–256.

136 Braune. see Boas (1910, reference 137).

137 Boas. Psychisch abnorme Zustände während der Schwangerschaft und ihre forensische Bedeutung. *Archiv für Kriminalanthropologie und Kriminalistik.* 1910;39:49–51.

138 Spire A. Psychose puerpérale. *Revue Médicale de l'Est.* 1911;43:289–297.

139 Bernard MPC. *Contribution à l'étude des psychoses puerpérales, de leur étiologie en particulier.* Thèse, Nancy; 1922.

140 Dupouy R. La confusion mentale puerpérale. *Consultation.* 1930;34:29–36.

141 Woddis GM, Robinson GA. Attempted suicide during the course of labour. *Medico-Legal Journal.* 1960;28:209–211.

142 Aresin L. *Psychopathologische, Psychiatrische und Neurologische Aspekte der Schwangerschaft.* Leipzig: Thieme; 1976.

143 Neale R. Attempted suicide in labour. *British Medical Journal.* 1976;i:321–322.

144 Anonymous. Délire consécutive à la parturition - suicide. *Annales Médico-psychologiques.* 1847;1:127–128.

145 Brière de Boismont A. Suicide pendant l'accouchement. *Bulletin de la Société Médicale de la Suisse Romande.* 1869;3:1–2.

146 Malins E. Preparturient insanity; suicide. *Edinburgh Medical Journal.* 1873;18: 1000–1003.

147 Neugebauer FL. Selbstmord einer Schwangeren durch Sprung aus dem 3 Stockwerk. *Centralblatt für Gynäkologie.* 1890;14:88–97.

148 Bumm D. *Grundriss zum Studium der Geburtshülfe.* Wiesbaden: Bergmmann; 1902. p. 175.

149 Haberda A. see v. Sury (1908, reference 150); 1905.

150 v Sury K. Beitrag zur Kasuistik des Selbstmordes während der Geburt. *Münchener Medizinische Wochenschrift.* 1908;55:1534–1536.

151 Weir JG. Suicide during pregnancy in London 1942–1962. In: Kleiner GJ, Greston WM, editors, *Suicide in Pregnancy.* Boston: Wright; 1984.

152 Winter F. *Die Wochenbettpsychosen.* Inaugural-Dissertation, Marburg; 1908.

153 Mauriceau F. *Observations sur la Grossesse et l'Accouchement des Femmes et sur leurs Maladies, et celles des Enfans Nouveau-nés.* Paris : chez l'Auteur; 1694.

154 Carus CG. Krankhaftes allgemeines Befinden als Folge der Geburt. In: *Lehrbuch der Gynäkologie.* Part II. Leipzig: Fleischer; 1908. p. 504.

155 Kamnitzer. see Freyer (1887, reference 8).

156 Montel E. *Contribution à l'état du shoc nerveux dans le post-partum.* Thèse, Paris; 1908.

157 Barth. Ein Fall von plötzlich nach der Entbindung entstandener *mania transitoria. Henke's Zeitschrift für der Staatsarzneikunde.* 1828;16:108–110.

158 Kipp. *Mania puerperalis transitoria.* Provinzial-Sanitäts-Bericht des Königlichen Medicinal-Collegiums von Westfalen (Münster). 1847;53.

159 Churchill F. *On the Diseases of Women including Diseases of Pregnancy and Childbed.* 3rd ed. Dublin: Fannin; 1850. p. 424–429, 526–528 and 733–742.

160 Samelson A. Delivery during sleep. *British Medical Journal.* 1865;ii:550.

161 Bertherand EL. Sur la syncope et la folie émotive des accouchées. *Annales de la Société de Médecine d'Anvers.* 1871;32 409–424.

162 Schwarzer O. see Becker (1926, reference 65).

163 Van den Bosch. Accouchement naturel; hémorragie; délire violent, guérison. *Journal de Médecine, Chirurgie et Pharmacologie.* 1880;70:456–463.

164 Vanverts M. Cas de folie puerpérale instantanée. *Journal des Sciences Médicales de Lille.* 1880;2:193–194.

165 Dörschlag O. *Beitrag zu den Puerperalpsychosen.* Inaugural-Dissertation, Berlin; 1886.

166 Manton WP. Puerperal hysteria (insanity?) *Journal of the American Medical Association.* 1892;19:61–62.

167 v. Krafft-Ebing R. see Sarrat (1911, reference 66).

168 Traugott. see Kirchberg (1913, reference 50).

169 Weinger MB, Swerdlow NR, Millar WL. Acute postoperative delirium and extrapyramidal signs in a previously healthy parturient. *Anaesthesia & Analgesia.* 1988;67:291–295.

170 Davis A, Yudofsky B, Quidwai S. Acute psychosis associated with butorphanol. *Journal of Neuropsychiatry and Clinical Neuroscience.* 1996;10:236–237.

171 Sieche A, Giedke H. Recurring short delirium with postpartum onset in two sisters. *Psychopathology.* 1999;32:325–329.

172 Kelso J. Nervous exhaustion dependent on and complicating the puerperal state with cases. *Lancet.* 1840;i:945–948.

173 Tott CA. Fälle von *melancholia attonita* bei Neuentbundenen. *Neue Zeitschrift für Geburtskunde.* 1844;16:187–190.

174 Steinberger, of Butzbach. Zwei Fälle von *melancholia puerperalis. Gemeinsame Deutsche Zeitschrift für Geburtskunde.* 1831;6:236–239.

175 Dretler J. Sur les psychoses puerpérales. *Semaine des Hôpitaux de Paris,* December 15, 1930;587–598 and December 30, 1930;623–630.

176 Ware CE. Puerperal mania. *American Journal of the Medical Sciences.* 1853;26:345–346.

177 Varges AW. Puerperal manie. *Zeitschrift für Medizin Chirurgie und Geburtsklinik.* 1857;11:451–461.

178 Curgenven JB. Bromide of potassium in puerperal mania. *Transactions of the Obstetrical Society of London.* 1867;9: 155–156.

179 Mayer CEL. *Die Beziehungen der krankhaften Zustände und Vorgànge in den Sexual-Organen des Weibes.* Berlin: Hirschwald; 1869.

180 Bretonville P. *Contributions à l'étude des psychopathies puerpérales.* Thèse, Paris; 1901.

181 Warburg B. *Über die im Jahre 1909 in der Kieler psychiatrichen- und Nervenklinik beobachteten Fälle von Generationspsychosen.* Inaugural-Dissertation, Kiel; 1915.

Section

4

Non-Organic Psychoses of Childbearing

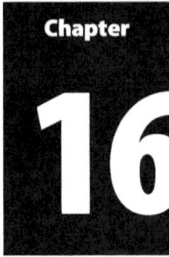

The Literature

16

Introduction

I have divided this analysis into six parts:

- Reviews, without data or case descriptions
- Surveys, which require location, source of data and time frame
- Long-term studies
- Investigations, which require comparison with a control group
- Case lore, with a description of the psychopathology and course
- Citation analysis of publications with references in the text or bibliography

Treatment trials will be considered later.

Reviews

The purpose of reviews (such as this monograph) is to find out what is known and to lay a foundation for future research. Their value depends on the number of publications reviewed, the inclusion of those written in foreign languages, and the quality of analysis and study. This literature includes more than 400 reviews, and it is obvious that this opinion on their purpose is not shared, because the median number of cited works is 9. Only one review[1] has more than 100 references; it covered 14 per cent of the existing publications.

To fulfil their function, reviews should augment previous work. An incomplete review is worse than worthless because it buries earlier work under a pseudo-literature, out of touch with the primary observations. For example, a recent 'review of postpartum psychosis'[2] cited 45 relevant works, all in the English language, none written before 1969 – about 2 per cent of the literature and only 10 per cent of the English language publications in the 35 years covered; although important details were missed, it has already been cited many times, presumably in the belief that it is authoritative. In 1930 Sir Thomas Lewis[3] wrote:

> There is little or no attempt of editors collectively to stem the tide of pseudo-scientific publication. By its mass it conceals work that has value; by its quality it undermines the general standard of accuracy in observation and thought.

The literature on the childbearing psychoses is spread over at least two centuries and published in many languages. Editors should immediately reject 'reviews' limited to recent publications in one language. Universities, when awarding doctorates, should insist on wide reading.

Surveys

These witness the occurrence of puerperal psychosis in a locality, estimate its frequency, and provide clues to its associations and aetiology.

There are *no surveys of puerperal psychosis in the general community*. There is also no information on the proportion of women who suffer puerperal episodes; we only know the proportion of pregnancies. Since all surveys are based on hospitalized mothers, all suffer from nosocomial bias.

Some 352 have so far been published. They include:

- A total of 36 obstetric surveys
- Various psychiatric surveys – from 201 asylums, 48 academic units and 7 mother-and-baby units; 42 have been population-based
- A total of 18 miscellaneous surveys: from private practice[4,5], out-patient clinics or general practice[6–8]; of fathers[9]; about post-abortion psychoses[10–12], sex ratios[13], maternal mortality[14,15], bipolar disorder[16,17] and suicide[18,19] and based on ultra-sound examination[20]

The United States has produced the most surveys (57), followed by Germany (54), United Kingdom and Eire (53), Italy (18), France (13), Denmark (11), India and Sweden (9), Holland, Poland and Switzerland (8), Australia and Hungary (7), Japan, Nigeria and Russia (6), Austria, China and Senegal (5), Brazil and Canada (4); Croatia, the Czech Republic, Norway, Tanzania and Venezuela (3); Algeria, Israel, Morocco, Pakistan, Saudi Arabia, Serbia, Slovakia, Slovenia, South Africa and Turkey (2); and Argentina, Bulgaria, Cameroon, Congo, Cuba, the Isle of Réunion, Niger, Portugal, Singapore, Sudan, Taiwan, Tunisia and the United Arab Emirates (one each).

Asylum Surveys

Since the advent of epidemiological surveys based on case registers, these have become obsolete. But they give some useful information, because state-of-the-art epidemiology can only document disorders in a particular place and time. The pioneers may have been Haslam[21] and Rush[22]. Haslam worked at the Bethlem Royal Hospital, and published *Observations on Madness and Melancholy* in 1809. He saw 80 cases between 1784 and 1794 (10 years). Benjamin Rush signed the Declaration of Independence and is considered the founder of American psychiatry; he established a mental hospital in Philadelphia and wrote *Medical Inquiries and Observations upon Diseases of the Mind* in 1812. Another early survey was that of Burrows[23], who kept private asylums in Chelsea and Clapham: he published data on 57 cases and tabulated details of each case. Macdonald[24,25], from the Bloomingdale asylum in Manhattan, published surveys in 1831 and 1847, tabulating data on 66 cases. Reid[26] collected data from 5 British asylums, and some maternity units. Gundry[27] collected data from 14 American asylums. Following these initiatives, asylum surveys have been published from 46 nations.

University Psychiatry Clinics

These date from 1811 (Heinroth's clinic in Leipzig). Until Anderson's Maudsley study[28], all were from Germany. Although universities often transferred patients to asylums, their rates are similar, so I have amalgamated data from asylums and university clinics. Table 16.1

Table 16.1 Proportion of female admissions related to childbirth

Period	Description	Percentage of female admissions
Up to 1900	57 asylum surveys, 2 university clinics	Mean 8.3, median 9
1901–1950	51 asylum surveys, 13 university clinics	Mean 5.2, median 4/5
1951–present	79 asylum surveys, 31 university clinics	Mean 3.3, median 2
	11 third world surveys	Mean 12.6, median 10

shows the proportion of female admissions to hospital, divided into three periods – before 1900, 1901–1950 and after 1950. I have considered surveys from underdeveloped nations separately because they have much higher maternal mortality rates, and a higher proportion of admissions related to childbirth.

After excluding that group, the table shows a striking fall in the percentage of female admissions, which could be due to

- 'dilution' by hospitalizing more women outside the reproductive range – surprisingly few surveys eliminated women more than 50 years of age
- falling birth rates
- the disappearance of some forms of puerperal psychosis

Some authors noted a fall in frequency during the time span of their own studies[29–34]. In two of them the fall occurred when the data were restricted to women of childbearing age[31,34]. These studies support the idea that the frequency of postpartum psychosis fell at the end of the nineteenth century. As an example, there is this detailed Danish survey[30]:

Between 1858 and 1895 (38 years), 2,088 women were admitted to Oringe Hospital, of whom 101 suffered from psychosis with onset less than six weeks after childbirth. The percentage was 7.9% in 1858–1860 (7/10 with infections), 5.5% in 1861–1865 (4/13 infections), 5.7% in 1866–1870 (8/15 infections), 5.6% in 1871–1875 (7/22 infections), 5.9% in 1876–1880 (9/23 infections), 2.2% in 1881–1885 (0/5 infections), 2.3% in 1886–1890 (1/4 infections) and 3.1% in 1891–1895 (2/9 infections). Thus there was a fall after 1880. There were 38 cases of infection, 35 occurring before 1880 and 3 in the next 15 years. Poulsen also gave figures for the frequency of puerperal fever, which fell from 0.6/1,000 population in 1862–1870 to 0.3/1,000 in 1881–1894.

Obstetric Surveys

These start with Elsässer[35] from Stuttgart, who surveyed 615 births in two years: in each year there was a case of infective delirium. They provide data of two kinds:

- They relate the frequency of psychoses to the number of births.
- They survey psychotic patients who may not reach the psychiatric hospital, because of early death or recovery.

Unfortunately, the data show too much variation to reach any conclusions; the problem is not the denominator (the number of births), but the numerator (the number of psychoses): some surveys measured hospital admission not psychosis, and 'psychosis' was defined in different ways. There are, however, four obstetric surveys of particular interest:

Weebers[36] gave details of 20 cases, obtained from 4,014 births at the Leyden obstetric unit: seven had infective psychosis, three eclamptic psychosis and one both infection and eclampsia.

Engelhard[37] studied 29 psychoses from 19,910 deliveries at the Utrecht obstetric clinic: six had transitory disturbances during labour, and ten eclamptic psychosis; there was no case of infective delirium.

Guzman[38] reported 106 psychoses from a maternity hospital in Caracas in 1965–1978 – one of the few studies from Latin America: 69 had somatic disease, including 42 with eclampsia.

Ndosi[39] reported 110 psychoses developing within six weeks of childbirth in Dar es Salaam in 1996–1998. This is almost the only study that gives an insight into what is happening in an African country with a high maternity mortality rate: 69 had organic psychoses, including 22 with falciparum malaria, many with other infections (three with AIDS), and 19 with gestosis.

These studies all show high rates of organic psychoses.

Population-Based Surveys

The pioneer population-based survey may have been a paper read by MacLeod[40], superintendent of the East Yorkshire asylum in Beverley (near Hull), in his presidential address to a local society: he examined the reports of the Lunacy Commissioners in 1878–1882 and related them to the number of births (3,537,580 in the five years). There were 1,794 cases of insanity. Since the population of England and Wales (1881 census) was 25,974,439, the incidence was .07/1,000 total population/year; the figure for females of reproductive age would be more than double, but this is still a very low figure.

Since then, 42 population-based surveys have been published, most of them from Britain, Denmark or Sweden. In 15 it was possible to calculate an incidence. Four obtained data from record linkage, and gave information on psychosis, not just hospital admission:

Kendell[41] studied admissions from Edinburgh in 1970–1981 (population 470,000 with 54,087 births). The results were presented for 16 trimesters – eight before and eight after the birth. The 3-monthly totals for psychosis were 7, 4, 4, 8, 8 (all before conception), 3, 6, 9 (during pregnancy), 89 in the 1st postpartum trimester (of which 51 in the 1st month), 17, 21, 10 (the rest of the 1st postpartum year), 15, 12, 9 and 8 (the 2nd postpartum year). The diagnoses of 120 women admitted within 90 days of the birth, using the Research Diagnostic Criteria[42], were 22 mania, 3 schizoaffective mania, 3 schizoaffective depression, 3 schizophrenia, one probable schizophrenia and 13 unspecified functional psychosis (45 in all); there were also 16 with depressive psychosis (hallucinations, delusions, incoherent or grossly thought-disordered speech, mutism or consistently bizarre behaviour) – thus 61 psychoses (1.13/1,000 births). The relative risk of admission with psychosis during the first postpartum trimester was 14.3.

Terp and Mortensen[43] used the Danish national register in 1973–1993 (population about five million with 1,270,117 births): 1,253 women were admitted with a hospital diagnosis of psychosis within 91 days of the onset of labour. Only 573 were first admissions (incidence 0.45/1,000 deliveries). Compared with the Danish population, they reported a relative risk of only 1.09; but there must have been something wrong with the denominator, because on page 524 (paragraph 3) they reported that 338 women were discharged from hospital in the 12 months before conception, that is, 85/trimester. With this baseline, 1,253 admissions in the first postpartum trimester amounts to a relative risk of 14.7 (the same as that obtained by Kendell). They found a relative risk for mania of 6.8 among mothers admitted within one month of the birth.

Nager[44] used the Swedish national register (population about 8.5 million) in 12 years (1986–1997), when there were 502,769 births: 339 *primiparae* had first admissions with psychosis within three months of the birth (0.68/1,000 births). In 2007 they extended the study to 29 years (1975–2003), when there were 1,133,368 births. The number of mothers admitted for their first episode of psychosis in the first postpartum trimester was 1,413 (1.2/1,000 births).

Munk-Olsen[45] used Danish record linkage data from 1973–2005: 28,124 women, with a history of psychiatric hospitalization, were divided into 10,218 mothers and 17,106 non-mothers: the highest risk of readmission was in days 10–19 postpartum (relative risk 2.7) and the lowest during pregnancy (relative risk 0.5). The highest risk of postpartum readmission was in those with bipolar disorder (relative risk 37): 27 per cent of mothers with this diagnosis were readmitted in the first postpartum year.

As a study of frequency, related to births, these figures offer no advantages over obstetric surveys, which have been available from the early nineteenth century and from 19 nations. But they all agree on a rate of about 1/1,000 births, with a much increased episode rate in the first postpartum trimester.

Other Surveys

There are seven mother & baby unit surveys. The large number of patients admitted with psychosis confirms that, in spite of a fall during the twentieth century, this is still a significant problem; 29 per cent of mothers admitted under my care in Birmingham had some form of 'puerperal psychosis'.

Parity

Many surveys give data on age, but differences can be related to parity. In the literature, 64 surveys have provided information (Table 16.2):

Table 16.2 Parity in the literature

Period	Number of surveys	Primiparae	Multiparae	Percentage of primiparae	
				Mean	Median
Before 1900	17	301	532	37%	36%
1901–1950	13	385	542	42%	42%
After 1950	34	1,189	1,299	48%	53/54%

These data, based on more than 4,000 mothers, show that the proportion of *primiparae* has increased during the last 200 years. Kendell's figures[41], typical of the modern era, indicate a relative risk of 2.0. These findings are consistent with the view that non-organic cases (which now predominate in Europe and North America) are more frequent in first-time mothers, but organic cases (which used to be common) may not have been. Since 1970, surveys have been reported from Africa, where the proportion of organic psychoses may be higher: they have a mean of 38 per cent *primiparae*, similar to the nineteenth century in Europe and North America.

Secondary Sex Ratio (Ratio of Infant Sexes at Birth)

Occasional cases in the literature have shown a preponderance of male children[46–49]. Taylor[50] studied the effect of pregnancy on 'schizophrenia' in 25 Puerto Rican women (33 pregnancies): prepartum psychosis almost invariably occurred with female infants, and postpartum with male infants; these extraordinary results have never been replicated. In pregnancies that resulted in a postpartum episode, an excess of females was reported by Melges[51] and Kendell[41] (65 per cent female, $p < .05$), while an excess of males was reported by McNeil[52]. In Robertson Blackmore's[53] study of 129 bipolar women, 55 per cent affected and 42 per cent unaffected pregnancies followed male births; but when they focused on mothers with both affected and unaffected pregnancies, the difference was not significant. A Swedish survey[54] of 1,413 first episode puerperal psychoses in 1,133,368 women found that the proportion of males was the same as the general population (hazard ratio 1.02); the findings of this enormous study are unlikely to be wrong.

Breastfeeding

It is widely believed that puerperal psychosis occurs equally often in lactating and non-lactating mothers, as first mentioned in the eighteenth century[55,56]. But data on breastfeeding are hardly ever provided in surveys: Macdonald[25] stated that 30/49 of his American cases, and Weber[57] 34/46 of his Russian mothers, were lactating at onset. Bergink[58] reported that 45/51 mothers who developed postpartum psychosis were breast-feeding, the same as in the contemporary Dutch population (88 per cent).

Clinical Studies

Diagnosis

Among the surveys there are many diagnostic analyses, using contemporary concepts, but without control groups. Some recent studies have compared these mothers with other female psychotic patients[59–63]. My series provides data from a larger number followed for a longer time, but three studies are of particular interest:

The Canadian study of Hays[64,65] reported a unique cluster analysis. He focused on 147 patients with a clinical diagnosis of 'schizophrenia'. All had routine but thorough clinical observations, plus an EEG; in 133 he interviewed relatives, and in 61 studied records. From 123 variables, he selected 51 for the cluster analyses. In the 1978 study, 35 per cent of patients fell into one of three clusters:

(1) sensitive ideas of reference
(2) atypical manic depression with catatonia, thought disorder, auditory hallucinations and bipolar disorder in the families
(3) puerperal schizophrenia ($N = 7$)

This puerperal group had onset within a few days of the birth, with thought disorder, catatonia, 'hectic mood changes', visual misrecognition, auditory hallucinations, and varying delusions. Two patients in this cluster, who were not puerperal, had a mother with puerperal schizophrenia and a recurrence after the 1st birth. The family study showed that puerperal schizophrenia was more common in the relatives of puerperal schizophrenics (9/39 episodes). In the second study, he compared groups 2 and 3 (10 and 9 patients): the most discriminating symptoms (favouring the puerperal group) were thought disorder, hallucinations and depression.

Our Manchester study[61] (described in Section 1) found 41 differences between puerperal patients and controls at $p < .01$. The largest differences were social withdrawal (19 puerperals *versus* 31 controls, $p = .0007$) and incompetence (19 *versus* 11, $p = .0008$). Also high were persecution (13 *versus* 24, $p = .003$), odd affect (14 *versus* 24, $p = .003$), systematized delusions (21 *versus* 35, $p = .004$) and auditory hallucinations (frequency 15 *versus* 31, $p = .004$), all more common in controls. Of the self rating scales 7/30 showed differences, including persecution ($p = .002$) and psychosis (p = .006), both higher in controls. This controlled study of psychopathology supported the presence of special features in puerperal episodes, and was one of the first to indicate a link with manic depression.

The Manchester study also collected data on 104 depressed postpartum patients using the same multiple information sources[66]. In a discriminant function analysis, a group of patients with early onset depressive psychosis had some special features: they were persistently depressed, but less hostile and angry, and showed normal animation as against sullen immobility, and a relative lack of sadness, anxiety and suicidal feelings. These symptoms were, perhaps, a manifestation of the depressed form of a bipolar illness. These patients made up 18/44 (41 per cent) of mothers who developed depression in the first two weeks.

In *Motherhood and Mental Health*[67] (pages 216–219) I summarized much evidence that some puerperal psychoses belonged to the modern rubric of manic depressive (bipolar) disorder. Some patients are obviously bipolar within the puerperal episode, switching from excitement and loquacity to morose taciturnity, as in this example[68]:

A 23-year old, five days after the birth, became excited and talked incessantly; she slept less than one hour at night. Ten days later she developed melancholic stupor, becoming mute and looking round with a vacant gaze; she had to be fed by stomach tube.

The switch can have a diurnal pattern. Among 195 mothers admitted to the Manchester mother and baby unit, 7 had mixed manic and depressive features. In others the bipolarity of the illness was seen in successive episodes. Several mothers developed depression with schizo-affective features, catatonia or mutism after one pregnancy, and manic excitement after another[69–71], as in this example from my series:

A mother became depressed thirteen days after giving birth to her 1st child: she was vacant, withdrawn and sleepless; she believed that the house smelt, that her hair was falling out and that she and the baby had deformities of the hands. Sixteen days after her 2nd birth she developed a manic illness so severe that she was secluded on many occasions.

Recent diagnostic analyses have shown that mania (as now conceptualized) is more common among new mothers than other female patients (Table 16.3):

Table 16.3 Episode diagnoses in puerperal patients

First author	Number of episodes	Number with mania or schizo-affective mania
Brockington (1981)[61]	58	25 (38%)
Dean (1981)[72]	24	9 (38%)
Schöpf (1984)[73]	33	11 (33%)
Meltzer (1985)[74]	90	35 (39%)
Klompenhouwer (1992)[75]	181	79 (38%)
McNeil (1986)[76]	14	6 (43%)

These studies agree on a frequency of 33–43 per cent manic episodes. These percentages are high, when compared with other women admitted to psychiatric hospitals. In the Camberwell 1st admission study[77,78], mania accounted for only 4–8 per cent of admissions (depending on the definition). Dean and Kendell[72] found that mania was more frequent in mothers admitted in the first postpartum trimester than other females (13 per cent *versus* 3 per cent, $p < .0001$). Why was this association not noticed before? The answer probably lies in the semantic shifts that have bedevilled psychiatry. Many puerperal manias have 'schizo-affective' features – disorders of the will and self, auditory hallucinations or mood-incongruent delusions. Studies conducted 40–50 years ago showed that, in terms of the course, genetics and treatment response, schizo-affective mania resembled mania[79,80]; mothers once considered to be suffering from 'puerperal schizophrenia' began to receive a diagnosis of mania.

But there are indications that puerperal mania is a severe variant, with unusual symptoms and an element of confusion. Table 16.4 summarizes some of this evidence.

Table 16.4 Puerperal and non-puerperal mania

First author	Features of the puerperal illness
Böszörményi (1974)[59]	17 Hungarian and 23 French Canadian cases were 'delirious-amentiform'.
Yogananda (1977)[157]	Comparing 30 postpartum with non-postpartum 'major disorders', the mothers had more confusion (6 *versus* none, $p = .011$) and perplexity (21 *versus* 4, $p < .001$).
Hays (1978)[64]	One of his clusters (see earlier discussion) was 'puerperal schizophrenia', which could be distinguished from schizo-phreniform bipolars.
Kadrmas (1979)[60]	Comparing 21 puerperal bipolar patients (with onset <6 weeks after the birth) with 136 bipolar controls, 13 (62 per cent) had Schneiderian 1st rank symptoms, compared with 38 (28 per cent, $p < .005$).
Brockington (1982)[81]	Comparing 21 puerperal and 11 non-puerperal manic or schizo-manic patients, the puerperals needed more supervision ($p = .001$), were more incompetent ($p = .006$), more confused ($p = .0005$) and, from speech transcripts, more loquacious and disorganized ($p = .0009$).
Katona (1982)[62]	Comparing 84 patients admitted within six months of the birth with a control group, puerperal mania had more delusions (12/18 *versus* 11/33, $p < .05$).
Wisner (1994)[63]	Childbirth-related psychoses scored highly on a factor with loadings on thought disorganization (0.56) and bizarre behaviour (0.53).
Oosthuizen (1995)[82]	Comparing 20 postpartum psychoses with 20 bipolars, the puerperal patients had more delusions of control (7 *versus* 1, $p < .05$), auditory hallucinations (11 *versus* 5, $p < .05$), lability of mood, perplexity and confusion (10 *versus* 4, $p < .05$) and flatness of affect (15 *versus* 4, $p < .001$).

Course

Episode Duration

The mean duration has fallen sharply in the last 75 years (Table 16.5). These durations are for psychosis. Robertson Blackmore[83] reported that many had prolonged post-psychotic depression, so that 52 per cent had symptoms for more than a year.

Table 16.5 Duration of non-organic puerperal psychoses

Generation	Mean duration
Before 1875	Unknown
1876–1900	5.7 months
1901–1925	7.2 months
1926–1940	7.1 months
1941–1950	4.2 months
1951–1975	2.3 months
After 1975	2.4 months

Relapses

A relapse is here defined as the return of symptoms not more than two months after recovery. The tendency of puerperal psychoses to relapse is one of their most interesting features – an ancient observation that has been almost completely ignored. Esquirol[84] was the first to describe it, 200 years ago:

> A 23-year old suffered from nervous disorders from her menarche. At 21 she married a general, and promptly became pregnant. Seven days after the birth, she became *furieuse*, but for only two days. She relapsed on the 25th day. *Délire furieuse* switched to stupor. In the 5th month her periods returned and, in spite of the death of her husband, she remained well.

This case is atypical in the extreme brevity of the 1st episode.

In the study of relapses in the literature, I have excluded the following:

The recurrence of a prepartum episode after the birth
Unusual cyclical disorders (see Chapter 19)
Runge psychoses (see Section 5)
Organic psychoses
Switches from mania to depression or *vice versa* in a continuous illness
Deterioration explained by an adverse event such as seizures or psychological trauma.

After these subtractions, at least one relapse was reported in 229 cases, with the following onsets (Table 16.6), related to the episode totals on Table 20.7 and 20.8 on page 207.

Table 16.6 Relapses in the literature related to onset

Episode onset	Number	Percentage
Post abortion[85,86]	3	3
Prepartum	9	9
Early postpartum	145	11
4–13 Week onset	37	9
Late onset	13	6
Weaning onset	3	8
Unknown onset	19	5

Table 16.7 Delay's[101] cases of relapse of puerperal psychosis

Presenting details	Course
Case 1: day 9 onset of a variable polymorphic state with alternation of depression and poorly systematized delusions of persecution	Recovery after 20 ECT, relapse with mutism, catatonia, delusions and excitement, requiring more ECT, followed by three more relapses at intervals of two months and three weeks, requiring further treatment by insulin comas and ECT
Case 4: on day 8 she was hospitalized with depression and ideas of cancer; she was disorientated, and could hear people speaking to her, and the cries of her mother suffering torture. Excitement alternated with stupor and catalepsy	After nine ECT her mind cleared. On day 43 her menses appeared and on day 48 she relapsed, and required 15 more ECT
Case 5: onset one month after the birth: she misidentified people and had hallucinations of people talking all the time. Hospitalized more than four months later, she was disorientated, and had visual and auditory hallucinations. She became excited and, six months after the birth, received ECT	She improved within two weeks, but relapsed a few days later. ECT was resumed. A state of excitement continued with persecutory ideas, and required treatment with insulin comas
Case 7: day 9 onset of excitement, laughing, crying and talking incoherently. Hospitalised on day 19 she was disinhibited, euphoric, shouting and dancing	With eight ECT she improved. About a week later she relapsed, recovered and was discharged five months after the birth
Case 9: two months after the birth she became disturbed and, after four months, was admitted to hospital with excitement, fugues, singing, joking, flight of ideas and complete insomnia	Two weeks later, after the reappearance of her menses, she calmed down. A month later she relapsed. After ECT, she was discharged eight months after the birth
Case 11: on day 6 she began to say that her husband wanted to get rid of her; she was being poisoned and persecuted by an unknown group. She was sleepless and refused food	Within a month, after five ECT, she improved. In the 6th week, her menses appeared, and she relapsed with delusional depression, requiring another five ECT
Case 12: on day 10 she became manic with flight of ideas, confusion, ideas of persecution and auditory hallucinations	At three weeks she improved. In the 2nd month she relapsed, with confusion and food refusal. With twelve ECT she improved, but, at three months, relapsed again. With more ECT she improved, but relapsed eight months after the birth
Case 15: on day 7 she became manic, with shouting, singing, familiarity and exuberance	Treated with ECT she improved. Her menses returned at two months, preceded by a relapse. She had several phases of excitation. She recovered nine months after the birth
Case 16: after a birth complicated by a fever of 40°, she became agitated, then sank into stupor, mutism and prostration. She claimed that her own child was dead, and this one was not hers	Treated with ECT, she lost her delusions. Five months after the birth her menses appeared, with a relapse of melancholic delusions and food refusal. She recovered with further ECT
Case 20: within a week of the birth she became depressed with delusions of guilt	Treated with ECT, she improved, but a month later relapsed with excitation. After 25 insulin comas she recovered

The nine prepartum cases included five with the relapse before the birth[87-90] and three that followed the postpartum continuation of a prepartum psychosis, so were in fact postpartum. There was the following Argentinian case[91]:

> A woman, whose father committed suicide, had a 3-month miscarriage in 1938, and normal births in 1940 and 1944. In 1950 she became clouded in the last month of pregnancy, with a poor memory for the birth. In February 1953 she again became clouded, excited and disorientated during pregnancy, this time in the 5th month; she responded to ECT, but relapsed. She gave birth in June and remained confused during the first month of the puerperium, recovered with ECT, then relapsed, with clouding of consciousness, disorientation, insomnia and incoherence. She responded to cortisone treatment.

This patient had a prepartum psychosis (2nd trimester onset) with a relapse, continuing into the puerperium, also with a relapse. Three mothers with weaning onsets had relapses[84,92,100]; one[92], summarized in Section 5, had several relapses.

Multiple Relapses

In the literature there were 23 episodes with two relapses, 12 with three relapses, 3 with four relapses, while 27 episodes were followed by multiple relapses of uncertain number or a periodic, phasic, alternating or remittent course. Ten mothers with six or more relapses all had evidence of a menstrual association, and will be summarized in Section 5. Four mothers, including one from my series, suffered from relapsing psychoses after two separate births[93-95].

Recognition of the Relapsing Phenomenon

In the search for the reason why this phenomenon is hardly ever mentioned, I examined case reports published by epoch and language group. There has been an increase in the frequency of reported relapses from 6 per cent before 1900, to 8 per cent in the next 50 years and 19 per cent since 1950; this increase can be explained by increased awareness of the phenomenon. The differences between language groups are striking: the lowest rates were reported by the Dutch (3 per cent): two large Dutch series[96,97], with a total of 61 non-organic postpartum psychoses, included only 2 with relapses; but recently Bergink[98] reported relapses in 12/64 cases (10 depressive and 2 psychotic). Britain and the Commonwealth also had low rates (4 per cent). In contrast, high rates were reported by American authors, starting with Macdonald[25]. Bower[99] reported that 17/39 (44 per cent) had at least one relapse. Almost half the reported cases are in the French literature, of which 55 were reported by six authors – Balduzzi[71], Sivadon[86] and Bourson[100] with 20 per cent; Fauré-Amiel[94] and Delay[101] with 50 per cent; and Cain[102] with 73 per cent. Delay's cases (summarized in Table 16.7) are of interest because, published in 1948, they preceded the introduction of neuroleptic drugs by Delay himself.

Differences between language groups can only be explained by under-reporting or over-reporting, and the first is more likely. Dutch, British and, to some extent, German authors either were ignorant of this phenomenon, or undervalued its importance. If the French observations are accurate, the frequency is much higher than is evident from the general literature.

The Cause of the Relapsing Phenomenon

Nowadays clinicians might be tempted to attribute a relapse to premature reduction of medication or poor compliance. But only 116/223 cases have been published since 1950, when Delay himself (with Deniker) was introducing chlorpromazine as a treatment for psychosis. Since non-compliance *cannot* be the explanation for many or most of these cases, one must find another. An explanation that springs to mind is the influence of menstruation. Until someone comes up with another reason for periodic relapses weeks and months after childbirth, this is the only hypothesis in the field.

It is obvious from Esquirol's first case[84], and many others, that episodes followed by a relapse are distinguished by the brevity of the first phase. Although the total length of the psychotic illness was longer (median 96 days *versus* 46 days), the first phase had a median of only 25 days, with 19 lasting less than three weeks. This raises the possibility that relapsing cases are a distinct variant of early onset postpartum psychoses. This is disproved by the fact that, in my series, 18 mothers had episodes of both kinds. The explanation must, therefore, be that the brevity of the first phase, with an interval of health, *allowed the relapse to be observed*. Unless there was a complete recovery, the clinician would not notice the phasic course. Thus, although a phasic course is common, and not due to treatment failure, it is probably even more common than the number of relapses suggests.

The Menopause

The menopause is often an indefinite and gradual event, as menstrual bleeding becomes irregular towards the end of the reproductive phase. Since puerperal psychosis commonly develops in the twenties, few women have been followed for long enough to observe its effect. There are eight published cases of postpartum or post-abortion psychosis with episodes after the menopause. The first two were described by Esquirol[103,104] (summarized below). One was described by Dupouy[105] and the other five by Robertson Blackmore[106], who reported that a patient became hypomanic within days of oöphorectomy.

Long-Term Studies

In the sixteenth century Ioannis Hess[107] from Noricum (now part of Austria and Slovenia) described the first patient followed beyond the index episode and with a postpartum recurrence:

> The wife of Hieronymus Schnitter, four years after her marriage, gave birth to a daughter and on the 4th day began to complain bitterly of sleeplessness and melancholy, and a little later became insane, and had to be put in restraints, but recovered. She became pregnant again the following year, but nothing is known about the postpartum period. In the 3rd year she certainly had a normal birth. Finally, in the 4th year, she gave birth again, and soon afterwards, just like the first time, became completely manic again.

Esquirol[103,104] followed two patients beyond the menopause. The first had 10 postpartum episodes and 2 in late life:

> A woman, whose mother and daughter were insane, and whose grand-child died in mania, was married at the age of 23 and had 13 infants. At 29, after the stillbirth of her 4th child, she had an episode lasting 18 months. Since then, after each birth, as soon as the milk came down, she became manic for a year. Sometimes the menses were suppressed, sometimes not. During these episodes she could neither sleep nor stop walking and talking, and was exasperated by thousands of hallucinations – auditory and visual. The last episode, at 45, was the most severe. At 50 she had her menopause. At 53, after her husband left for the army, she had another episode lasting six months with hallucinations and paroxysms every two days. After this, each autumn and spring she suffered from compulsive trembling

for some days. At 59 she had another episode, with hallucinations and the need to walk and run; she was ill for eleven months. She then developed dementia (case 9).

The second had 13 postpartum episodes, followed by non-puerperal episodes before and after the menopause:

> A woman, whose sister suffered from puerperal psychosis, was married at the age of 25. At 26 she gave birth to her 1st child, after which she suffered from furious mania until her 2nd pregnancy, which was normal. She had 12 further pregnancies, all with hard labours, after which she was insane for 4–6 weeks. At 39 she had an attack of apoplexy followed by hemiplegia. At 47 she suffered a severe febrile illness that was followed by furious mania lasting five months. At 50 her menses ceased. At 51 her husband died and she was imprisoned. This was followed by mania from which she recovered after a month (case 2).

In this entire literature, only 194 cases were described and followed for more than 10 years: 79 of them were reported by six authors – Visscher[97] (22), Daseking[108] (16), Bonse[109] (14) and Schröder[110], Beckmann[111] and Van Steenbergen[96] (9 each); only one of the theses that have made the greatest contribution has ever been cited, and that by one Dutch author. Karnosh and Hope[112] also followed 20 cases long term, but the details were presented in a schema, without a narrative description.

Other 'follow-up studies' have provided numerical data, without individual details. The first was published by Jolly[113] from Halle:

> He selected 79 patients, nine admitted during pregnancy, 55 postpartum and 15 in the 'lactation period'. They were followed for at least 10 years, through the records and by a questionnaire sent to the relatives. No information was given about the index diagnosis, which at that time would have included some organic psychoses. Of the puerperal patients, 29 recovered, 20 suffered continued illness or defect, and six died. Recurrences occurred in 6/45 who had further children, a low figure that includes prepartum, infective and lactation cases. The most interesting finding was that 20/51 children (on whom they had information) died while their mothers were in hospital.

These 'follow-up studies' have three main purposes:

- To research the prognosis
- (Closely allied to this) to establish a kraepelinian diagnosis
- To give information about recurrences related to later pregnancies. This requires an index group narrowly focused on well-defined puerperal psychosis, followed beyond the next pregnancy, preferably by interview and a study of the records.

Prognosis and diagnosis will not be considered here, because there is much other evidence. As for recurrences, the literature includes 50 follow-up studies, but many have been poorly conducted, using index cases that are not well defined, and inferior methods of follow-up. Table 16.8 summarizes 11 of the better studies. There are too many differences between them to attempt a meta-analysis. The older studies had surprisingly low recurrence rates, probably because of the inclusion of a wider range of diagnoses. One can conclude that there is a substantial risk (at least one-third) of a recurrence after one puerperal episode. The results from my series will be given later.

There are also studies focused on bipolar women, observing the effect of pregnancy and birth. The pioneering study was Norwegian[127].

> They followed 82 parous patients with 'manic depression': 51 had no puerperal episodes in 158 births, and 74 non-puerperal episodes; 31 had puerperal episodes (52/93 births) plus 29

Table 16.8 Some follow-up studies

First author	Number followed, onset after the birth	Duration of study in years	Recurrences/ pregnancies	Comment
Arentsen (1968)[195]	168 onset <6 months	6–30	16/114 (14%)	This included 15 organic psychoses, 30 depression and only 9 mania
Protheroe (1969)[115]	114 onset <6 weeks	5–40	30/149 (20%)	61 had further pregnancies, 25 one recurrence, 3 two recurrences and 1 three recurrences
Platz (1988)[116]	18 mania or schizo-affective disorder, with matched controls	3–15 (mean 9)	2 /14 (14%)	This also provided information on the number and duration of non-puerperal episodes
Dean (1989)[117]	79 (29 with other bipolar episodes and 19 bipolar patients with no puerperal episodes)	3–29 (mean 9)	29/80 (36%)	
Klompenhower (1992)[75]	93	Mean 11.6	15/36 (42%)	12 had one recurrence and 1 had recurrences after four births. There is information on suicides
Schöpf (1992)[118]	119	3–33 (mean 22.7)	21/57 (37%)	19 had one recurrence, 2 had two recurrences. There is information on suicides
Pfuhlmann (1998–2000)[119–121] Lanczik (1994)[122]	21 cycloid psychosis, onset <6 months	Mean 12.5	11/15 (73%)	Two recurrences were prepartum
Terp (1999)[123]	1,173 hospitalized with psychosis, onset <91 days	Mean about 10	80/388 (21%)	This reports the readmission rate
Robling (2000)[124]	64 onset <6 months	17–28 (mean 23)	10/34 (29%)	38/64 had an index admission of depression
Garfield (2004)[125]	66 onset <6 months	10	10/13 (80%)	31/66 did not have an index diagnosis of psychosis
Robertson 2005[126]	103	9	31/54 (57%)	Mothers who relapsed, not pregnancies
Robertson Blackmore (2013)[83]	116 onset <6 weeks	12	31/57 (54%)	Plus 4/10 with more than one additional birth

non-puerperal episodes, and 13/22 who had further children had puerperal recurrences. Only eleven had a history of mania, and only eleven were hospitalised in the puerperium (all with depression).

This was evidence of a special group of 'manic depressive' women particularly liable to postpartum depression.

Thirteen other investigations have studied the effect of childbirth in bipolar patients. Three had postpartum depression (not psychosis)[128–130]. The findings of 10 others are summarized in Table 16.9.

These studies all show evidence of a high rate of postpartum episodes in bipolar or cycloid women. There are two additional findings:

- The rate is even higher if there are both puerperal and non-puerperal episodes[131]; for a replication of this finding, see page 214.
- Pregnancy has a protective effect[135]; this requires replication. There is no doubt that bipolar episodes do recur during pregnancy: Viguera and her team[139–142] measured the frequency of prepartum episodes: 22/42 women, who discontinued lithium, had a recurrence before the birth, but even those who continued prophylaxis had recurrences – 10/37[141] and 3/10[518]; in a study[142] of 1,120 pregnancies in 621 women with 'bipolar 1' or 'bipolar II' disorders, 23% had prepartum episodes. Bergink[58] also reported that 10/41 bipolar women (most of whom were taking prophylactic medication) had a recurrence during pregnancy.

Investigations

These compare mothers with postpartum psychoses with a comparison series, either normal mothers or women with other psychoses. They are discussed under the headings of stress, obstetric variables, laboratory studies and genetics. I have omitted 13 investigations, covering psychological tests, parental attitudes and the quality of interaction with the infant.

Stress

Several investigations have studied 'life events': all found no evidence of increased adverse events or difficulties in the recent past[143–146].

Single parenthood is, other factors being equal, relatively stressful. Esquirol[104] was the first to note a possible association: 29/92 of his sample of women admitted to the Salpêtrière were single, but his series was not confined to postpartum psychoses. Tetlow[147] and Kendell[41,148] have found significantly more single mothers, but others[58,149–151] found that more were married. If this had been a consistent finding, it would have required confirmation in a study of the general population, because single parenthood could influence the decision to admit a mother to hospital.

The greatest stressor in the puerperium is loss of the child. Three studies have reported an association with severe mental illness leading to hospitalization – 7 per cent of bereaved mothers *versus* 3 per cent in other mothers[152], 4.7 per cent *versus* 1.1 per cent[153] and 9 per cent *versus* 2.7 per cent[154]. Nager[54] found a hazard ratio of 1.58, but this did not survive adjustment for prior psychiatric hospitalization. Hellerstedt[155] reported a four-fold increase following foetal death (2.8 per cent *versus* 0.7 per cent, $p < .01$): most of these deaths occurred early, associated with prematurity, low birth weight and congenital abnormalities, although these were not significantly increased in the mothers with postpartum episodes.

Table 16.9 Bipolar follow-up studies

First author	Patients	Findings
Reich (1970)[131]	20 parous women with a history of mania, studied in St Louis in 1964–1967	14/46 (24%) pregnancies were followed by episodes (11 manic). Six births occurred in women who had both puerperal and non-puerperal bipolar episodes: all had another postpartum episode
Akiskal (1983)[132]	206 depressed out-patients in Memphis	Change to bipolar occurred in 20% after a mean of 6.4 years; 7/12 who became bipolar had a postpartum episode, compared with 1/16 who did not ($p < .01$, sensitivity .58, specificity .84)
Kendell (1987)[41]	Edinburgh record linkage study	Of 10 previously admitted with a manic or circular illness, 3/14 births were associated with a puerperal admission (21%)
McNeil (1988)[133]	Cohort study of 88 pregnant women with non-organic psychosis followed for one birth	15 had cycloid and 15 'affective' index episodes (most bipolar). 14/30 (47%) of pregnancies in women with cycloid or affective psychosis were followed by postpartum episodes
Wehr (1988)[134]	51 'rapid-cycling' patients (four or more episodes/year)	41 were parous: 16 had postpartum episodes and 9 began with a postpartum episode
Grof (2000)[135]	From a four-nation database of bipolar lithium responders, 28 women became pregnant	Three nine-month periods were compared, (1) before pregnancy and in childless controls, (2) during pregnancy, (3) postpartum. Before pregnancy there was 0.43 episode lasting 6.1 weeks, during pregnancy 0.14 episode lasting 0.9 weeks, and postpartum 0.68 episode (seven women, 42% manic) lasting 12.2 weeks. Only 4/28 women had a prepartum episode, all depressive, all in the last five weeks with average duration less than one week
Jones and Craddock (2001)[136]	As part of a family study, they studied 152 parous bipolar women	81/313 births (26%) were followed by an episode within six weeks: 58/152 (37%) women had at least one puerperal episode; 11 others had a prepartum affective episode, and 6 had a manic episode between six weeks and six months post partum
Akdeniz (2003)[137]	72 parous bipolar Turkish women (retrospective analysis)	23/252 pregnancies were affected. During pregnancy, there were 11 episodes (4 depressive, 7 manic). Within a month of childbirth there were 26 episodes (17 depressive, 9 manic); 16 followed the birth of the 1st child
Robertson Blackmore (2006)[53]	129 bipolar or schizo-manic women who suffered an episode within four weeks of childbirth	167/242 (69%) births were followed by an episode
Di Florio (2013)[138]	980 'bipolar 1'	326 (33%) women had a history of an episode of mania, hypomania or depressive psychosis within six weeks of the birth. Of 1,404 pregnancies, 60 (4%) were complicated by an episode during pregnancy and 640 (46%) within 12 months of the birth

The only study that disagreed with this increased rate is Kendell's[41]: he found foetal loss in 5.8 per cent mothers admitted, *versus* 3.1 per cent controls; but only one of seven mothers who lost a baby had a psychosis. The effect might be due, at least in part, to grief rather than psychosis.

Obstetric Variables

The main studies are those of Paffenbarger[152,154,156], Jansson[153], Kendell[41,148], Robertson Blackmore[53], Nager[54], Bergink[58] and Hellerstedt[155]. Kendell's[41] and especially Nager's stand out because of their much larger control series (54,087 and 1,133,368 normal women). Robertson Blackmore's study[53] compared affected and unaffected pregnancies, using the mothers as their own controls. These studies have addressed as risk factors multiple births, pregnancy complications (anaemia, hydramnios or antepartum haemorrhage), pre-eclamptic toxaemia (PET), delivery complications, Caesarean section, gestation period, birth weight, postpartum complications and miscarriage rates.

No one has found that multiple births are associated with puerperal psychosis. Only Hellerstedt[155] found an increase in pregnancy complications (22.4 per cent *versus* 15.8 per cent, $p < .05$). As for PET, Paffenbarger[152,156] found more hypertension, but Kendell[41] found less PET in psychotic mothers (6.8 per cent *versus* 10 per cent), as did Hellerstedt[155]; Bergink[58] reported pre-eclampsia in 3/51 (5.9 per cent) compared with 1.9 per cent in 7,000 normal mothers and Nager[54] found a hazard factor of 1.19, so this association is small, and disputed. Prematurity and low birth weight were identified as risk factors by Paffenbarger and Jansson[153], but Kendell[41] found the same gestation periods and birth weights, as did Hellerstedt[155] and Robertson Blackmore[53]. Nager[54] found that 'small for gestational age' had a hazard factor of 1.46, so this effect is also small and disputed. Kendell[41] found an association with Caesarean section (17 per cent *versus* 8.4 per cent, $p < .05$[148]; 17.5 per cent *versus* 9.6 per cent[41]). Hellerstedt[155], Bergink[58] and Robertson Blackmore[53] found no association. Nager[54] found that this was the only factor that survived all adjustments, with a hazard ratio of 1.31, so there is evidence of a weak effect, which could be due to surgery rather than childbirth.

The effect of birth complications is also disputed. Kendell[41] studied six (malpresentation, long labour, perineal tears, haemorrhage, sepsis and anaemia) and found that 5/6 were less frequent in psychotic mothers, the other having the same frequency. Hellerstedt[155] examined a similar list, with the same result. Nager[54] reported on anaemia, malpresentation, haemorrhage and obstetric trauma: they all had hazard ratios below 1.0. Robertson Blackmore[53], using multiple regression, found an association ($p = .022$), which was confirmed in 53 mothers who had both affected and unaffected births ($p = .016$), but it was not possible to single out specific risks. Hellerstedt[155] found an increase in puerperal complications (infection, thrombosis or lactation difficulties): these were present in 5.0 per cent of those with a postpartum episode and only 3.3 per cent of the others ($< .05$). I have found no other data on these variables.

Kendell[41] found a reduction in miscarriages (4.1 per cent *versus* 16.3 per cent, $p < .05$). Jansson[153] found no difference in historic abortions (22.6 *versus* 21.7 per cent), but reduced miscarriages (4.9 per cent *versus* 9.7 per cent) and increased terminations (15.2 per cent *versus* 10.2 per cent) in the follow-up period. My findings are given on page 213.

There are therefore no agreed and confirmed obstetric risk factors.

Laboratory Studies

The literature includes 28 biochemical and neuroscientific investigations. These began in 1857 with the detection of protein in the urine – before it was realized that eclamptic psychosis was a distinct form of childbearing psychosis. Since then there have been measurements of haemoglobin[158], blood urea[159], body weight[160], EEG measures[161], urinary catechol and indole amines[162], prolactin[163], oxytocin[164], CSF endorphins[165–167], milk proteins[168,169], gonadotrophic and sex steroid hormones[170,185], calcium[171], cholesterol and triglycerides[172], REM sleep[173], CSF chromatography[174], CT scans[122,175–177], sleep diaries[178] and several markers of immune system dysregulation[58]. These diverse measurements have all been published by a single research team, without replication of any positive findings.

Several teams have examined the dexamethasone suppression test. Singh[179], who studied 7 patients and 4 control groups, found that it was raised, but not more so than in normal postpartum women. Eberl[180], who studied 6 patients, found that 3 were non-suppressors. Paykel[181], who studied 11 patients and matched controls, found that the mean post-dexamethasone cortisol was 4.9 *versus* 1.9 in controls ($p = .014$), with 3 non-suppressors.

Several have studied thyroid function. Nomura[182] studied 15 patients with puerperal psychotic depression, and found reduced tri-iodo-thyronine (T3) ($p < .05$). Later, the same team[183] studied 15 patients with puerperal psychosis, 10 with postpartum depression and 10 normal women: thyroid stimulating hormone (TSH) was raised in puerperal psychosis (3.9 *versus* 2.7, $p < .05$), and thyroxin (T4) was lowered (6.6 *versus* 7.7 and 8.4, $p < .05$); the greatest change was in T3, which was also lowered (93 *versus* 108 and 143, $p < .001$). Stewart[184], who studied 30 puerperal psychoses and 30 controls, found the opposite: TSH was low (2.1 *versus* 3.7 in the early stages), while T4 (154 *versus* 144) and T3 (0.23 *versus* 0.22) were slightly raised; these changes were corrected within a month, and none was statistically significant. Paykel[181] studied TSH-releasing hormone stimulation of TSH and found no significant differences. Meakin[185] found no abnormalities in thyroid hormones in 10 women at high risk of recurrence, followed into the puerperium. Bergink[58] studied 31 puerperal psychoses and 117 controls: 6 patients (19 per cent) and 6 controls (5 per cent) had evidence of auto-immune thyroid disease ($p = .019$), 3 of whom had thyroid dysfunction; 3 more developed this during the next nine months ($p = .02$); this interesting finding requires replication by another group. There are no agreed findings on thyroid dysfunction.

Under this heading is research on dopamine supersensitivity, which was initially hailed as a breakthrough:

In 1991, a team from the Institute of Psychiatry[186] used apomorphine challenge tests to measure the increase in growth hormone (GH) – a sign of dopamine sensitivity. They followed 15 pregnant women at high risk of puerperal psychosis, matched with 15 controls: after childbirth, seven remained well, six developed puerperal psychosis and two developed postpartum depression. For growth hormone peak minus the average baseline before injection of apomorphine, controls averaged 3.40, high risk mothers who remained well 1.73, those who developed puerperal psychosis 3.71 and those who developed postpartum depression 16.22. Merging the last two they obtained a mean of 6.74 which was significantly raised ($p < .05$). This was immediately challenged[187]. The response was that one mother "just failed to meet criteria for hypomania" and the other unexpectedly and impulsively attempted to kill her 8-week old infant. In 1995 Meakin[185] reported an attempt to replicate these findings: 10 women at high risk of puerperal psychosis were compared with 19 normal mothers; three high-risk mothers, who became ill, had *sub-sensitive* GH responsiveness. In 2003, the London team[188] replicated their study in bipolar women: the results were shown in table II of the paper: 17 who remained well had a mean growth hormone response of 5.93, and 12 who became ill 5.34. Thus it has been confirmed that early onset puerperal bipolar disorder is not associated with increased dopamine sensitivity. The error was due to a clinical misclassification.

Genetic Studies

It was noticed early in the history of puerperal psychoses that there was often a family history of mental illness. There are some remarkable family pedigrees:

> In five generations of a family, nine members suffered from psychosis. The frequency, and transmission by both males and females, indicated that this involved an autosomal dominant gene. Five affected members were female, and three had postpartum episodes. These were fulminant psychoses with confusion or delirium, amnesia for the episode, depressed or elated mood, hallucinations, delusions and bizarre behaviour. They had a favourable outcome[189].

> In another family, eleven members suffered from schizo-affective psychoses. Ten were women, of whom four had postpartum episodes. Two were mother and daughter, and one had two puerperal episodes[190].

These studies illustrate the tendency of puerperal psychosis to run in families. The next shows the additional effect of consanguinity:

> In a Walsall family, an incestuous father-daughter relationship led to the birth of several children. One daughter had puerperal bipolar disorder and corneal macular dystrophy (an autosomal recessive). A second had two episodes of puerperal psychosis. A third, who also had congenital eye disease, immolated herself during a puerperal episode. A fourth daughter, not the father's child, suffered only from depression. Thus all three daughters, born from incest, suffered from puerperal episodes[191].

Another family raises the possibility of an association with an inherited disease:

> A family was afflicted with Coffin-Lowry syndrome. This is a form of learning disability, with facial and skeletal anomalies; it is due to mutations of the *RPS6KA3* gene on the short arm of the X chromosome; the gene makes a protein involved with intracellular signalling. Two of the less severe female cases (a mother and a daughter) suffered from mental illness. The mother had two early puerperal manic episodes. The daughter also had bipolar disorder, and was admitted eight months after childbirth[192].

There have been several large family studies. Since these have, to some extent, been superseded by molecular genetic investigations, they will be summarized briefly.

> Protheroe[115] studied the mothers of women who suffered episodes within six months of childbirth: 2/386 births were followed by puerperal affective disorder.

> Thuwe[193] studied the children of 47 women who suffered episodes within six months of childbirth: they had significantly more mental illness than matched controls.

> Whalley[403] compared 17 mothers with puerperal psychosis with 20 bipolar women who remained well after childbirth: the relatives of both groups had puerperal episodes (2/90 and 3/90 births).

> Schöpf[118] studied 80 women with 1st episode psychosis, starting within three months of childbirth (34 depressed). There was a high morbidity risk in the 1° relatives, especially for affective and schizo-affective disorders. The relatives of patients who also had non-puerperal episodes had higher rates than those whose episodes were limited to the puerperium (30/252 *versus* 2/112, $p = .01$). Of the 16 parous psychotic female relatives, 6 developed a puerperal episode.

Dean[117] studied 51 mothers with episodes limited to the puerperium (starting within two weeks of the birth), 33 with both puerperal and non-puerperal episodes, and 19 bipolar women without puerperal episodes: the highest rates of mental illness were found in relatives of those who had puerperal episodes only (38/134), followed by those with both (18/82). These findings contradicted those of Schöpf[118]. Bipolar women who remained well after childbirth had significantly less mental illness.

Jones and Craddock[194] also studied bipolar women with children – 9 who suffered a puerperal episode and 16 who did not. The number of 1° relatives with mental illness was 7/46 and 1/87 ($p = .008$).

In the last 15 years, Craddock and Jones have used the national register of several hundred mothers (Action on Puerperal Psychosis), collected by Jackie Benjamin, to study large numbers of mothers by molecular genetic techniques. These are their main findings:

In a study[194] of 152 parous bipolar women, 27 had a family history of puerperal psychosis in a 1° relative: 20/27 (74%) had puerperal episodes themselves, compared with 38/125 (30%) who did not have a family history. The number of births followed by psychosis was 28/49 (57%), compared with 53/264 (20%). This is evidence that the puerperal trigger is inherited separately from bipolar disorder. Evidence of a different kind, supporting this finding, is offered on page 223.

They also studied the concordance between parous sisters: In 16 pairs, both had puerperal psychosis, in seven neither had it, while two pairs were discordant ($k = 0.67$, $p = .001$).

Coyle[196] studied the serotonin transporter gene, comparing 97 women who suffered puerperal psychosis with 97 controls from a general practice: there was evidence that this gene was involved ($p < .003$). But there was no such evidence for oestrogen receptor genes[197,198] or tumour necrosis factor alpha[199]. Robertson[200] also studied serotonin genes, comparing 165 mothers who suffered a bipolar episode within six weeks of childbirth with 77 parous bipolar women who remained well in the puerperium: they found no difference in the frequencies of two polymorphisms at the 5HT2A gene. In 2007, after a number of gene probes drew blank, they found a genome-wide significant linkage signal (LOD score 4.07) on chromosome 16p13, and possibly 8q24[201].

These studies require replication.

Case Lore

In spite of the large number of surveys, follow-up studies and investigations, this review has discovered few findings, if any, confirmed by other research teams. One reason for failure is the use of heterogeneous patient groups. It is the task of nosology to discover and define homogeneous groups, based on symptoms and course. The nosologist searches intuitively for patterns, which can be proposed as clinical entities, and submitted for validation. In an attempt to improve the homogeneity of groups in this area (and to look for causal clues), I have returned to the *incunabula* – the case descriptions – and have examined all the cases that I could find.

I set certain boundaries. I rejected:

- Many patients who suffered from depression without psychotic features, even when depression was severe, with suicidal or filicidal acts. Depression was accepted only if accompanied by stupor, catatonia, delusions or other psychotic features.
- Cases in which the description was too brief to identify psychotic phenomena. I was more tolerant of brevity if there was an obvious organic cause.

- Cases with evidence of a chronic psychosis present before conception
- Cases with onset more than one year after childbirth (except those claimed to complicate weaning).

This yielded the 4,029 cases mentioned in Section 1. These data are subject to all sorts of bias, especially publication bias and (since almost all were admitted to mental hospital) Berkson bias[202]. But they are the best source for establishing a provisional classification.

The number of cases of postpartum psychosis (all forms) published in each epoch can be seen in Table 16.10.

The main contributors can be seen in Table 16.11.

Table 16.10 The number of cases of postpartum psychosis (all forms) published in each epoch

Before 1850	286
1851–1875	298
1876–1900	668
1901–1925	889
1926–1950	869
1951–1975	534
After 1975	475
Total	**4,029**

Table 16.11 Main contributors

France, Belgium and Suisse Romande	1,155
Germany, Austria and Northern Switzerland	870
USA	460
UK and Eire	451
Italy	315
The Netherlands	180
Poland	107
Denmark and Norway	104

The remaining cases (fewer than 400) have been published by 30 other nations, none of which contributed more than 50.

These figures show:

- We have a debt to French and German authors, who have contributed more than half.
- During the last 50 years, there has been a fall, not entirely explained by the reduction in organic psychoses. This has occurred despite the establishment of mother & baby units in Western Europe and Australasia, which have given specialist teams a golden opportunity to observe unusual occurrences.

Theses have contributed 1,194 cases – 734 from French *thèses*, 315 from German *Inaugural-Dissertationen,* and the rest from Argentina, Holland, Senegal and 10 other nations. Table 16.12 summarizes the largest series.

Table 16.12 Series with more than 50 cases[a]

Year	Author	Number of cases	Publication
1933	Sivadon[86]	57	Paris thèse: *Les psychoses puerpérales et leurs séquelles*
1958	Bourson[100]	60	Strasbourg thèse: *Contribution à l'étude des psychoses puerpérales*
1949	Visscher[97]	65	Groningen thesis: *Generatie-psychoses en hersenstam*
1903	Widerøe[250]	66	Norwegian survey from Rotvold Asyl, Trondheim
My series		321	Obtained from Manchester and Birmingham, 1975–2001

[a] This is an enumeration of puerperal psychosis. Some larger series included cases without psychotic features; for example, Knauer[69] had a complete series of 70 cases, only 49 of which qualified.

The results of my study of more than 4,000 cases, together with my own series, form the substance of the present analysis.

Citation Analysis

The psychoses of childbearing, first recognized at the dawn of medical science, provide an opportunity to study the growth and spread of knowledge. For this purpose I carried out a citation analysis. The assumption is that authors cite what they have read. Doubtless there are scholars who scorn to exhibit their erudition, but many or most authors, if only to underpin their statements, cite works they have obtained, unless they consider them trivial. The corollary – that they have carefully read what they have cited – is by no means true: citing a publication certainly does not mean that it has been studied.

Indices

I noted the number of citations made, and received, for each article, book or thesis and used them to derive the following indices:

(1) A measure of scholarship, based on mean citations made by various language groups (with the number of publications in that language as the denominator)
(2) An index of linguistic isolation or arrogance, based on the proportion of citations in the author's language (with the number of publications that have at least one citation as the denominator)
(3) An index of recognition or neglect, based on the number of citations received
(4) For individual works, an index of international acclaim, based on the number of citations by other language groups

This reports the analysis of more than 2,200 publications on the psychoses of childbearing. It is convenient also to report here the analysis of more than 350 publications on menstrual psychosis. Omitted are more than 400 publications of puerperal psychosis and more than

100 of menstrual psychosis, which I failed to obtain, or whose reference lists were missing; I also omitted my own publications.

In the literature on puerperal psychosis,[a] the median number of citations was only 6, mean 9 (0.3 per cent of the literature). Only 11 authors cited more than 10 per cent of publications up to one year before their own[1,36,203–211], with Marcé (1858)[203] at the top of the list (19 per cent); since Dazzi's[211] thesis, no publication (apart from my own) has cited more than 10 per cent of the literature. The corresponding figure for menstrual psychosis is median 2, mean 4.7 (1 per cent of the literature); 10 authors cited at least 20 per cent of the prior literature[212–221] with Berthier[212] (21/41 = 56 per cent, of which 17 were French) and v. Krafft-Ebing[218] (54/103 = 52 per cent, of which 28 were German) at the top of the list. One can safely conclude that there is room for a more complete review.

Citation Fraud

There are two remarkable examples of cheating. Lallier's bibliography[205] listed more than 280 references – approximately 44 per cent of those published. Born in 1865, he was only 27 years of age, and would have had but a few years to collect this literature. There are various points to make:

- The number of references, and proportion of works published, was much higher than that of any other nineteenth century writer.
- The French language was fourth by frequency (52 references) after German (75), British (68) and American (59). It is unusual for authors to cite foreign works more often than their own.
- Few Frenchmen cited American works, and only one cited as many as three. Lallier cited 59 (out of 99 published by 1891), which is almost as many as Boyd[222] (63), writing 50 years later. He cited some I was unable to find after searching for more than 30 years, with the help of inter-library loans and friendly American libraries. Indeed, his list included two American papers[223,224] said not to exist in the United States.
- In the text he cited only two American works[24,225].

A few years later Castin[226] went further: his bibliography included more than 400 works, including 104 American articles (much more than has ever been cited by an American); in the text he mentioned 46 articles including 2 American. There can be no doubt that these authors copied titles from one of the American inventories that had recently appeared – probably the Index Catalogue of the Surgeon General (which appeared in 1885). A bibliography is not a list of works known to exist – it is testimony to the scholastic activities of the writer. Lallier and Castin's bibliographies are a species of academic fraud. Their significance here is that they underline the fact that citation lists exaggerate the reading that has been done.

A Comparison of Language Groups

Table 16.13 compares some language groups in order of the mean citations made by publications on childbearing and menstrual psychoses.

---

[a] More detailed results are given in *What Is Worth Knowing about 'Postpartum Psychosis'*.

Table 16.13 Citations by language group

Language group	Psychoses of childbearing			Menstrual psychosis		
	Mean citations		Proportion in own language, %	Mean citations		Proportion in own language, %
	Made	Received		Made	Received	
Italian	15.5	2.4	16	5.8	0.9	2
Dutch	14.5	4.3	7	6.0	1.5	3
Nordic	9.3	8.7	4	2.2	6.6	10
French	8.1	6.7	47	2.7	3.9	73
German	7.6	6.6	32	5.7	2.7	87
Japanese	6.5	1.8	19	6.6	4.0	31
British Commonwealth	5.2	7.3	67	2.4	2.3	57
American	4.4	5.6	45	3.6	3.0	80

These results conceal large differences:

- In the literature on the psychoses of childbearing, French theses made the most citations (27) and other French works the least (3.7).
- There was a sharp drop in German citations received after 1914.

They show, however:

- A low level of scholarship: even the highest rates are low (27 cited works is a small number for a thesis); medians of 6 and 2, with means of 0.3 per cent and 1 per cent of the literature are extremely low.
- This is especially true of the Anglo-Saxon nations.
- More than 60 per cent of publications on childbearing psychoses cited by British Commonwealth nations were in the English language. As for menstrual psychosis, German, American and French authors all made more than 70 per cent of citations to publications in their own language. There has been a general failure of Anglo-Saxon, French and (before 1914) German authors to cite works from other languages. Italian, Dutch and Nordic nations were more scholarly and less arrogant.

International Acclaim

Only three publications had more than 100 citations from other language groups – Kendell[41] (112 including American), Esquirol[227] (144 – available in the English translation) and Marcé[203] (161). The international acclaim received by the Scots author Campbell Clark[228] is interesting: his study of infective delirium received 62 foreign and only one British citation. Widespread international recognition of a paper ignored in Britain was also true of another British writer, Donkin[229], who received 19 foreign and no British citations. As for menstrual psychosis, v. Krafft-Ebing's work is most cited, with 87 in all; he is the only author to receive more than 20 citations from non-German authors, and has even been cited twice by American authors, but never before by an

Englishman. It would be justifiable to regard citing v. Krafft-Ebing as a marker for scholarship; no one who has not read his work can claim a knowledge of this subject. But it has been forgotten by some German authors[230-234], and, since 1925, has been cited only 12 times.

Under-Cited Works

There is a long list of important publications which have received few citations. They include a dozen pioneering or sedulous studies of organic psychoses, including the first descriptions of parturient[235] and postpartum delirium[26], postpartum stupor[237,238], six major articles on eclamptic psychosis[239-244], Kalbag and Woolf's account of cerebral venous thrombosis[245], a Venezuelan obstetric survey[38] and the Japanese description of hyperammonaemic psychosis[246]. Two of the best French theses, by Breton[247] on chorea psychosis, and Collet[248] on rapid births, have received one and two citations, respectively.

As for non-organic psychosis, Osiander's marvellous descriptions[249] have received 15 citations (9 German, 3 French, 2 Dutch and 1 British). The two largest series, by Visscher[97] and Wideroe[250], received 1 and 5 citations. Van Steenbergen-van-der-Nordaa's superb thesis[96] received only 3 citations (1 Italian and 2 Dutch), and 2 massive case series[108,109], with description of all cases and long follow up, have never been cited. Delay's[101] unique investigation by serial uterine biopsies has been cited 30 times, but only 15 times by French authors, among 149 published in that language since 1950; French psychiatrists came under the influence of psychoanalysis, and this promising line of research petered out.

In the literature on menstrual psychosis, some important German works have been neglected, especially Mendel's[251] – the first case established beyond reasonable doubt - with five citations; Wollenberg's[252] description of mid-cycle psychosis, with seven (all German); and Ewald's[253] remarkable case with 54 episodes, with five. Our paper[254] on premenstrual relapse of puerperal psychosis should perhaps have been cited by more than six authors, none of whom were British. The paper by Horwitz and Harris[255], the only American paper to cite v. Krafft-Ebing's works as well as Brière de Boismont[256], has been cited once (by an Italian author). Half of the 38 Japanese papers have never been cited by a non-Japanese author; they include Yamashita's[257] *Periodic Psychosis of Adolescence*, which has been translated into English.

Comment

Literature reviews should not be delegated to students, not only because they lack the experience to interpret what they read, but because it takes years to obtain publications scattered in obscure journals and university libraries. With few exceptions, senior investigators have set a bad example. To illustrate this, I have chosen distinguished scientists, one each from four nations.

> Siemerling, Professor at Kiel, inspired at least 19 theses on subjects related to puerperal psychosis, and wrote six reviews. The most extensive[258] cited 81 publications – about 8 per cent of those published by that time; 80 per cent of his citations were to German authors, who were responsible for one-third of the literature. It is not surprising that the scholastic standard of the Kiel theses fell below that of other German universities, and only one cited a foreign paper. Siemerling's approach to literature had something of the arrogance now shown by Anglo-Saxon authors, since English became 'the language of science'.

Delay, Professor at the Salpêtrière, was perhaps the most distinguished psychiatrist of his generation. With Deniker he introduced chlorpromazine to clinical psychiatry. In the 1940s he published a unique study of the hormonal basis of puerperal psychosis. But, of his six publications, only one[259] had 20 citations (1.5 per cent of publications by that time), of which 12 were to French authors, who had contributed less than one-quarter of published works.

The Americans Thomas and Gordon[260] published a paper entitled 'Psychosis after childbirth: ecological aspects of a single impact stress'. This stands out among more than 40 American reviews published since 1950, 75 per cent of which have no citations in any language except English. Whatever these authors meant by 'single impact' (because childbirth, a single event, has many impacts), their review was based on 59 relevant references (4 per cent of the literature then published), of which 48 were in the English language. Although American libraries are the best stocked in the world, no American working on 'puerperal psychosis' has more than scratched the surface of this literature.

Kendell, much lamented since his early death in 2002, was a psychiatrist of worldwide reputation. His series of epidemiological studies are landmarks in the study of puerperal psychosis. His six papers have been cited more than any other author's (bar none), and his 1987 paper ranks third after those of Marcé and Esquirol in international acclaim. His article with the most cited articles[261] had 20 references relevant to 'puerperal psychosis' (1 per cent of the literature), all (including Esquirol) published in English.

Symptoms

In *Motherhood and Mental Health*[67], describing the symptoms of puerperal psychosis, I wrote:

> Almost every psychotic symptom is found in these psychoses. The delusions cover the whole gamut of morbid ideas … Verbal hallucinations, thought insertion, echo phenomena, thought broadcasting and 'made' impulses occur, often accompanied by ideas of control or possession. Catatonic features … and catalepsy have been emphasized as particularly common.

This general statement can be amplified by the study of more than 4,000 cases in the literature and my series.

The first characteristic symptom to be mentioned was one that does not appear in modern operational definitions – rhyming. Hoffman[262] observed an insane mother, who talked day and night, mainly in rhyme. Osiander[249], describing in detail his first patient with *mania lactea*, wrote:

> Her delirium took the form of a stream of rhyming nonsense, declaimed to hymn tunes. She spoke and sang (in a loud melodic voice) always in rhyme. Senseless rhyming could continue for many hours, in which she did not for a moment stop talking or rhyming. She incorporated any objects on which her gaze happened to fall; this was done with astonishing rapidity.

A footnote gives an example of her rhyming madness and its mechanism:

> Hölle [Hell], Hölle, Delle [a hollow], Delle
> Du verdammter schwartzer Gselle [You damn black fellow],
> Lass mich du mein Kind erretten [Let me save my child]
> Von des Teufels *ofen* Ketten [From the Devil's *stove* chains]

At that moment her gaze fell on the black stove, and this was inserted into her rhyme.

In the discussion, it was made clear that she had never previously attempted to write poetry. He cited the Latin writer Petronius (27–66 A D) who referred to *furentis animi versification* [the versification of the raging mind] found in high fevers. Clinicians would now probably regard this as a feature of manic speech. But only one of nine mothers in the literature[263] had an unequivocal non-organic psychosis. All the others, including Osiander's, had much evidence of infection. This is another example of a rhyming case, in which there were several indications of infective delirium, and none to favour a non-organic psychosis[36]:

> A 26-year old gave birth to her 1st child. It was a difficult delivery that required some assistance. On day 4 she complained of headache and pain in the back and limbs. Her temperature reached 40.5°. By day 10 she was delirious: she was excited, spoke only in rhyme, sang and only occasionally recognized bystanders. She did not know where she was, who was with her, or whether it was summer or winter, day or night, and she had visual hallucinations. By day 18 she was improving.

In my series, this symptom was noted in two mothers, one with mania and one with a cycloid psychosis. Thus 'rhyming madness' can occur in both organic and non-organic cases.

Another early symptom to be reported is enhanced intellect, as in this eighteenth century case[264]:

> She was continually speaking and shouting incoherently with frightful fantasies. She raved with awful shouting and cursing, hitting out, scratching, biting and spitting on people. It required 3–4 people to keep her in bed. Particularly at the height of the illness, the energy of her mental powers was remarkable: her understanding and judgment was sharpened in an astonishing way.

In Osiander's discussion, he cited ancient and contemporary literature on patients who acquired special powers when mentally ill, starting with Plato, who wrote that an ignorant man, Tynnichus of Chalcedon, composed beautiful hymns. His second case of *mania lactea* has been translated in Section 1; briefly to recapitulate,

> No actress in the world, not even a Garrick, would better her indescribable originality . . . in all the finest nuances of muscular movement.

Three other authors mentioned this symptom. Scott[265] described a mother who became ill on day 7: she started reciting, with astonishing accuracy and rapidity, parts of scripture and hymns. Arnold[266] described a mother with a mammary abscess: her incessant and rambling speech was interspersed with snatches of poetry, which was remarkable for its elegance of expression. Brooke[267] described a woman with puerperal mania: there was an exaltation of her intellect – she was composing *impromptu* and singing jingling verses, many of them remarkably bright and witty, a feat that was beyond her in her normal state. This clinical manifestation is not included among the defining features of mania, but perhaps it should be. One mother in my series had a heightened ability to answer quiz questions and crossword puzzles; there was much evidence of a Donkin psychosis, but this symptom might favour puerperal mania.

Osiander's patient also showed "an extraordinary acuteness and sensitivity of sensation". Several mothers in my series described this enhanced perceptual quality – colours unusually bright or vivid, the world in brilliant Technicolor and exceptionally beautiful, noises louder, or a heightened sense of textures. This is a cardinal symptom in the ecstasy phenomenon described by Anderson[268], but occasionally occurs in mania.

Denial of pregnancy or birth is common. There is an extensive literature on denial of pregnancy in women who are not suffering from psychosis. I summarized this in *Motherhood and Mental Health*[67], pages 65–68, but there have been at least a dozen works published since then, especially Wessel's *Habilitationsschrift*[269]. In women with severe psychosis, as in those with severe learning disability, there may be unawareness of their pregnant state and of parturition. Morel[270] had experience of 12 women suffering from 'imbecility' or 'idiocy'.

> Most of these unfortunate women give birth either with complete indifference, or without understanding their situation.

Worthington[271] wrote,

> A remarkable feature of the insanity of pregnant women is the almost utter absence of suffering during labour.

Imperviousness to all stimuli (external or internal) is a feature of catatonia, a disorder now rare, but common in the nineteenth century. Unnoticed birth has also been reported in neurosyphilis[272–273], and von Economo's encephalitis (see Section 2). It can occur in depressive stupor or prepartum melancholia[274]: labour pains failed to arouse these patients from their apathy, and the infant's cry could be their first inkling of what had happened. Two patients shook their heads in disbelief when told they had given birth, and two gave a delusional interpretation of labour pains – dogs gnawing the intestines[275] or a snake inside[273]. Bamford[276], reviewing 97 pregnant women admitted to Rainhill Hospital (1883–1933), wrote,

> In many instances labour has been so sudden in onset and precipitate in character that the medical and nursing attendants have been taken unawares, and this has resulted in perineal tears of various degrees.

Here are three examples, two from the literature and one from my series:

> A melancholic patient developed anasarca, and also had amenorrhoea, very common in the insane. In the infirmary she thanked the physician for visiting and said she had suffered a severe attack of colic, which was relieved by passing urine. They found a full term infant next door, still enclosed in its amniotic sac. She never realised she had given birth[277].

> A melancholic woman went to the toilet and cried out. She was standing on the seat, held back by the umbilical cord attached to an infant, whose head was engaged in the pan. It could not be pulled out. The apparatus had to be dismantled, and the head delivered from below. The infant survived[248].

> A Yemeni woman in her 2nd pregnancy presented with insomnia at 23 weeks gestation. At 27 weeks she was suspicious, perplexed and overactive; she heard voices and had delusions of surveillance. She believed the President of Yemen would visit her, the television was watching her and police were photographing her and the family. After ECT she became bright and cheerful and was hugging and kissing the staff. But she relapsed into stupor. At 5.30 am she was rubbing her abdomen. Staff pulled her trousers down and found the baby's head had already appeared. She did not realise she had given birth, and refused the baby offered to her[67].

Ten mothers in my series did not believe they had given birth, or had similar delusions, such as that they had never been pregnant.

Another characteristic symptom is the changeling delusion. There are five cases in the literature, and two in my series, in which the mother believed the infant had been swapped for another[101,278–281]. The Capgras delusion has been reported by four authors[282–285] and in one of my series ('people were not real, but carbon look-alikes'). Silva[285] described a woman with a prepartum psychosis, who believed that her husband had been replaced by a stranger; her teenage son and daughter had died and been reincarnated, all possessed by the devil; and that a second set of children were living away with her real husband. Two patients had a combination of Capgras and changeling delusions[282,284]:

> A 23-year old, whose mother had four postpartum episodes, became depressed in the 9th month of her 2nd pregnancy, with mutism, food refusal and the hallucination of a dictaphone reading a register of her sins. She misidentified doctors, nurses and patients. She began to believe that her husband had been replaced by a double, her eldest son by a man transformed into a 3-year old boy, and her youngest son by a changeling. She threw herself in front of a car, resulting in multiple fractures.

> A mother gave birth to her 2nd child; 24 hours later she became agitated, and expressed the idea that she had two husbands. She knew the man caring for her children was not her husband. She also believed her child had been switched with another in the nursery. After ECT she recovered with no memory of the psychotic experience.

A mother in my series had a combination of Capgras and Fregoli syndromes:

> During an episode of puerperal mania, she said she had given birth to six children, or even 13, "because her husband had super sperm". She was picking up other mothers' children, with the delusion that she was mother to all the babies. She believed she was still pregnant and requested a scan. She was preoccupied with a man called Chris (a dead friend). She believed the doctor was Chris, having the same smile. Her husband was dead; he and her mother were doubles, with subtle differences in manner and voice. Some of the nurses were doubles or imposters, and two of them were Chris. She recognized schoolfellows and workmates from her early life. A medical student was identified as Prince Charles, and another as herself – or her other spirit; for two weeks she greeted this student with the words, "You are me, aren't you!"

The nihilistic Cotard delusion was noted in three mothers in my series. The beliefs included having no organs – stomach, heart, intestines – or no limbs, head, eyes, blood, circulation, soul or emotions. One mother believed her head was made of cardboard, another that her brains were leaking through her nose, another that bits of her had died away, another that her nose and lips were falling off, and another that her vagina and anus had fused and her organs rotted. A mother said she was covered in faeces, her bones were heavy and fragile, her insides rotting, her neck blown up; she had no pulse, was dead and her body corrupting.

One patient had a delusional erotomanic relationship with the doctor[286] and, in my series, there was this case:

> A mother suffering from a postpartum cycloid episode heard the voice of "Lisa" telling her what to say and do. (Her husband explained that Lisa was an ex-girlfriend he had known for a short time eight years ago, before he met his wife.) She announced that she knew he was having an affair with Lisa. When a female doctor asked who Lisa was, she said, "It's you. You had sex with my husband and then fertilized me last night". She often mistook this doctor for Lisa. She thought she was pregnant with Lisa's twins; she often spoke about them, and answered hallucinatory comments – "Yes, I'll keep them, don't be stupid – I wouldn't do that. I love children".

Other unusual delusions include Ekbom's syndrome[287], also found in one of my series, poisoning the child with breast milk[288], and the placenta lodged in her throat[289].

Catatonia is often reported, including automatic obedience[290] and catalepsy (maintaining uncomfortable positions)[291]. Churchill[292] graphically described this example of catatonic stupor:

> A patient of Dr Lever, who had been the life of the household, light-hearted and gay, sat wherever she was placed, neither turning her head or eyes to one side or the other – a living automaton. There was life, but no mind. Her chiseled face seemed cut in alabaster. She recovered after the birth.

Stereotypic movements have been described[293,294]:

> A 19-year old gave birth to her 1st child, and was admitted to hospital within a week: among many other symptoms, her motor behaviour was most curious. On one occasion, she stretched herself stiffly on the bed, so strongly that the bed timbers creaked, with her tongue stuck out. She stood on her head, her feet against the wall. She pushed her tongue in and out a hundred times with great speed. She was grimacing and making stereotypic movements for hours.

> A mother in my series, during an episode that followed her 2nd birth, walked with her knees bent and arms sticking out, then repeatedly stood up and sat down. She lay on the floor for five minutes with her head raised, as if by a pillow, and maintained awkward positions of her limbs. She had 'seizures', when she became hypertonic, with eyes staring, shaking but with no spontaneous

movement, responsive only to pain; her arms were flaccid, her reflexes brisk with increased tone in her legs, but the Babinski sign was negative. Neurologists found no evidence of brain damage, with a normal skull X ray and CAT scan.

As for *automatisme mentale,* Gooch[295], Arnold[266] and two in my series described echo phenomena, such as echolalia or echopraxia. Another mother[296] said that someone was controlling her thoughts and repeating them, so that everyone who was not deaf could hear them. Others described command hallucinations[69,297]. A mother in my series heard a voice saying she had to sacrifice her daughter; she could also hear her thoughts out loud, as an echo.

Self-mutilation was described by Rocher[204]: his patient extracted two teeth and a fistful of hair, then several more teeth.

Folie-à-deux: Bürgi's[298] patient believed that God would punish her for letting her employer down, and her husband fully supported these ideas.

Erotic or nymphomanic behaviour is one of the notorious features of puerperal mania, as seen in this mother from my series:

A mother suffering from postpartum mania spoke frankly about previous affairs and abortions, and criticised her husband's sexual performance. She wanted to dress up in her wedding clothes and go through the ceremony again. She frightened the milkman by suggesting the baby was his. Though normally troubled by feelings of ugliness and sensitive about her weight, she walked about in the nude. She believed the doctor was her husband's brother, merely playing at being a doctor. "You're so handsome, (name), and I love you, and I know you love me. I know you want me, because I am so beautiful. Don't let anything come between us". She got up and kissed him on the lips. When he was performing a physical examination, she said, "You just watch my arse. I know you are dying to get your hands on me". She was considered too dangerous for the Mother & Baby unit and was transferred to an intensive care ward, where she was found in bed with another patient.

Non-Organic Psychoses of Childbearing

Classification

18

The *International Classification of Diseases* (ICD)

In the 7th revision[299], chapter 5 (mental disorders) devotes 300–309 to psychoses, but makes no mention of postpartum psychosis, not even in 308 (psychoses of other demonstrable aetiology) or 309 (psychosis, not otherwise specified). But it could be classified in chapter 11 (complications of pregnancy, childbirth and the puerperium), where 688.1 (on page 200) had puerperal psychosis, or various synonyms such as insanity after delivery. There was no mention of menstrual psychosis in chapter 5, but in chapter 10 (the genitourinary system), 634 on page 189 has 'mental disorders'.

In the 8th revision[300], postpartum psychosis was given a special category (294.4), with the qualification that restricted its use to a minority of cases:

> Statistical data have been of little value because some psychiatrists classified their cases according to the type of mental disorder present, while other psychiatrists classified them under the general class of puerperal psychosis. Users of this classification are strongly advised to do the former, and to use the sub-category 294.4 (psychosis associated with childbirth) only in the rare cases when a specific diagnosis of the psychotic state is not possible.

Category 294.4 was defined as follows:

> Psychosis associated with childbirth (excludes psychosis of any type classifiable to 295–298 arising during the puerperium): this category includes only unspecified psychoses which have occurred within six weeks (42 days) following delivery. Every effort should be made to specify the condition, in which case it should not be included here. Sections 295–298 'specify' schizophrenia, affective psychoses, paranoid states and other non-organic psychoses.

Many psychiatrists, however, ignored these restrictions; for example, Edinburgh psychiatrists diagnosed 30/71 mothers admitted within nine days of childbirth as suffering from puerperal psychosis 'in ignorance or defiance of the request in the British glossary to avoid the term'[148].

With the 9th revision[301], puerperal psychosis lost this precarious status. No mention was made of it. It was, however, possible for clinicians to use a category in the obstetric section (648 'other current conditions in the mother, classifiable elsewhere but complicating pregnancy, childbirth and the puerperium'), one of whose subcategories (648.4) dealt with 'mental disorder', but this coding was not mentioned in the offprint of the chapter on mental disorders (chapter 5) used by most psychiatrists, which contained no instruction to code any physical disorders present. In consequence, few psychiatrists knew of the possibility, and it was of little value in identifying puerperal psychosis for epidemiological research. Nevertheless, in the South-East Thames region, 83/142 cases were identified from the returns of the Department of Health and Social Security by the use of the code 648.4[74].

The 10th edition[302] included, in its introduction, a paragraph giving instructions for recording more than one diagnosis, with the exhortation

> Clinicians should follow the general rule of recording as many diagnoses as are necessary to cover the clinical picture.

There is a paragraph about puerperal illness, which reads:

> This category is unusual and apparently paradoxical in carrying a recommendation that it should be used only when unavoidable. Its inclusion is a recognition of the very real practical problems in many developing countries that make the gathering of details about many cases of puerperal illness virtually impossible. However, even in the absence of sufficient information to allow a diagnosis of some variety of affective disorder (or, more rarely, schizophrenia), there will usually be enough known to allow diagnosis of a mild (F53.0) or severe (F53.1) disorder: this subdivision is useful for estimations of workload, and when decisions are to be made about provision of services.

> The inclusion of this category should not be taken to imply that, given adequate information, a significant proportion of cases of postpartum mental illness cannot be classified in other categories. Most experts in the field are of the opinion that a clinical picture of puerperal psychosis is so rarely (if ever) reliably distinguishable from affective disorder or schizophrenia that a special category is not justified. Any psychiatrist who is of the minority opinion that special postpartum psychoses do indeed exist may use this category, but should be aware of its real purpose.

F53 has four subcategories – F53.0 'mild' (which includes postnatal depression not otherwise classified), F53.1 'severe' (which includes puerperal psychosis not otherwise specified), F53.8 'other' and F53.9 'unspecified'. F53 reads:

> Mental and behavioural disorders associated with the puerperium, not elsewhere classified. This classification should be used only for mental disorders associated with the puerperium (commencing within six weeks of delivery) that do not meet the criteria for disorders classified elsewhere in this book, either because insufficient information is available, or because it is considered that special additional clinical features are present which make their classification elsewhere inappropriate. It will usually be possible to classify mental disorders associated with the puerperium without using these special codes by using two other codes: the first is from elsewhere in chapter V indicating the specific type of mental disorder (usually affective F30–F39) and the second is 099.3 (mental diseases and diseases of the nervous system complicating the puerperium).

These recommendations are strengthened in ICD-10's *Diagnostic Criteria for Research*[303], which states that category F53 should be used in research 'only in exceptional circumstances'.

> Mental disorders associated with the puerperium should be coded according to the presenting psychiatric disorder, while a second code (099.3) will indicate the association with the puerperium.

Essentially this is a return to ICD-8, with the addition of a reminder to use multiple codes, which allowed epidemiologists to identify cases, whatever their symptomatology.

ICD-10 introduced an innovation by recognizing 'acute polymorphic psychotic disorder'.

> This was an acute psychotic disorder in which hallucinations, delusions, and perceptual experiences are obvious but markedly variable, changing from day to day or even from hour to hour. Emotional turmoil, with intense transient feelings of happiness and ecstasy or anxieties and irritability, is also frequently present. This polymorphic and unstable, changing clinical picture is

characteristic, and even though individual affective or psychotic symptoms may at times be present, the criteria for manic episode, depressive episode or schizophrenia are not fulfilled. This disorder is particularly likely to have an abrupt onset (within 48 hours) and a rapid resolution of symptoms; in a large proportion of cases there is no obvious precipitating stress. If symptoms persist for more than three months, the diagnosis should be changed: persistent delusional disorder or other nonorganic psychotic disorder is likely to be the most appropriate.

A variant had 'typical schizophrenic symptoms'. This was intended to include *bouffée délirante* and cycloid psychosis.

The 11th revision (ICD-11) will be released in 2017.

Evidently the experts of the World Health Organization regarded the diagnosis of schizophrenia, affective psychoses and paranoid states as 'more specific' than puerperal psychosis.

The American *Diagnostic and Statistical Manual*

The American Psychiatric Association decided to develop its own *Diagnostic and Statistical Manual*. In the 1st edition[304], there was no mention of postpartum disorders. The 2nd edition[305] had a category 294.4, with instructions similar to those of ICD-8:

Almost any type of psychosis may occur during pregnancy and the postpartum period and should be specifically diagnosed. This category is not a substitute for a differential diagnosis and excludes other psychoses arising during the puerperium. Therefore this diagnosis should not be used unless all possible diagnoses have been excluded.

The next edition[306], which is 494 pages long, mentioned puerperal psychosis only once, on page 203, under 'psychotic disorders not elsewhere classified'. This section included schizophreniform disorder, brief reactive psychosis, schizo-affective disorder and atypical psychosis; this last was defined as a residual category for cases in which there are psychotic symptoms 'that do not meet the criteria for any specific mental disorder'; it included monosymptomatic delusions, transient auditory hallucinations, menstrual psychosis, brief schizo-phreniform psychosis and postpartum psychosis. The reference to puerperal psychosis was followed by the words 'that do not meet the criteria for an organic mental disorder, schizophreniform disorder, paranoid disorder or affective disorder'.

DSMIII, however, broke new ground in providing a multi-axial framework, and two of its axes could be used for the puerperium. Axis III dealt with physical disorders, but without a specific recommendation to code childbirth. Axis IV dealt with 'psychosocial stressors', and here 'becoming a parent' was mentioned; but it was not the type of stress that was coded, only its severity on an 8-point scale. In the guidelines, pregnancy was given as an example of a moderate stressor, and the birth of a child as a severe stressor.

An interim revision[307] appeared a few years later. It made no mention of puerperal psychosis in the index, nor in its list of 300 diagnoses. 'Atypical psychosis' was to be used in a similar way to DSMIII. The section explaining 'psychosocial stressors' made the distinction in axis IV between 'acute events' and 'enduring circumstances': abortion and 'being a single parent' were given as examples of moderate stressors and 'birth of the first child' as a severe stressor. Examples indicated that the nature of the stressor should be stated in addition to the severity rating.

In the 4th edition[308], postpartum psychosis had a section in the chapter on mood disorders entitled 'postpartum onset specifier'. The specifier 'with postpartum onset' could be applied to various mood disorders or to a brief psychotic disorder, if onset was within four weeks of the birth. This was helpful in most cases, but it did not deal with the large minority of puerperal psychoses that are cycloid or schizo-phreniform. 'Brief psychotic disorder' did not cover their symptomatology; it was restricted to illnesses with a duration of less than a month, and was contraindicated if criteria for schizo-affective disorder were met.

In the multi-axial system, complications of pregnancy, childbirth and the puerperium could be coded under axis III (630-376). Psychosocial and environmental problems, associated with pregnancy, could be coded under axis IV, though they were not specifically mentioned.

The 5th edition[309] was published in May 2013. On page 152 there is a paragraph in the section on bipolar and related disorders headed 'with peripartum onset':

> This specifier can be applied to the current or, if the full criteria are not currently met for a mood episode, most recent episode of mania, hypomania or major depression in bipolar I, bipolar II and brief psychotic disorders, if onset of mood symptoms occurs during pregnancy or in the four weeks following delivery.

I understand that this 'specifier' is in the text of axis I, not a separate axis.[a]

A disorder mentioned by Hippocrates, one of the first psychoses to be mentioned in medical history, does not appear in the index.

Comment

In my view, it was a strategic error to attach so much importance to the clinical syndrome, as against the context of the illness (indicating, potentially, causation), such as childbirth and other circumstances; it seems likely that a single aetiological agent or pathogenetic process can result in a variety of clinical manifestations (as in the genetic concept of pleiotropism).

The influence of the *International Classification of Diseases* and the *Diagnostic and Statistical Manual* has been unhelpful. It has been difficult to identify puerperal psychoses for epidemiological purposes, and the absence of the *imprimatur* of the World Health Organization and the American Psychiatric Association has depressed research and the provision of services. As Dr Hamilton wrote, in a letter to the Task Force on Nomenclature and Statistics of the American Psychiatric Association:

> During most of the 19th century, almost every physician in the Western world knew that there was such a thing as puerperal psychosis, and that it had to be handled with special care. By contrast, for the past half-century, since the category of puerperal psychosis was abolished, identification and treatment of these cases has been casual, if not negligent.

I recommended[310,334] the rigorous implementation of the biaxial diagnosis, suggested 50 years ago by Essen-Möller[311]; his axes were 'syndromatic' and 'etiologic'; but aetiology is speculative, and I would replace this by contextual association. It should be mandatory for all psychiatrists to code both clinical syndrome and obstetric context. The clinical syndrome would be in terms of local and contemporary concepts, and would cover all psychiatric disorders, not just psychosis or mood disorders. The obstetric context would code onset after abortion, each trimester of pregnancy, parturition, the first three weeks of the puerperium, the next two months, weaning and menstruation. This would replace confusion by clarity and, in Essen-Möller's words, provide epidemiologists with a 'greater richness of possible combinations'.

---

[a] I thank Professor Yonkers, Chair of an advisory workgroup, for advice on this point.

Chapter

Clinical Forms

19

The Scope of This Chapter

In 1972–1975 I worked with the late Professor RE Kendell on the classification of the psychoses. This research resulted in 16 papers published in high-impact peer-reviewed journals (one of which has received more than 100 citations[77]), and visiting professorships in the University of Chicago (1980–1981) and Washington University in St Louis (1981). It provided the need, time and opportunity to read widely. The concepts used in the present work are derived, not from the ICD or DSM classifications, but from the nosological literature; they differ from current practice especially in the use of the psychogenic and cycloid concepts.

Non-Psychotic Disorders

Before considering any form of non-organic psychosis, one must cast an eye on disorders that are not 'psychoses', but occasionally cause diagnostic problems. These include reactions to traumatic births (post-traumatic stress disorder and complaining disorders), anxiety and obsessional disorders, depression and 'bonding disorders'. They have been eliminated from the literature analysis, but, in my series, a few mothers with a diagnosis of 'puerperal psychosis' may have been suffering from one of these other disorders.

Post-Traumatic Stress Disorder

It is now known that a traumatic birth, with its agonizing pain and loss of control, sometimes with a fear of imminent death, can be followed by flashbacks, nightmares and a high-tension state lasting for weeks or months[312]. My series included this mother:

> A Roman Catholic woman became pregnant before her marriage to the child's father. The pregnancy caused a family row. Five years later she gave birth to her 3rd child. After the birth she was sterilized by tubal ligation, but was still conscious when the operation began. Following this ordeal she had, when falling asleep, visions of the surgeon in white boots and a green overall approaching with a knife. She shouted to her husband to take the knife away, and fell into a daze for 20 minutes. The same happened when she awoke the next morning. She was completely normal between attacks. Someone had told her she would go mad after sterilization, and she felt terrified. Admitted to the mother & baby unit, she would sit in a daze for 15–20 minutes, then burst out, "Go away" – clearly in response to these images. She was discharged after five days, and had completely recovered 2–3 weeks later.

Seen before Bydlovsky's classic description, this was misdiagnosed as puerperal psychosis. It is a typical post-traumatic stress disorder.

Complaining (Querulant) Disorders

Pathological complaining is based on the idea that unpardonable injury has been sustained through actions that most people would not consider culpable. These disorders resemble paranoid disorders, but the nature of the idea (about malpractice, not facts) does not meet the accepted criteria for delusions. In *Motherhood and Mental Health*[67], I drew attention (pages 154–156) to their occurrence after childbirth, which is an event so important in a woman's life that mistakes or misunderstandings can lead to lasting recrimination. One woman complained of 'a high technology delivery', another of 'not being treated as a human being', another of humiliation by procedures involving the most intimate part of her body. One complained that her husband had ruined her life by suggesting the wrong name for the baby. The querulant behaviour could be extreme – haranguing the midwives night after night with 'unmitigated hatred', fantasies of burning down the hospital, and, in all cases, impaired child care. In this literature there was one case[313]. Neuroleptic agents are not the right treatment – they respond to psychological techniques aimed at shifting the focus to child care and normal activities.

Anxiety Disorders

After childbirth, a mother can experience overwhelming anxiety, either because of her responsibility for the fragile newborn (puerperal panic[314]), or because of threats to its survival (for example, the pathological fear of cot death[315]). In *Motherhood and Mental Health*[67], I described (on page 158) a mother who became so agitated that she had to be restrained:

> She was screaming and shouting, and chuntering on about nothing in particular, not logical at all, with no train of thought, her mind elsewhere. She was unable to absorb instructions or undertake a single task. She had no idea of the day or time. Reassurance and medication had no effect, but, after six days on the mother & baby unit, with the gentle support of the nursing staff, she became a competent mother.

It is easy to see how this could be misdiagnosed as a psychosis. In my series there were three other examples. This is one of them:

> A gentle and charming woman, who as a child required the support of her *younger* sister when shopping, gave birth to her 1st infant. The baby was colicky, and she became anxious about breastfeeding. She developed palpitations and feared that she was about to have a heart attack or die of cancer. She tried to control her anxieties by writing copious and repetitive notes – "I must get well", "Help yourself to health"; soon these bits of paper were all over the place. She felt unable to cope, settle to anything, relax or sleep. Her brain was working overtime and friends noticed that she was overtalkative. Flowers in the garden were very bright, and she played the piano better than before. Committed to hospital, she sat with her teeth clenched and muttering. She felt confused and unable to concentrate, and her speech was incoherent. Staff considered her to be excited, overactive, overtalkative, deluded and disinhibited. She settled quickly, and was discharged after three weeks. Reunited with her baby, she relapsed. She worried that it would stop breathing, and developed a phobia for the infant, which had to be removed by family members. She was treated with ECT and discharged after six weeks, but suffered from panic attacks for several months. During the next 27 years she had several other episodes of severe anxiety. For example, when one of her children left home to attend university, she became 'worked up and tense'; 'everything was jumbled' and she was 'switching from one thing to another', rather like her postpartum state.

This was probably an anxiety disorder, not a 'puerperal psychosis'.

Bonding Disorders

Mother–infant relationship disorders, involving emotional rejection of the infant, are more frequent, and have more serious long-term effects, than postpartum psychosis. Psychoanalysts have occasionally invoked this relationship in the cause of the psychosis: Zilboorg[208,316], who regarded 'postpartum schizophrenias' as 'castration complexes of the revenge type', described depressed patients with bonding disorders under the heading of 'schizophrenic reactions to childbirth'. In the Manchester series[61], 2 of 56 mothers with 'puerperal psychosis' had severe bonding disorders. In my series there were 2 mothers who suffered from depressive psychosis with prominent rejection of the child.

Psychogenic Psychosis

This is a concept developed in Nordic psychiatry[317–319]. The essential idea is that the onset, content and course of the psychosis (usually depressive, sometimes paranoid) are all determined by an extremely stressful event. The treatment of choice is psychotherapy.

Post-adoption psychoses, discussed in *Motherhood and Mental Health*[67] (page 26) are presumably psychogenic: there are eight in the literature[320–325]. They were reviewed by Trixler and Jádi[323], who found three examples among 230 postpartum psychoses; this is one:

> A 21-year old had a prolonged abnormal grief reaction after the death of her father. She and her mother pretended he was still alive, leaving the home untouched 'as he would have liked it' and even laying a place for him at table. When, at the age of 39, she began the process of adopting a 5-year old boy from an orphanage, this reawakened her grief and she took the child to see the grave. Her thinking became more and more troubled, and she started looking for her father, believing he was still alive somewhere. She was admitted to hospital after asking a policeman if he had seen him. She was in a dreamlike state and reported hearing her father's voice. After her recovery, the process of adoption continued.

Psychogenic psychosis also occurs after abortion, with 15 published cases[326–331], 6 following criminal abortions. In Edelberg and Galant's Russian study[329], 4 had psychotic features and 6 followed terminations, some of greatly desired children; an example is summarized on page 186. Here is another example of delusional depression following a miscarriage in a woman who had a criminal abortion long ago[327]:

> A 33-year old with three living children suffered two miscarriages in a year. Shortly after the second she expressed the idea that she would be arrested because, at the age of 19, she had brought on a miscarriage with strong spirits. She believed this child was still held in fragments, and would have to be cut out. She was anxious and hallucinated and made a suicide attempt. With treatment she recovered in two weeks.

This is from my series:

> A 26-year old Irish woman, who for three years had been drinking a bottle of wine or sherry every night, plus whisky, presented in a domestic crisis. Her marriage of only 2½ years had ended because of her husband's violence. She had a termination of pregnancy without his consent. The pregnancy was planned, and she had named the baby. She became depressed, and heard the voices of neighbours 'taking the mickey', and felt everybody was referring to her. She was admitted to hospital, but was still depressed six months later.

Psychogenic psychoses also occur after full-term pregnancies. In the literature, there are 22 examples. The most common source of stress (eight cases) was seduction and desertion, usually associated with an out-of-wedlock conception; another 7 followed the death of the baby or another much-loved child. The less common stresses were illegitimate pregnancy itself, destitution, incest, unwanted marriage, domestic violence and conflict with the mother-in-law. The following psychosis, with a theme of persecution, developed after desertion during pregnancy[87,203]:

> A 22-year old was seduced and brutally rejected. The man threatened to throw the baby out of the window. She immediately became mentally ill – would not eat and could not sleep. Admitted to hospital, she was agitated, oblivious to her surroundings and 'plunged in a sort of ecstasy', repeating the words, "Adolf, do not throw the baby out of the window". She was totally absorbed by these obsessive memories and by the frightful spectacle her imagination presented. She recovered in two weeks, but relapsed, and 'saw' three men sent by Adolph to kill her. Incidents like this continued until she gave birth. The neonate soon died, and she recovered.

The next case, with a theme of guilt, occurred in an incestuous relationship[204]:

> A woman lived for five years in concubinage with her brother. Their first three children died. After a 4th pregnancy, she gave birth to a daughter, whom she loved, but she also died. Profound grief developed into melancholy: she never spoke, except to reply very slowly to questions. She heard God's voice ordering her to repent; her incest left her unworthy to live and she refused food. She wounded her head with a pair of scissors. She was transferred to an asylum.

In this case from Dakar, the theme was querulant[332]:

> A 28-year old, for four years a postulant nun, had a miscarriage, then became pregnant again. Her fiancé renounced her, and she left home to live alone, out of touch with her family. After an obstructed labour, she was delivered by Caesarean section of a stillborn child. She refused to accept the loss of the child and pursued her case against the maternity hospital. The 'plot' involved police and hospital staff. She even wrote to the President of Senegal. After hospital admission and ECT, she was still not well. She said that God would judge the matter.

In my series, there were eight examples of episodes considered psychogenic. One was published in *Motherhood and Mental Health*[67], but is recapitulated here because it draws attention to the stressfulness of infant rejection, and demonstrates cure by psychosocial events after resistance to other treatments:

> An immigrant mother became depressed during her 3rd pregnancy, with delusions and auditory hallucinations, but none of the ideas that developed after the birth. Treated with ECT, she went into premature labour, and gave birth to an infant weighing only 1.5 lb. She seldom visited the neonatal intensive care ward, and failed to develop maternal feelings. She formed the idea that a healthy infant, born to an acquaintance a few doors up the street, was her own baby. She 'remembered' travelling in this neighbour's car during the pregnancy, and feeling a tearing sensation in her abdomen, after which it felt empty. Obviously the baby had entered this woman's belly. She could hear it calling (in Urdu), "Mummy, take me home". She went round and insisted on the return of 'her' baby, claiming that the infant in intensive care belonged to the neighbour. ECT and neuroleptic agents had no effect, but when her husband threatened her with divorce, she visited her child, rapidly bonded and lost her delusional ideas.

Here are three other cases. In the first, severe depression with delusions of reference was fully explained by the circumstances:

After seven years of childless marriage, a woman became pregnant. Her husband had already left for two months to live with another woman; he spent every evening away from home and was drinking heavily. He did not want the baby, and did not believe it was his child. He demanded a termination, and continually taunted her about the pregnancy. After the birth of an infant that resembled her husband, she was distressed by his lack of interest. Within two weeks she became agitated and weepy, saying she had sinned, and was going to die. Everyone knew about her and the television referred to her. She lost two stones in weight. Admitted to hospital, she gave a timid and mouse-like impression. She felt a failure and was very worried whether her husband would support her. But during the admission she showed concern about the child, and improved.

Another mother, elsewhere described as a failure of lithium prophylaxis (page 231) suffered from bipolar disorder, but, at the age of 54, developed a sensitive psychosis, *after her daughter gave birth to her first grandchild*:

She was upset because the midwives knew about her puerperal illness, and were looking at *her* confidential medical records. This was the trigger. "It opened a door that I had closed firmly. It brought back what I had put in the back of my mind". She became withdrawn, blank and retarded, with minimal speech. Her sleep was poor, she lost weight and was frightened to go out. She became 'increasingly paranoid about the safety of her younger daughter'. She refused medication and was not admitted to hospital. One session with a counsellor was enough and she recovered.

Finally there is this classic example of a psychogenic psychosis:

A 35-year old suffered from infertility. She became pregnant after her 7th *in vitro* fertilization, and 3rd intra-uterine injection of spermatozoa. She had a threatened abortion four weeks later. She was anxious throughout the pregnancy, feeling "100% responsibility to deliver a baby at term". At 36 weeks gestation the couple visited Birmingham for a golfing weekend. She suffered a premature rupture of membranes, and gave birth to a son weighing 6 lb 13 oz. She was extremely anxious during labour, so much so that a midwife had to stay on several hours beyond her shift to calm her. On day 3 the baby was transferred to special care with jaundice and respiratory problems. A junior doctor informed her that he was seriously ill and was not expected to live. On day 6, on waking, she was unable to move her limbs. Falling asleep again, she felt her body moving, as on a wave, and saw a woman standing at the foot of the bed: she had white hair and was smartly dressed in a red jacket with green and blue checks; she explained that she was looking for someone whose name began with S, the initial letter of her own name and the baby's. She leapt out of bed and appeared in the corridor, agitated and crying, carrying the baby. She was afraid of a lady in red, who kept appearing and disappearing, wanted to harm her baby, and would certainly return to take him. "I feel her now". She spoke in a low voice so that the lady would not be able to hear. This lady was not a physical person and did not use doors. She searched all the rooms on the unit, prepared a detailed set of rules for visitors, and asked her family not to tell this woman her address. Her husband was admitted to support her, and she improved spontaneously without neuroleptics, but, after discharge, relived the whole thing repeatedly. She recovered and remained well in the next 14 years.

Since the diagnosis of psychogenic psychosis involves judgments about personality and circumstances, not just identification of symptoms, it is made with a lower level of confidence than most other diagnoses. Nevertheless, these cases are important because they have a radically different cause from other 'puerperal psychoses'. Abortion, pregnancy and birth often occur in circumstances of turmoil, and there may be others, if one knew all the circumstances in which depressive psychoses developed.

Depressive Psychosis

In many cases reported in the literature, the psychopathological details were sketchy: in 66 per cent of episodes, the only possible diagnosis was 'psychosis, unspecified'. It was, however, usually possible to recognize the presence of a depressive syndrome. Depression is common, especially in women of childbearing age, whether infertile, pregnant, puerperal, involved in child care or menopausal. Such cases have only been included if 'psychotic features' were present – usually delusions, mutism or stupor. In the literature, the number of depressive psychoses was 569 (20 per cent of non-organic psychoses). In my series, there were 76 cases (16 per cent). An important issue is how many of these are manifestations of bipolar disorder. This is discussed later in this chapter.

Fürstner's[274] Postpartum Hallucinatory Disorder

An assistant at the prestigious Charité hospital in Berlin published one of the best-cited papers, with the title *Über Schwangerschafts- und Puerperalpsychosen* [On prepartum and postpartum psychoses]; it has 156 citations in 15 languages, including 100 by German authors. He reported a survey and observations on 34 personal cases, of which 5 were prepartum, 21 puerperal and 8 'lactational'. He supported Marcé's observation that puerperal psychosis broke out either between days 10 and 12 or at 4–6 weeks, with a free period between. He was aware of the difficulty in distinguishing *Fieberdelirien* from puerperal mania, which depended mainly on somatic signs or a close correspondence between the timing of delirium and the fever. He thought he could distinguish a *bestimmte Kategorie* [clear-cut category] that differed from the usual form of mania. This was the *hallucinatorische Irresein der Wöchnerinnen* [postpartum hallucinatory disorder] for which he is famous. The disorder had two phases, followed by convalescence:

- The *tobsüchtig* [raving] *Initialstadium*. After a brief prodromal phase there was the acute onset of frightening hallucinations (visual or auditory).
- *Stupidität* sometimes with catalepsy.

He gave three examples of this two-phase psychosis, one that started on day 3, and two with onset in the fifth and sixth weeks. The hallucinatory experience was not described in much detail in any of them. In spite of its renown, few clinicians have employed this concept. Ripping[289] could not identify any examples among his 29 cases. Only five surveys reported substantial numbers – 12/68 cases[333], 18/21[335], 52/100[336], 63/100[337] and 23/45[338]. As for cases described in detail by other authors, I can only find two in the entire literature[339,340]. I have never seen a mother who followed this biphasic course and began with intense hallucinations. In my view, the *hallucinatorische Irresein der Wöchnerinnen* is not a helpful contribution to the nosology of the postpartum psychoses.

Amentia

This term was introduced by Meynert[341], in an article entitled '*Amentia, die Verwirrtheit*', which emphasized the cardinal symptom of intense confusion – a dream-like state. This was similar to acute delirium (then usually fatal), but ran a benign course. Like Fürstner's *hallucinatorische Irresein*, it usually started with hallucinations, followed by either mania or catatonic stupor. It could be idiopathic or symptomatic (especially of epilepsy). He gave 21 illustrative cases of varying length, one of which (case 6 on pages 41–43) had some evidence of menstrual timing. No case was related to childbearing, although Fürstner had signalled its frequency in the puerperium. His 112-page article, which contains much anatomical speculation, distinguished it from melancholia, mania and paranoia. This concept has been widely used in this literature, not only in Germany[339,342,343], but also in Russia[344], Poland[345], the Netherlands[96,97], Italy[346], Croatia[347], the Czech Republic[348] and Slovakia[349]. Later experts, such as Kraepelin[350] and Runge[339], regarded these cases as variants of infective delirium. The concept, therefore, seems to be a precursor of both symptomatic and cycloid psychoses, and does not discriminate clearly between organic and non-organic cases.

Bipolar Disorder

In 1854 Falret (*folie circulaire*) and Baillarger (*folie à double forme*) introduced the noso-logical concept that later became known as 'manic depressive insanity'[351]. Later Angst and Perris divided the depressive component into bipolar and unipolar varieties[352]. In the 1970s, there was a revision of the boundary between schizophrenia and manic depression: previously catatonia, some forms of verbal hallucinosis, disorders of the will and self, and delusions of control were considered specific for 'schizophrenia', but it was realized that they also occurred in mania, and this enlarged the bipolar spectrum. This group of disorders has a high heredity, and a variety of biological triggers – not just childbirth, but also seasonal changes, surgical operations, various pharmaceutical agents and steroid therapy. There is a common theme of contrasting energy levels, which suggests a disorder of an arousal system, either at cortical level or in the core of the brain.

A problem in the classification of the psychoses is the absence of clear boundaries. The psychopathological keyboard has few notes – mood disorders (euphoria, depression, anx-iety, anger, suspicion, perplexity), various delusional themes, various types of hallucination, catatonic symptoms and various forms of 'defect'. Multivariate analyses tend to find that patients lie on a continuum. But this is not true of bipolar disorders. Using the criterion of 'an area of rarity', it has been possible to show that they are distinct. A multivariate study[353] involved 302 patients, 'lifetime diagnoses' over a study period of nine years with a mean of five episodes, psychopathology condensed by maximum likelihood factor analysis, and canonical variate analysis: canonical variate functions were generated in one (randomly selected) half, and validity tested in the other half. The analysis was repeated 10 times with different criterion groups, and each time bipolar patients were distinct. Except in one analysis, when cycloid patients were also distinct, the other patients lay on a continuum that extended from defect states to psychotic depression. Although it does not have its own rubric in ICD or DSM, the concept of bipolar disorders is one distinct category in the nosology of the psychoses.

At present the diagnosis depends on the typical 'manic' syndrome – euphoria, excessive energy, reduced need for sleep, distractibility, loss of inhibition, accelerated thinking and loquacity, sometimes with increased libido, recklessness and grandiose ideas. But, taken one by one, none of these symptoms is specific. States of excitement (with reduced need for sleep) occur:

- In normal people reacting to challenging events and circumstances
- In religious experiences
- In organic psychoses, such as infective delirium (see page 25)
- In chronic psychoses with grandiose delusions, which sometimes have phases of excitement similar to mania

- In neurological lesions, especially affecting the frontal lobes
- During intoxication with a variety of drugs

High activity and speech pressure occur under extreme emotion, especially anxiety and anger. As for euphoria, there are many normal causes. Anderson[268] described an ecstatic syndrome psychopathologically distinct from mania. Thus, the diagnosis of a manic episode requires more than a single symptom – it requires a cluster of symptoms, interpreted within the context of the patient's life. The recurrence of similar episodes, or depressive psychosis, consolidates the diagnosis, but single manic episodes are vulnerable to misdiagnosis, as in this example from my series:

> A 19-year old gave birth to her 1st child. Six weeks later she became hyperactive, with limitless energy, insomnia and overspending. A diagnosis of puerperal mania was made. But this patient was a rebellious teenager with convictions and a cruel streak, who abused cannabis, amphetamines, barbiturates and Ecstasy. She later showed much evidence of a chronic psychosis.

When 'schizo-affective' mania, often seen in the puerperium, was annexed to the bipolar group, it became clear that there was a link between non-affective postpartum psychosis and bipolar disorder (see pages 138–139). The link has since been confirmed by several population-based surveys[43,45,354,355]. The idea has taken hold and, in the last 25 years, the concept 'puerperal bipolar (or affective) disorder' has tended to replace 'puerperal psychosis'. In the literature, however, only 263 (10 per cent) non-organic psychoses had a recognizable bipolarity. In my series the number was higher. I distinguished between

- 48 mothers who showed switches between mania and depression (or *vice versa*) within the episode, or had both manic and psychotic depressive episodes at some time in their lives (manic depressive cases)
- 38 with recurrent mania (including episodes unrelated to reproduction)
- 43 with single manic episodes
- 21 with depression, with minimal bipolar features

Of the 48 manic depressive mothers, 8 presented with a depressive psychosis related to childbearing, and were shown by long-term study to suffer from bipolar disorder – one from the Manchester series, 2 from the Birmingham series and 5 from the Roper series; all had later puerperal manic episodes except one, who had two episodes of postpartum depressive psychosis and one unrelated manic episode.

The proportion of patients with unequivocal bipolar disorder (129/314)[a] are similar to figures published in the literature (Table 16.3 on page 138). At 41 per cent, its predictive value (the square of this proportion) would be negligible (17 per cent).

Cycloid (Acute Polymorphic) Psychosis

At the beginning of the twentieth century Wernicke[356] developed the idea of motility psychosis in opposition to Kraepelin's two-entities principle. In the 23rd *Vorlesung* of his *Grundriss der Psychiatrie*, he described two patients who had *hyperkinetischen Mobilitätspsychose*, one of whom became ill 10 days after childbirth; the other had two brief premenstrual *Tobsuchtsanfälle* [bouts of raving].[b] The idea was developed by Kleist[357] and

---

[a] This total excludes 7 cases mentioned in earlier publications, whose records were missing.
[b] I thank my friend Mario Lanczik for drawing this description to my attention.

Leonhard[358], who used the term 'cycloid' to cover endogenous psychoses that are neither schizophrenic nor manic-depressive; in his *Auftheilung der endogenen Psychosen* he subdivided them into motility, confusion and anxiety-elation psychoses. In 1974 Perris[359] developed the idea, and proposed this definition:

Syndromes with affective symptoms (mood swings) and two or more of:

- confusion of various degrees (from slight perplexity to gross disorientation) with agitation or retardation
- paranoia-like symptoms (delusions of reference, influence or persecution) and/or hallucinations not syntonic with mood levels
- pan-anxiety associated with ideas of reference
- motility disturbances (hypo- or hyperkinesas) as illustrated by Leonhard
- occasional episodes or states of ecstasy

The course is of recurrent episodes with complete remission, without defect.

In ICD-10[302], the name was changed to 'acute polymorphic psychosis', emphasizing the unstable and rapidly changing clinical picture, with several types of hallucination or delusion, not meeting criteria for mania or depression – a definition different from that of Perris. The concept has not been widely accepted: it is not mentioned in DSM, is hardly known in Britain, is controversial in Germany, and is used mainly in Sweden and a few other European centres. By June 2014, PubMed listed only 189 publications under this title (a ratio of one paper on cycloid to nearly 600 papers on 'schizophrenia'). Nevertheless it is not rare: it applies to about 10 per cent of psychotic patients – approximately half that of 'schizophrenia'[360]. It has a clinical value, enabling clinicians to identify benign psychoses that respond to ECT and lithium. In 1980, I had the privilege of working with Perris when he applied his concept to 233 patients studied with Kendell; thus I learned the diagnosis by apostolic transmission. In the resulting paper[360], we raised the possibility that cycloid psychosis was a variant of manic-depressive disease – the third form in which this (hitherto) bipolar disorder can present.

It is relevant here because some have claimed that puerperal psychosis has its own specific clinical features. Apart from 'lewd and erotic manifestations', the specific symptoms most frequently mentioned are confusion, bewilderment and perplexity, which are among the cardinal symptoms of cycloid psychosis. In surveys of postpartum psychosis, all those who use the concept have found a substantial minority of cycloids – 13/27 in Berlin[361], 16/120 in Edinburgh[41], 36/130 in Switzerland[118] and 28/58 in Würzburg[122]. Among the 4,029 reported cases, however, I could find only 14 clearly described[90,339,345,356,361–370], of which 3 were recurrent[90,369,370]. This is an example described by the patient herself[368]:

At the age of 20, a medical student had her 1st episode of mental illness: the diagnosis was 'catatonic schizophrenia' and she was treated with ECT. At 28 (by then a general practitioner) she gave birth to her 1st child. On day 9 she became overactive, talked incessantly and was convinced that she and her husband were going to die. She alternated between catatonic withdrawal and rambling speech with hidden meanings. Admitted to hospital, she seemed in a trance. She was restless with some posturing and grimacing. Her mood was labile, perplexed and bewildered. She mistook other patients for friends or relatives. Sometimes she thought she was at home, at other times in the maternity hospital. She said the floor was covered with broken glass and drawing pins, and her foot was bleeding. She became suspicious, believing she could hypnotise other patients. She sometimes maintained a position for an hour, at other times wandered aimlessly, ritualistically kissing people and objects. In retrospect she recalled believing she was the Madonna, and that people were trying to kill her. She recovered within four weeks.

The concept of cycloid psychosis shares with 'schizophrenia' the lack of a central and unitary theme, and there will be the same difficulty in reaching an agreed definition. But some acute psychoses have delusions without a persistent paranoid state, and manic or depressive symptoms but no complete or lasting manic or depressive syndrome; in addition there is perplexity or confusion and/or catatonic symptoms. These patients cannot be given a diagnosis of mania, depressive psychosis, mixed manic-depressive psychosis, paranoid psychosis or schizophrenia without violence to the definitions, emphasizing certain symptoms and ignoring others. These are the patients diagnosed as cycloid in my series.

Primed by my work with Perris, I expected to find a substantial number. I was unsure whether they would be a separate group, with their own special characteristics, or linked to bipolar disorder. In those followed long term I was curious to know whether any suffered from later manic or bipolar episodes. I grouped the mothers with a cycloid diagnosis, under four headings:

- 12 with single cycloid episodes
- 6 with recurrent cycloid episodes
- 30 with cycloid and manic features in the same episode ('concurrent')
- 36 with some episodes manic or bipolar, and some cycloid ('serial')

These results came as a surprise. The total number with cycloid features was 84 (27 per cent), compared with 129 (41 per cent) with substantial evidence of bipolar disorder. The number with a combination of cycloid and bipolar features far outnumbered those with cycloid alone (66 *versus* 18). Followed long term, it became clear that these mothers exhibit, in different episodes, a bewildering variety of clinical pictures, bipolar and cycloid episodes completely intermingled. Thus, the idea of a distinct form of puerperal cycloid psychosis is untenable. Instead there is a large group of mixed (concurrent or serial) manic and cycloid patients.

The following mother illustrates a concurrent manic/cycloid episode. After her first baby was born, her 'confusion' was so marked that a symptomatic psychosis was suspected, but she had a normal electroencephalogram and her relapse was hypomanic:

A religious woman, with an unhappy childhood, married a man 38 years her senior, and became depressed when he died from a subarachnoid haemorrhage. She then married a man 31 years her senior. After a pregnancy complicated by pre-eclamptic toxaemia, she gave birth to her 1st child. Within four days she developed Ekbom's syndrome, believing her skin was infested by parasites. She appeared slow, tired and dreamy. She worried about blood spreading from the crucifix on the wall. Admitted to the mother & baby unit, she was tired and dishevelled, with slow monotonous speech. She believed she was in another part of Britain and misidentified staff as relatives. She was disorientated in time and could not recall recent events. She then became overactive – her thoughts racing, running up and down the ward smashing things. A diagnosis of an acute confusional state was made, supported by an erythrocyte sedimentation rate of 81 and leucocyte cell count of 13,400/mm^3, possibly due to cystitis, and toxaemia (BP 130/90, with ankle and leg oedema), but her EEG was normal. Within a fortnight she recovered, but then relapsed (24 days after the birth, and four days before her 1st postpartum menses). She became overactive, talking long & loudly, laughing a lot and expressing the belief she was being monitored by listening-in equipment and magic eyes. She soon recovered, but suffered from depression for three months. Later she had a second postpartum episode with similar features, and, in the next six years three more episodes, unrelated to reproduction, with some catatonic features. Between episodes she returned to normal.

Among the 25 mothers with serial cycloid and manic episodes, there were many examples. The mother described in Clinical Gem 29.1 in on page 322 had two cycloid episodes at 16 and many manic episodes later in life.

Comment

- The nosology of cycloid psychosis is controversial and difficult, both in theory and in practice – in theory because the concept is not well accepted, and has rival definitions, in practice because the identification of cycloid features might be unreliable. But it has been noticed from the beginning that the clinical picture of puerperal psychosis is often unusual, and there is an extensive literature on its relation to cycloid psychosis, or other non-kraepelinian categories such as 'undiagnosed functional psychosis'[41,118,148,371]. The problem cannot be swept under the 'bipolar' carpet. If these nosological issues are considered to be important, this conundrum could be addressed by a multi-rater diagnostic study, using the polydiagnostic technique pioneered by Kendell.

- With the limitation that the diagnoses were made by one rater, the idea mooted in the 1982 paper[360] is supported – there are not two, but three, presentations of 'bipolar disorder' – mania, melancholia and cycloid. This combined group needs a name. Best would be an adaptation of Baillarger's *folie à double forme* – this is *folie à triple forme*; but this is a rather lengthy French term. The English equivalent would be 'tripolar disorder', but the planet has only two poles. *Faute de mieux* I have chosen the term 'bipolar/cycloid group'. The combined group includes 214 cases (68 per cent of my series, predicting 46 per cent of the variance).

- Merging these two groups will not affect current practice, because many researchers, whose ideas on classification are kraepelinian, by selecting certain symptoms and discounting others, are already massaging these cases into a single 'puerperal affective' group. But accepting this idea will have wider implications for the classification of the psychoses. In the 1970s, there was a seismic shift of 'schizo-affective' patients from schizophrenia to bipolar disorder. There would be another *terramoto* if the cycloids were added to manic-depression.

Depression with Minimal Evidence of Bipolar Disorder

In addition to mothers who manifest a full manic or cycloid syndrome, there is a small group of depressed mothers who have some but insufficient evidence of bipolarity. In my series there were 21 of them, falling into the following groups:

- Eleven had subclinical hypomanic episodes at other times, for example, lasting a single day.
- Five had a single hypomanic symptom, without other elements of the syndrome. In four this was overactivity, as in this example:

  A sensitive person troubled by guilt, suffered from bouts of depression, one during pregnancy and one starting in the 4th week after one of her births; she had 'boundless energy' when moving into a much-desired new home.

In another it was elevated mood:

> A mother suffering from a paranoid psychosis, summarized on page 244, after her arrest and transfer to a secure forensic unit, felt "overwhelming euphoria and peace". She "was in a place of safety. The nurses were angels sent to protect her".

- Two mothers had brief periods of elevated mood immediately after delivery ('postpartum pink'), as in this example:

> After the birth of a much-desired first child, a mother was "on cloud 9, over the moon, sleepless, rushing around, garrulous and bubbly", but only for two days, after which she became depressed.

According to recent reviews[372,373], 'postnatal euphoria' is found in 10–18 per cent of mothers. Several studies have shown that these mothers have an increased incidence of depression a few weeks later; but there have been no longitudinal studies reporting later bipolar/cycloid episodes.

- Six mothers became 'high' after ECT. Here are two examples:

> A Yemeni woman (already summarized on page 160) developed a prepartum depressive psychosis; the first sign of parturition was the emergence of the infant's head from the birth canal. After ECT, she became elated and overtalkative; for 12 hours she was singing, giggling, and sexually inappropriate, hugging and kissing strangers.

> A mother of three children suffered six episodes of depression, with delusions and hallucinations, in 15 years. Five weeks after one of her births, she developed a psychosis with grandiose and religious ideas, auditory hallucinations and morbid jealousy. Three times she became elated after ECT.

Five of the 125 bipolar/cycloid mothers, who received ECT, also developed hypomania afterwards. All these 'hypomanic' states were brief. If ECT can restore a person in a profound state of melancholy to normal mood, it might also, on occasion, overcorrect, not necessarily implying the existence of a bipolar diathesis.

In addition to these 21 depressed mothers, there were 6 with a paranoid psychosis, 3 with schizophreniform disorders (discussed later), and one with recurrent brief psychosis, who had some evidence of bipolarity; for example, a mother had two early onset episodes of paranoid psychosis, each with a relapse, and occasional racing thoughts and overactivity. The inclusion of this group of 31 mothers, whose diagnosis in most cases required long term study (not a single episode), would bring the total bipolar/cycloid group to a maximum of 245 (78 per cent of the series), predicting 61 per cent of the variance. But there can be no certainty about their inclusion, and it is unwise to risk increasing heterogeneity.

Paranoid Psychosis

Paranoid psychoses are disorders in which the psychotic symptoms are limited to delusions. They were rare in this literature – only six, two with early[86,332] and four late postpartum onsets[96,105,374,375]. But 29 women presented with morbid jealousy: this had onset at all stages of the reproductive process – in all three trimesters of pregnancy, and early or late in the first postpartum year. Some became morbidly jealous as part of a complex psychosis and some as the sole symptom. Saunders[376] described a woman who had four pregnancies: after each birth she became depressed, with feelings of being neglected by her husband and delusions of his infidelity.

In contrast to the dearth of published cases, there were nine mothers in my series with paranoid disorders. In some, their personalities and circumstances were compatible with an understandable paranoid process, as in this example:

A woman, always a loner, met a young man, who killed someone, who (he thought) was making improper advances to her. She was pregnant and, when she lost the baby at six months, interpreted this as a punishment. Her boyfriend was imprisoned, but she was already again pregnant. When she bled at six months this was another punishment. For a year people had been hostile, laughing at her, thinking she was mad and silly – an idiot and a bitch. Sometimes they said she should die. After improvement she was discharged to a hostel where there were arguments and outbursts. People, including the staff, were muttering about her, and organizing against her. They had a key to her room, and had tampered with her radio and TV. She threatened to cut another girl's throat.

In others the course in some respects resembled a bipolar/cycloid episode: the next patient, who also had evidence of a paranoid personality, had two relapses, and became high after ECT:

A woman was self-conscious at school and often played truant. She several times left her employment after taking offence at supposed criticism. At 20, after giving birth to her first baby, she became depressed. She looked in the mirror and could see there was something wrong with her face – it was puffy, her hair had changed horribly and she could see the Devil in her. Her baby was blue – it would starve and die. In the street everyone was staring at her and criticising her. She improved, but relapsed four months after the birth. After ECT, she became slightly elated (her husband said unusually so) and more sociable, and could think more clearly. A month later, in the premenstrual period, she relapsed again and became mute. During the next five years she became possessive, and accused her husband of infidelity. After divorce, she developed morbid jealousy with a new partner. At 25 she gave birth to her 2nd child. The illness began after the baby had bowel surgery. She believed her baby's operation was part of an experiment, and that the Gestapo were after her. She heard voices commenting on her actions and believed people could read her thoughts. She recovered five months after the birth.

Schizophrenia and Schizophreniform Disorders

'Schizophrenia' is a word with many meanings, which vary from time to time and country to country. At present it is used for a heterogeneous group of chronic polymorphic psychoses. None of its 'characteristic symptoms' is specific. The psychoses of childbearing start abruptly and hardly ever run a chronic course; patients who are already ill at the conception of the child are excluded. But some patients will escape this exclusion for various reasons:

- They may stop prophylactic drugs because they become pregnant or wish to breastfeed.
- They may default from treatment, and come to the staff's attention on the maternity ward.
- The history and onset of their illness may be obscure.

Unless the records of previous episodes are obtained and studied, such cases can mistakenly be diagnosed as prepartum or postpartum psychosis, as in this example:

A woman born in Pakistan, whose mother had a diagnosis of schizophrenia, obtained a university degree. At 27, after her marriage, she developed delusions of poisoning, and hallucinations like a radio in her head that she could not turn off, describing her actions. Others could hear what she was thinking, and forced her to think about her father's death. She recovered with neuroleptic treatment, but was not compliant with prophylaxis. She became pregnant, unwillingly, and, at 36 weeks, had a recurrence, which responded to olanzapine. After a Caesarean delivery, she did not believe the baby was her own – indeed she had never been pregnant. She refused to care for the child, whom she threatened to kill. With medication she recovered. Five years later she became pregnant again. After another Caesarean delivery, she denied her marriage, refused to own the baby and told her elder child she was not its mother. Followed by the home treatment team, she was inactive, staying in bed most of the time.

In addition to these misclassified patients, three of my patients suffered from episodic illnesses with prepartum or postpartum episodes, and a course somewhat similar to bipolar/cycloid cases: they responded to ECT with full recovery, and tended to relapse, with menstrual effects. But their salient symptoms were 'mental automatisms' such as verbal hallucinosis or inserted thoughts, as in the next example:

A woman, whose mother spent years in an asylum, was reared by friends and relatives. She was a sensitive, touchy person. At the age of 19 she gave birth to her 1st child. Within two weeks she became depressed and heard a voice saying "You are a bitch, causing your husband all this trouble". She was agitated, muddled and confused, but not disorientated. In hospital she was afraid the junior doctors would make love to her. She felt the menacing presence of a boyfriend, who attacked her years ago – he would get her sooner or later, and his friends were looking for an opportunity to kill her. With ECT she recovered, relapsed (78 days after the birth) and recovered again three months after the birth. In the next five years she suffered two further episodes of depression accompanied by ideas of reference, or voices in her head. At 30 she gave birth to her 2nd child. On day 14 she became agitated, and left home because there was a smell of death. She had delusions about her mother-in-law, who could look into her eyes and know what she was thinking; she could hear this lady's voice, saying, "You'd better love me". The baby was the Devil and the television was talking about her. With ECT she improved, but relapsed twice (two and four months after the birth). In spite of the failure of her marriage, she remained well for 15 years. After an early menopause, she had three further episodes. At 46 she presented with the complaint that she was living in a plastic world – her son was not her own, and her son-in-law was abusing her grandchildren; she soon recovered, but relapsed twice. At 47 she became restless, agitated and suspicious: her loved ones were turning against her. She telephoned her children expressing her fears for their imminent deaths; her new partner was collaborating with the Devil. At 51 she again became violent to family members: she believed she was an alcoholic lesbian, and was being controlled by her son-in-law. She had racing thoughts and slept only four hours. She was dashing from one end of the ward to the other in bare feet. She spent a whole year in hospital with a diagnosis of chronic schizophrenia.

These three cases, and some of the paranoid disorders mentioned, raise the possibility that the bipolar/cycloid group might also present with paranoid or schizophreniform symptoms; but this is an innovation that the psychiatric community is at present in no shape to tolerate.

Unusual Cyclical Disorders

The tendency of puerperal bipolar disorder to relapse, on an approximately monthly basis, was discussed in pages 140–142. But several authors have reported cycling with a different time base. Meschede[377] reported this case:

The illness began in the first postpartum week with a 5-day cycle of acute confusion and *Tobsucht*, followed by a day of sleep and normal behaviour. Fourteen months later she was admitted to the Königsberg asylum. The alternating course continued for 26 months, after which she recovered. Ten years later she had a recurrence and was readmitted for another 18 months, again with a cyclical course, first on a 3-day, then 4-day and then 5-day basis, by which time she had one day of *Tobsucht*, one day of sleep and three days rest.

Another mother had 10 relapses on a short time base during the early puerperium[378]:

> A 30-year old, who suffered from a brief *Nervenfieber* at the age of 20, was delivered of her 1st child by forceps. On day 3 she became euphoric and garrulous. On day 12 she was anxious and restless, sensing that her end was near. This passed off, but returned the next evening (1st relapse). She recovered and was well for some days. On day 18 she had a recurrence of anxiety, euphoria and confused ideas: laughter and crying rapidly succeeding each other (2nd relapse). On day 20 she had a 3rd relapse, this time with delusions that followed each other like lightning; it lasted 2–3 hours. On day 22 she had a 4th relapse, taking the form of religious themes and nocturnal restlessness, followed by exhaustion. On day 24 she had her 5th relapse, with *Tobsucht*. The 6th relapse on day 26 was the worst: she let out a stream of obscenities, which (a modest woman) she had never spoken before, and scratched and bit anyone within reach. The 7th relapse on day 28 was milder, taking the form of a tiresome humour, with less confused thinking. The 8th relapse on day 30 was mild – she had a sense of pressure below, as if she was about to give birth. The 9th relapse on day 32 and the 10th and last on day 34 were no more than an abnormal chattiness and cheerfulness.

Two mothers have developed a diurnal pattern. Dickson[379] described a mother who was dejected and listless in the morning, and furiously manic in the evening. This is the other example[380]:

> A 30-year old gave birth. On day 3 she suddenly fell into frightful raving: she no longer wanted to know her husband and child, leapt out of bed, smashed a window, tore her clothes and tried to destroy everything in the room. The next day she lapsed into stupor, out of which she could only be wakened with difficulty. In the first 14 days this switching from disturbance to calm appeared at irregular intervals, and then developed an intermittent pattern, in which attacks of raving started every evening at 11 pm and lasted until daybreak. With treatment, stupor changed to sleep, but the raving continued. She was treated with opium and quinine, and, after an unstated time, recovered.

Bromocriptine Psychoses

The argoline derivative 2-bromo-α-ergocriptine, a dopamine D_2 agonist, was developed in 1968 to block the release of prolactin[381], and has been used since 1978 in a dose of 5–7.5 mg/day to inhibit puerperal lactation. Since then 14 postpartum episodes have been reported, associated with its use[382–393]. In a 15th case[394], the mother became overactive before bromocriptine was prescribed. The onset, where known, was early in the puerperium. In 8, the clinical picture was typical of mania, and another had a bipolar course, starting with depression[391]. In 3 it was atypical[387,392] (including one with a seizure[388]), and, in one, depressive with 'voices' telling her to destroy the baby[385]. In 6, duration was short – one week or less in 5 and 17 days in the 6th. Two mothers recovered after withdrawal of bromocriptine without other treatment[384,385]; but other episodes have lasted up to two months, and required much treatment, in one case ECT. Two mothers suffered previous manic episodes, including steroid-triggered episodes[390,393]. One had a family history of psychosis[390].

In my series there was one possible example:

> A 24-year old was delivered of her 1st child by Caesarean section because of a suspected foetal facial cyst. She was treated with bromocriptine 5 mg/day. She felt excited because the baby was normal. On day 4 she began to behave strangely and became increasingly anxious, overactive, emotionally labile and disinhibited. She was talkative and cheerful, and gave a running commentary on her actions. Admitted to hospital, she was confused and perplexed; she did not

know the day of the week. She was unable to think clearly, and spoke little, with slow and deliberate answers. The possibility of a toxic delirium secondary to bromocriptine was raised; it was stopped and she was treated with chlorpromazine. She rapidly recovered, but, a month later, was 'over the top' for two days. She remained well in the next 32 years.

Chateau[395] wrote a thesis on *psychose puerpérale et bromocriptine*, with nine case descriptions. In three of these, a mother *recovered* one to two days after bromocriptine was prescribed.

It is clear that bromocriptine can trigger postpartum episodes, perhaps only in mothers with a bipolar diathesis. It can also trigger episodes in other circumstances, as described in the treatment of parkinsonism[396], acromegaly[397,398] and prolactinoma[399]. Serby[400] reported that psychiatric complications required withdrawal of bromocriptine in 5/66 cases. This trigger may be unrelated to that provoking early postpartum bipolar/cycloid episodes.

Lifetime Diagnoses

Table 19.1 summarizes the lifetime (longitudinal) diagnoses in my series.

Table 19.1 Summary of the lifetime (longitudinal) diagnoses in my series

		Manchester series	Birmingham series		Roper series	Total
			Mother and baby unit	Others		
Bipolar/cycloid		56	64	30	64	**214**
Depressive psychosis	Minimal bipolarity	4	7	3	7	**21**
	No bipolarity	10	17	8	4	**39**
Other psychosis		12	13	8	7	**40**
Total		**82**	**101**	**49**	**82**	**314**[a]

[a] This omits seven mothers from earlier publications on whom I had no records.

The 40 'other psychoses' comprised

- 16 with organic psychoses (13 Donkin, 2 infective, 1 epileptic)
- 8 with paranoid disorders
- 9 with 'schizophrenia' (chronic paranoid hallucinatory psychoses, hebephrenia, auditory hallucinations as the sole symptom)
- 7 others – psychogenic, pseudopsychosis, recurrent brief psychosis, recurrent postpartum stupor and misdiagnosed PTSD

None of these can safely be included in the bipolar/cycloid group.

These results demonstrate the problem of heterogeneity in samples of non-organic childbearing psychoses. Even if mothers with minimal evidence of bipolarity are included, the inclusion of unrelated disorders would obscure all but the most prominent findings.

Chapter

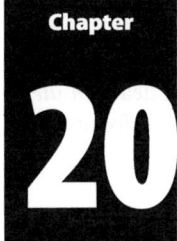

Episode Onset

Recurrent Episodes Associated with Childbearing

It has been known since the sixteenth century that puerperal psychosis can recur. The literature contains many examples of mothers with multiple episodes, to which I can add a good many more (Table 20.1).

When there is no information on onset, the only contribution multiple episodes make is to support the general tendency to recur, which is one of the best-founded and widely known facts about puerperal psychosis.

When episodes begin in the same time frame, it supports the existence of a specific causal factor, acting at that stage of the reproductive process; this becomes more convincing if the mothers are followed long term, and their episode rate is known, and low enough to exclude sporadic attacks.

When mothers have multiple episodes with onsets during different phases, this is evidence of the interdependence of triggers. If this occurs more often than can be attributed to the sharing of the same (bipolar/cycloid) diathesis, it indicates, not necessarily the same aetiology, but shared components in the cause or pathogenesis. These cases are considered further at the end of this chapter, under 'Matrix of Associations'.

The *International Classification of Diseases* and *Diagnostic and Statistical Manual*, in so far as they mention childbearing psychoses, specify only postpartum or 'perinatal' onsets. This analysis covers nine onset groups – post-abortion, prepartum, short gestation, parturient, day 1, early postpartum, weeks 4–13, later postpartum and weaning onsets.

Table 20.1 Multiple episodes of psychosis related to childbearing

Number of episodes	The literature	My series
Unknown	4	None
Two episodes	334	110
Three episodes	74	22
Four episodes	20	3
Five episodes	10	None
Six episodes	5	
Seven to thirteen episodes	6	
Total	**453**	**135**

Abortion

In the literature, 'abortion' can include miscarriage, ectopic pregnancy, hydatidiform mole, medical termination, criminal abortion and 2nd trimester births after foetal death *in utero*. Here it covers all of these, except short gestation births. Abortion can be followed by organic, psychogenic and bipolar/cycloid episodes.

Organic Psychoses

The first case (an infective delirium) was reported by Hippocrates[401] (page 8). The literature reports 48 organic psychoses, with a wide variety of causes: 23 were infective (16 after a miscarriage, 5 after a criminal abortion and 2 uncertain), 13 Wernicke–Korsakow psychosis (10 after termination and 3 after a miscarriage), 3 chorea psychoses, 2 water intoxication after oxytocin was used to terminate the pregnancy, and the rest rheumatic, encephalitic or of unknown cause. Engelhard[37] described a Donkin psychosis following a 2nd trimester termination. Dupouy[105] described recurrent visual hallucinosis, 1 episode following a miscarriage and the other during pregnancy.

Non-Organic Psychoses

Few surveys even mention post-abortion psychosis. Of the nine that do, between 0.6 and 9 per cent of patients admitted with 'postpartum psychosis' had an abortion, not a full term birth. More recently, several surveys from the Maghreb or West Africa have reported a higher proportion[402,404–406]: three from Senegal had 8 per cent, 12 per cent and 15 per cent post-abortion cases. A Venezuelan study[38] reported that 6 per cent followed abortion. A Brazilian study[407] focused on 30 patients from Rio de Janeiro, who had 86 deliveries and 11 *abortos*: the psychosis rate was 33/86 (38 per cent) for births and 4/11 (36 per cent) for abortions.

Two British studies[10,12] claimed that post-abortion were much less frequent than postpartum episodes, but their information was second-hand from doctors. Several population-based studies have used Danish registers. Somers[11] studied the admission rate following abortion: it was above the level in the general population; for example, women in the 3rd decade had a relative risk of 1.85 for admission after abortion, with 85 per cent for psychosis. David[408,409] found that the post-abortion rate (1.84/1,000) was higher, not only than that of the population (0.75/1,000), but also than that of women giving birth (1.2/1,000). Munk-Olsen[410] followed 78 Danish women with a diagnosis of bipolar or schizophrenia-like disorder for 12 months after an induced abortion, and found a relative risk of psychiatric readmission of only 1.12–1.20. Di Florio[411] interviewed 873 bipolar women about 25 years after their first episode: 19 per cent suffered mania or a psychosis after a live birth, and 5 per cent after a miscarriage or termination; there were 10 post-abortion episodes after 196 abortions (about 50/1,000) – less than the postpartum rate, but much higher than the frequency of postpartum psychosis in the general population.

Roldan[412] conducted a cohort study:

> She followed, through the psychiatric and general practice records, 33 women who developed mania before the age of 25, with the 1st episode at a mean of 19 years. The duration of study ranged from 3.5–25.5 (mean 11.4) years: 271 episodes of illness were studied (about eight episodes/person). The base rate for new episodes was high – a mean of 0.16/trimester (1 every 18 months).

Fifteen women remained nulliparous and 18 had a total of 13 pregnancies and 13 abortions, of which 2 were miscarriages and 11 terminations. The number of episodes in each trimester was:

The trimester preceding conception	6/26
The 1st trimester of pregnancy	2/26
The 2nd and 3rd trimesters of pregnancy	1/13
The 1st postpartum trimester	5/13 (38 per cent)
The 1st post-abortion trimester	9/13 (69 per cent)

After abortion there were five manic episodes, with onset 3, 4, 6, 8 & 8 weeks after the event (all rather late); the other four were depressed. The post-abortion rate was higher than the postpartum rate.

The most detailed study[354] was conducted in California:

This group studied 41,442 women who gave birth and 15,299 who had a termination. Over a 4-year period, 253 women, who gave birth, and 181, who had an abortion, were hospitalized – a post-abortion rate 1.7 times the postpartum rate ($p < .0001$). The figures for psychosis were also higher – 176 (4.2/1,000) *versus* 126 (8.2/1,000). Those for bipolar disorder were 14 & 17 ($p = < .01$). The highest odds ratio was found for the first 90 days, when the post-abortion rate was 2.6 times as high as postpartum rate. But there are problems with these data: only 56/434 admissions occurred within six months of the event, and there was a surprisingly low rate of postpartum admissions (0.36/1,000 births). The post-abortion rate (16/15,299) was at the level usually reported for postpartum psychosis. The data, however, do show higher rates for bipolar episodes after abortion, than after childbirth.

In my series, 95 mothers were known to have had an abortion: 54 had one, 28 had 2, six had 3, two had 4, three had 5, one had 6 and one had 18 abortions – 175 in all. Of these, 108 were miscarriages (before the 20th week), 62 terminations, 2 mole pregnancies, and 3 ectopic pregnancies; One termination was probably illegal; 20/95 (21 per cent) of mothers who reported abortions had post-abortion episodes, and 24/175 (14 per cent) of the abortions were followed within three months by episodes. This is much less than the frequency of recurrent postpartum episodes: of 223 mothers who had at least one more birth 123 (55 per cent) had additional postpartum episodes, affecting 146/358 (41 per cent) additional births. But the rate after abortions was much higher than in the population (1/1,000 births).

Case Lore

In the literature, 99 patients suffered non-organic post-abortion psychoses (108 episodes): 40 were known to have followed a miscarriage, 23 a termination, and 11 a criminal abortion. One was associated with a mole[413] and 4 with ectopic pregnancies[108,414–416]. This is a post-ectopic episode; post-operative psychosis is an alternative diagnosis[108]:

A 26-year old, with one child, had an extra-uterine pregnancy. Ten days after surgery, she became confused and incoherent. She developed ideas of persecution, attacked a nurse with scissors, and ran out into the street naked with her child. Admitted to hospital, she was disorientated in time and place, had ideas of sin, and heard voices mocking her, as well as horses and pigs swearing. She misidentified one of the nurses as her sister. She was ill for four months, with phases of improvement and deterioration. She remembered little of her illness, and refused to believe she was in a mental hospital.

The diagnoses are compared with other onset groups in Table 20.7 on page 207.

There were six cases in which pregnancy was terminated in mothers with a history of puerperal psychosis[417–422]; this complication was so well known 100 years ago that Chrobak[423] warned against termination in such women: he had repeatedly seen mental illness after the termination.

Psychogenic Psychosis

Abortion is a major stressor, and can lead to lasting grief, guilt and shame; in these powerful affects, psychogenic psychoses take root. Edelberg and Galant[329] described 10 post-abortion psychoses, 4 with psychotic features. This is an example, with some features of pathological grief:

> A 22-year old childless woman had a 3-month abortion. She believed herself a criminal, and had dreadful dreams of her child's reproachful eyes; she tried to avoid falling asleep to escape them. But these visions began to appear during the day, whenever she was in the dark. She recovered with psychotherapy, and six months later became pregnant again, and became a happy mother.

This is an example of a post-abortion paranoid psychosis:

> A 58-year old suffered from recurrent depression. After a criminal abortion, involving her son, she came to believe that the police were taking action against her and her family. Reference was made to her crime in the newspapers, sermons and people's behaviour. She was admitted trembling with anxiety, with a pulse rate of 184. She became mute, refused food and had to be tube-fed. Five months later she died unexpectedly from cerebral venous thrombosis, presumably an independent complication[330].

Serial Post-Abortion Episodes

The first hint was by Justus de Berger[424] in a brief Latin statement:

> I have learned of a 20-year old, who suffered, like her mother, four months after her last menstrual period: she twice emitted a foetus and suddenly became insane, but it did not last long.

Only three other cases have been reported with recurrent episodes limited to abortion[412,425,426]. But others, who had postpartum episodes as well, had more than one post-abortion episode: Capelle[296] described a patient with two post-abortion and one postpartum, and Mahe[422] two post-abortion and four postpartum episodes. The most impressive is Steinmann's[343] first case, also reported by Schwingenheuer[365]:

> A 25-year old, whose brother had a diagnosis of schizophrenia, had a puerperal episode at 21, and post-abortion episodes at 22, 23 and 24, each lasting about three months and marked by confusion and flight of ideas. She was admitted for another episode five weeks after a 4-month miscarriage: she manifested silly euphoria, unmotivated laughter, unstoppable pressure of speech, incoherence, verbigeration and hand-clapping. Schwingenheuer reported only three post-abortion episodes, but a further unrelated episode at the age of 30.

Thus she had three or four post-abortion episodes and one postpartum episode in nine years, during which she had only one (reported) non-reproductive episode. This would be highly significant statistically ($p = .0002$), but Steinmann's description was limited to a schema, without narrative details, and Schwingenheuer's was also brief.

Four mothers in my series had two post-abortion episodes, and, since all were followed long term, it was possible to calculate the probability that they were not sporadic. One had four abortions, only two of which were followed by psychosis, and six unrelated episodes (p = .19). This is the second, who had one episode of early onset puerperal psychosis, three abortions (all followed by episodes, but one in the form of sub-clinical depression) and one unrelated episode in 37 non-reproductive trimesters (p = .011 for the two psychotic episodes):

> A 22-year old became depressed, followed by a phase of exceptional well-being, when she was 'on a high', active and energetic, and slept little. At 28 she was pressured into a termination, and became depressed, but not at a clinical level. In the following year she had another termination: although upset, she felt high with lots of energy and a reduced need for sleep; she had hundreds of thoughts running through her mind, saw visions of colours and had a heightened sense of textures. After treatment in hospital, she became depressed, with the delusion that she was a witch, and God was punishing her for the abortion. She recovered after three weeks. At 31 she had a 12-week miscarriage: three days later she became depressed, forgetful and restless, and was unable to sleep or eat; she felt surrounded by impressions of death, as a punishment for the abortion. At 32 she was delivered by emergency Caesarean section of her only child: on day 6 she appeared confused and perplexed, with jumbled speech. She had a heightened sense of colours and textures, and saw visions of colours, sometimes in the form of a rainbow. She heard a woman's voice speaking in her head. She felt the pain of a million people, like that of inmates in a concentration camp. On admission to hospital she was dishevelled, perplexed and distractible. Her mood was labile – smiling, laughing and tearful. She recovered in three weeks and was followed for another two years.

The third had one full term pregnancy and two abortions, all followed by episodes, although there are no details of the first. She had nine unrelated episodes in 54 non-reproductive trimesters (p = .04):

> A 23-year old, with a history of three manic episodes, had an incomplete abortion: about three months later she was admitted again, but there are no records and no diagnosis. In the following year she had a miscarriage or termination of an 8–9 week pregnancy: two hours later she became high with increased activity and reduced sleep; she lacerated her hand smashing windows. On admission she was low and retarded, then elated with pressure of speech. Nine years later, after five more episodes of depression or mania, she became pregnant, and gave birth in the 2nd trimester to an infant weighing less than 2 lb. Within a day or two she became manic and, ten days later, was slain by the child's father.

The fourth was followed for 33 years after her first psychotic episode; she had four full-term pregnancies and two abortions. She had two or three postpartum and two post-abortion (or post-operative) episodes; but she also had at least 15 unrelated episodes in 114 non-reproductive trimesters (p = .02):

> A 23-year old abused ethanol and developed *delirium tremens*. At 25 she gave birth to her 1st child: on day 3, she became anxious, restless and sleepless, then 'very high'; she believed there was a conspiracy with hidden cameras and tape recorders. She recovered in six weeks. The following year she gave birth to her 2nd child: after the birth she felt high and energetic, but did not come under treatment. At 27 she had a 12–14 week miscarriage and required two operations for dilatation and curettage (D & C): she became agitated and depressed, with insomnia and loss of weight; she was almost mute, frightened of everything, and had feelings of persecution and premonitions of death. At 28 she had a 12-week miscarriage, and again required a D & C (under anaesthetic): one month later she was sleepless, and, when her menses returned, stayed up all night, drinking coffee, playing

music and writing to old friends; she became confused and could not tell whether she was dreaming or awake. At 30 she gave birth to her 3rd child: the illness began the day *before* she went into labour, with panic and hallucinations. After the birth she was high for 10–11 weeks, then depressed and suicidal. Two years later she gave birth to her 4th child, without complications. During the next 20 years she had numerous bipolar episodes.

Lack of Post-Abortion Episodes

Three mothers in my series had numerous abortions (4, 6 and 18) without an episode. The extreme example is Clinical Gem 20.1, which illustrates several points. Four of her pregnancies were affected by prepartum or postpartum psychosis, and two were followed by menstrual episodes; one episode followed a short gestation birth, and she may also have had a Runge psychosis (see pages 320–321). None of her 18 miscarriages was followed by an episode.

Mole Pregnancies

In my series, two mothers developed psychoses after the removal of hydatidiform moles. Since they both suffered an episode within three months, and no other mothers reported a mole pregnancy, this is significantly more frequent than post-abortion psychosis (p = .02). Both had a stable background, suffered two episodes of puerperal psychosis and later episodes unrelated to reproduction. One has already been published[427]. This is the other:

> A 29-year old gave birth to twins at 26 weeks gestation; both babies died. On day 5, she became overtalkative, disinhibited and labile in mood – varying between inconsolable grief and elation. She had pressure of speech, and was punning with clang associations and flight of ideas. She also had hallucinations of sounds responding to her thoughts. On admission she was disorientated in time, place and person. She improved, then relapsed, became depressed and finally recovered six months after the birth. Two years later she gave birth for the 2nd time: on day 3 she developed insomnia, giggling, rhyming, punning, racing thoughts, hallucinations of muttering and tapes running, and persecutory ideas. She was disinhibited and overactive, but recovered in two weeks. Two years later she miscarried at 11–12 weeks, and was found to have a mole pregnancy. This was followed by a milder manic episode, with onset a few days or some weeks later. She had more energy, her mind was 'whizzing', and she was giggly, rude, off-hand and inappropriate. She was committed to hospital, recovered and then relapsed, swearing and shouting, screaming, and disinhibited, with elevated mood and pressured speech. She finally recovered four months after the event. The following year she gave birth to her 2nd child. With lithium prophylaxis she remained well. In the next 16 years she had ten episodes of mania or depression, unrelated to reproduction, unless menstrual.

No other author has reported such cases, but Girot de Dinan[413] described this case of a psychosis associated with a mole pregnancy *before* it was removed:

> A woman became more and more tormented by vague anxieties. She began weeping for no reason and had ideas of morbid jealousy. Gradually this was replaced by indifference and her intellectual faculties changed: she was speaking incoherently, making slanderous reproaches and threatening suicide. She was suffering from uterine haemorrhages and eventually expelled a mole. Since then she enjoyed perfect health, without the least memory of her former state.

Clinical Gem 20.1 Multiple Triggers but Not Miscarriage

A woman whose sister suffered from bipolar disorder lost her mother, at 22 months of age, in a vehicle accident. She had an unhappy childhood, reared by a drunken father and unkind stepmother. She was scapegoated and abused emotionally, physically and sexually. But an aunt gave valuable support, and she later became an excellent mother and worked for many charities. Her psychiatric history began in childhood with a conduct disorder, anorexia nervosa and parasuicide. Later she developed washing rituals. At 18 she had the first of many miscarriages. She gave birth to five children. Each of her full pregnancies had a psychiatric complication. The first (at 22) was followed by nine months depression. The second (at 23) was followed by severe depression, with onset on day 12 and delusions that she could read people's thoughts and was suffering from poliomyelitis. During her 3rd pregnancy (at 26) she became ill at six months gestation – her mind racing and continuously overactive. After the birth, on day 3, she heard God's voice and came to believe she was an angel, could heal the sick, transmit thoughts, change the world and save human kind. She felt fine, and managed on an hour of sleep. She saw her dead mother, and heard the voices of her mother and mother-in-law (also deceased). Admitted to hospital, she developed ideas of persecution: a nurse had broken the baby's leg, they were all out to harm her, and a thermometer was a knife. The world was about to end. Voices told her to kill her 3-year old as a sacrifice, and she was interrupted in the act of suffocating her. She improved, then relapsed with every menstruation, becoming psychotic for a few days before or on the first day of menstrual bleeding; she kept a record and the intervals were exactly 28 days; treatment with oestrogens and a progestin brought some improvement. At 29 she became pregnant again and, at 30 weeks gestation, began to feel mentally ill, but did not consult. After the birth, again on day 3, she developed a 4-day psychosis – she required only a few minutes sleep and thought the birds were singing backwards and her dog was talking to her. At 30 she was pregnant again and, after premature rupture of the membranes and an antepartum haemorrhage, gave birth at 25 weeks to a child weighing less than 2 lbs. On day 3 she developed racing thoughts. It was up to her to stop the end of the world by shouting "Amen!" and raising her hand; so she did so, louder and louder until she was screaming, and there were nurses and doctors everywhere. Admitted to hospital she improved, but again suffered menstrual relapses – for two days before each menses she had 'a slight psychosis' when she used to think people on the television were using sign language, and God was giving her instructions. She continued to have miscarriages to a total of 18. During one of her brief pregnancies, at six weeks, she had a 4-day psychosis, in which she believed the baby was conceived by the Devil, and heard frightening voices; two weeks later she miscarried. She had two unrelated bipolar episodes, but was well when seen 20 years after her first puerperal episode.

Multiple Episodes with Other Associations

The proportion of post-abortion psychoses that occurred as part of a recurrent sequence (40 per cent) is higher than that for any other onset group except weaning onset. Associations with other onset groups are shown in the Matrix of Associations (page 209).

In *Motherhood and Mental Health*[67], I was impressed by the association between puerperal and post-abortion episodes (pages 91–93), and concluded that there was "a *prima facie* case for the association between abortion and acute manic or cycloid psychoses in susceptible women". Whether or not this conclusion has survived a more detailed analysis will be discussed in Section 6 (page 359).

Pregnancy

The literature contains many accounts of psychosis during pregnancy, which has attracted interest from early days, for example, in this seventeenth century report[428]:

> In 1668, in Frankfurt am Main, a 35-year old, mother of four or five children, consulted the physician. She told him that, whenever she became pregnant, she lost control of her mind: she laughed and became garrulous, with disturbed and disgraceful conduct. Eventually her husband and relations recognized this as a sign of pregnancy. After the children were born she recovered her reason, spoke in a composed and appropriate way, treated everyone with dignity, decorum and kindness and performed her womanly duties excellently.

There are many publications devoted entirely or substantially to prepartum psychosis. A total of 611 cases have been reported, as summarized in Table 20.2:

Table 20.2 Prepartum cases in the literature

Onset	Organic	Non-organic	
		Single episodes	Multiple episodes
1st trimester	38	63	6
2nd trimester	72	79	4
3rd trimester	61	101	4
Unknown	33	38	112[a]
Total	**204**	**281**	**126**

[a] In most cases, the trimester of onset was unknown; or a mixture of 1st, 2nd and 3rd; or a combination of prepartum and other reproductive onsets.

Organic Psychoses

Two organic psychoses are particularly associated with pregnancy – chorea psychosis, complicating *chorea gravidarum*, and Wernicke–Korsakow syndrome, complicating pernicious vomiting. Both can occur after a birth or abortion, but usually present during pregnancy, more commonly in the 2nd trimester (23/53 chorea psychosis and 48/89

Wernicke–Korsakow syndrome). Eclamptic and Donkin psychoses can also start before the birth, usually in the 3rd trimester (23/29 cases). Other causes include cerebral venous thrombosis (3), anti-NMDAR encephalitis (3), hyperammonaemia (3), epilepsy (4), water intoxication, *delirium tremens* and AIDS encephalitis (1 each) and 22 miscellaneous cases of unknown cause or incidental to the reproductive process.

Non-Organic Cases

A total of 103 surveys gave the number of pregnant women admitted to hospital, compared with those admitted within three months of childbirth. In total, 1,961 women were hospitalized during pregnancy and 13,030 after childbirth – a prepartum/postpartum ratio of 14 per cent (median) and 15.2 per cent (mean). These figures cover three trimesters; the number admitted per trimester is more than an order of magnitude less than those admitted in the first postpartum trimester.

Thirty-six surveys gave other information. Omitting civil state and diagnosis (much affected by epoch and locality), heredity (of little value without interviewing relatives), recovery rates (affected by diagnosis and available treatment), previous episodes (only twice reported), and recurrences (on which there is much information from case lore), the following are of interest:

- Age. Three surveys reported that the pregnant patients were older than those with postpartum psychosis: Holm[429], who compared 26 prepartum with 58 postpartum, had only 3 below the age of 30, 9 aged 30–34 and 14 above the age of 35, *versus* 20, 18 and 20. Reinhardt[430] reported a mean and median of 30–35 *versus* 20–30 for postpartum. Paffenbarger[156], who compared 72 prepartum with 242 postpartum, found 44 below 30, 17 aged 30–34 and 11 older *versus* 158, 56 and 28, thus 39 per cent aged 35 or more *versus* 25 per cent. But Jolly[431] disagreed, stating that they were younger (mean 28.5 *versus* 30)

- Parity. All surveys have agreed that the ratio of *primiparae* to *multiparae* was lower in prepartum psychosis[203,430,432–434]. Most striking were the findings of Pedler[435], who had no *primiparae* among 9, Holm[429], who had only 2/26 *primiparae*, and Quensel[436], who had 1/17 *primiparae*. Holm reported that 11/26 were in their fifth pregnancy. Paffenbarger[156] stated that prepartum patients averaged 3.4 pregnancies, compared with 2.5 for postpartum patients

- Trimester. 23 surveys gave information, with much variation. The total numbers were 92 in the first trimester, 86 in the second and 113 in the third. Paffenbarger's[156] study dwarfs the others, with 27 in the first, 24 in the second and 21 in the third trimester (evenly distributed)

- Incidence. Several modern studies have calculated an incidence. Paffenbarger[156] gave 0.5/1,000 births (compared with 1.9 for postpartum), Kendell[148] 0.22/1,000 births, and Munk-Olsen[355] 0.53/1,000 births admissions. These are all surprisingly high, considering that the frequency of postpartum psychosis is only 1/1,000 births. But an even higher figure was reported in a Swedish record linkage study[17]: in 1987–2001, 62,306 women gave birth to their first child: 287 were admitted to hospital during pregnancy – 4.6/1,000 births; although women are admitted to hospital for reasons other than psychosis, these findings support the frequency of prepartum psychosis.

Epidemiological surveys can be subject to nosocomial bias, which may be important in pregnant women. It is possible that the threshold for admission is raised, especially towards the end of pregnancy, when admission to an obstetric ward may be preferred.

Case Lore

The total number of non-organic cases, reported in the literature, is 407 (281 with single episodes and 126 with multiple episodes). This can be compared with 2,084 postpartum cases (1,211 early onset, 399 4–13 week onset, 215 late onset and 259 unknown onset); that is 20 per cent of those with postpartum onset, a somewhat higher ratio than found in surveys. As shown in Table 20.2, the number of episodes rises with each trimester (especially single episodes). As shown in Table 20.7 (page 207), the average number of episodes per trimester (146) is greater than that of post-abortion psychosis (108) and late postpartum (78), but much less than that of early (5,629) and 4–13 week onset (531) postpartum groups.

In my series, 57 mothers had 71 prepartum episodes – 15 with first trimester, 15 second trimester and 39 third trimester onsets, plus 2 of unknown onset. This is an episode rate of 23/trimester, similar to post-abortion episodes, and only 8 per cent of the number with onset in the first postpartum trimester; but this ratio may be low because most British mother & baby units in the past did not admit pregnant patients. Among the 57 mothers, 24 presented with a prepartum episode and 33 with postpartum psychosis, among whom 6 gave a history of prepartum episodes and 27 developed prepartum episodes during a later pregnancy. The episode diagnoses are compared with those of other onset groups in Table 20.8 (page 207).

Precocious Early Onset Episodes

Sivadon[86] briefly described this case:

> A 19-year old, with a history of a previous episode of 'dementia praecox', developed confusion, terrifying onirism, anxiety and mutism in the 3rd trimester. The next day she gave birth. Nine days later she was admitted to hospital (case 96).

Three mothers in my series had similar experiences: one may have had a Donkin psychosis; one suffered two cycloid episodes, which started two days after, and three days before her children were born[438]; and one, who had serial post-abortion episodes (summarized on pages 187 and 189) had an episode starting the day before she went into labour.

Serial Prepartum Episodes

To the 126 cases of recurrent psychoses in the literature that included prepartum episodes, I can add 29 from my own series, making 155 in all. A surprisingly large number had serial prepartum episodes. Five authors made general statements reporting 4[431], 5[227,434], 7[69,439], 9[46] or 12[440] prepartum episodes, without giving details. Another 30 had details on timing: 14 had all the onsets in one trimester (6 in the first trimester, 4 in the second trimester and 4 in the third trimester). To these can be added 6 cases with at least two prepartum episodes, as well as postpartum episodes[90,203,322,361,370,441,442]. Evidence for a specific prepartum trigger requires that patients be followed long term, so that the frequency of psychotic episodes can be estimated. There are five in the literature, and eight in my series; but I had to exclude one (summarized Clinical Gem 20.1 on page 188), because, with 18 miscarriages, she was pregnant for 32 trimesters. I also excluded two others, who had five pregnancies and so many unrelated episodes that their prepartum onsets were at chance level, and I excluded a mother who claimed three prepartum onsets, but was thought to be an unreliable informant. In the remaining nine, I noted the length of study, number of pregnancies and abortions, and number of episodes unrelated to childbearing, and estimated the probability that the prepartum episodes were sporadic: in four cases the probability was in the range 0.06–0.09[361,370,443]. The remaining five – two from the literature and three from my series will now be summarized.

The first[444] had one full pregnancy and two miscarriages in seven years: given three prepartum and two unrelated episodes, $p = .03$, or for three first trimester episodes, $p = .004$; but the social circumstances were so adverse that an alternative diagnosis of pseudo-psychosis – a series of emotional crises – is just possible:

> A 25-year old single woman gave birth to two children, both of whom died within ten weeks. Pregnant for the 3rd time, she became depressed and wanted to drown herself. Admitted to hospital, she was restless, talked day and night and thought that knocking on the window meant that her two children were still alive; later she developed catalepsy and heard voices saying she would be killed. After the birth she recovered. The following year she became anxious about another pregnancy, and started running about aimlessly, wringing her hands. Admitted to hospital, she was making stereotypic movements, hopping like a frog, weeping and singing, and smearing faeces; she heard voices and was intermittently energetic and over-active. She recovered and had a miscarriage. After some months she became pregnant again. She had two seizures and was unconscious for a time. Admitted to hospital she laughed, sang and wept, talked monotonously with flight of ideas, saw ghosts, tore her clothes, and awaited investigation by the police. She expected to be married, but, after a letter to the boyfriend was returned undeliverable, became disturbed and aggressive, wanted to strangle herself and ran about aimlessly. At four months gestation, the pregnancy miscarried, but the illness continued, with restlessness, shouting and cursing, stereotypies, obscenity and aggression to the nurses. In the next four years she had two similar episodes unrelated to pregnancy.

The second[322] had two full pregnancies and six episodes in eight years – three prepartum, one postpartum and two unrelated; for prepartum episodes, $p = .04$:

> A mother of two became pregnant for the 3rd time. In the 1st trimester, she developed an acute psychosis with manic features. During the next six years she had two similar acute episodes. In 1977 she became ill again when two months pregnant (no details), and again in the 9th month; this continued and a few days after the birth she presented with insomnia, labile mood, hyperactivity, a confusional–delirious picture and phases of mutism. She had audio-visual and caenesthetic hallucinations and memory difficulties: she mistook the sex of the baby; she felt the baby inside her, and the pains of labour. Some days later her menses reappeared and she immediately recovered with complete amnesia for the episode.

The third had two full-term pregnancies in 13 years. She had two, perhaps three, prepartum episodes, one of which continued after the birth (after a gap of five days), together with three unrelated episodes. If the two admissions during her second pregnancy were separate episodes, $p = .02$; there is an alternative diagnosis of a chronic psychosis.

> An 18-year old was admitted with restlessness, social withdrawal, auditory and visual hallucinations, passivity phenomena and thought disorder, and given a diagnosis of 'schizophrenia'. Five years later, she presented with ideas of reference and 3rd person auditory hallucinations. At the age of 27, when nine months pregnant, she suddenly became euphoric, sleepless and overactive. She could not control her voice – "It was someone else's voice; I could hear the voice talking

through me". On the obstetric ward, she was disorientated, running about, laughing and shouting, with pressure of speech and flight of ideas. She improved then relapsed. After a forceps delivery, she remained well for five days, then suddenly lay on the floor talking to God. She was disorientated in time, and became hyperactive and overtalkative, with religious themes. Her mood was labile – angry, elated or tearful. She recovered within a month. The following year she stopped her medication, and began to neglect her housework and baby. She was receiving messages about her husband's sexual behaviour and a former boy-friend. Readmitted, she was unkempt, and spoke nonsense. She was labile in mood, cheerful, suspicious and hostile, with ideas of reference and persecution. She recovered. Three years later, she became pregnant again. During this pregnancy she suffered two episodes in succeeding months, each leading to hospital admission with a diagnosis of 'schizophrenia'. Six months later she gave birth to her 2nd child, and remained well.

The fourth had three full pregnancies and the first trimester of a fourth in 16 years. She had two postpartum and three or four prepartum episodes, together with five unrelated episodes. If the last episode had onset in the first trimester, $p = .008$, if the onset was before conception, $p = .047$.

A Jamaican woman came to Britain at the age of 12. At 19 she was admitted in catatonic stupor; she was hearing voices, believed she was Anne Boleyn, and was disinhibited sexually. At 22 she had three more acute episodes, and was admitted to hospital after running naked down the street, believing she was being stalked by ghosts. She recovered and was married. At 30, when 8½ months pregnant, she again developed 'catatonic excitement' – went berserk, angry and agitated, shouting and swearing. After the birth, on day 2, she became manic: she was abusive, had pressure of speech and flight of ideas, sang, laughed and exposed herself, and started a fire. She recovered within two months. Two years later, in the 3rd month of her 2nd pregnancy, she became manic – overactive, abusive and disinhibited, with pressure of speech, flight of ideas and grandiosity. She recovered and had a new episode at six months of the same pregnancy, with manic symptoms and 3rd person auditory hallucinations. She recovered a month later. After the birth, on day 11, she was readmitted – abusive and aggressive, elated and laughing, with pressure of speech. Treated with Depixol, she remained well for three years. After stopping the prophylaxis, she became ill, lay in bed, would not leave the house and spoke nonsense. Five months later she became pregnant. At 11 weeks gestation, she was readmitted, overactive, disinhibited and socially intrusive, with pressure of speech. The records ended at this point.

The last mother was a strange woman, who may have suffered from dysmorphobia in early life and was hoarding soft toys in late life. She had two pregnancies in 36 years, both with prepartum episodes. Recurrence was not due to stopping treatment. For manic episodes, $p = .047$.

At the age of 25, a woman had a mandibular osteotomy to reduce the length of her chin. At 28, she became depressed and, five months pregnant, switched to mania: she was restless and sleepless, talking non-stop about the Queen Mother's birthday celebrations; she was up all night telephoning people about this great event. She recovered with ECT and remained well after the baby was born. During her 2nd pregnancy, at four months gestation, she again became manic – not sleeping, euphoric, talking non-stop, obsessed with gold and silver, and again with the Queen Mother's birthday celebrations. She had a 'mad urge' to clean and tidy cupboards. After the birth she remained well. She had eleven other episodes in 36 years, of which seven were manic. When seen at 64 she was hoarding soft toys, and the disorder in the home suggested Diogenes syndrome.

The calculations are only approximate and there are difficulties in defining episodes. None of these cases had highly significant statistical associations.

Multiple Episodes with Other Associations

The association of prepartum with postpartum psychosis has already been reported in the literature[58,438]. One must distinguish between postpartum psychoses that are merely a continuation of a prepartum episode, and new postpartum onsets. In the literature, a rough count showed that 74/142 with onset in the third trimester, 42/108 in the second trimester and 14/99 in the first trimester continued into the puerperium. In my series, 36 continued after the birth (2 with first trimester, 6 second trimester and 28 third trimester onsets) and 22 recovered before the birth (7 with first trimester, 6 second trimester and 9 third trimester onsets). Occasionally there was a brief return to normal after parturition, as in the preceding example and two other instances in the literature[433,434]; these could, perhaps, be separate early postpartum onsets. It is not true, as we claimed[438], that the postpartum episode always occurs first: in 16 the prepartum episode was first, in 13 of which the postpartum episode may have been the continuation of the same illness, although there appeared to be an interval of health.

But the associations are not confined to prepartum and early postpartum occurrences – they involve all phases of the reproductive process, as will later be discussed under Matrix of Associations (page 209). The evidence for a specific prepartum trigger will be wrapped up, after considering the bipolar/cycloid series, in Section 6 (pages 359–360).

Short Gestation Births

These are defined as second trimester births and fifth and sixth month abortions. Extreme prematurity (birth before 28 weeks gestation) occurs in about 0.5 per cent of pregnancies[446]. All forms of psychosis may occur in these circumstances.

Organic Psychoses

Of 35 cases in the literature, 16 have been organic, as first mentioned by Hippocrates (see page 8). There are three other cases of infective delirium, six of eclamptic or Donkin psychosis, one of combined infection and eclampsia, three of Wernicke–Korsakow syndrome, one of chorea psychosis and one of cerebral venous thrombosis. Some followed a foetal death *in utero*, and one a termination of pregnancy because of life-threatening maternal disease.

Non-Organic Psychoses

The others were non-organic – 10 single episodes, and 7 recurrent. To these can be added 6 from my series – one single episode and 5 recurrent; this is a relatively large number, since we wrote a paper on the subject[447]. One followed a five-month criminal abortion, and 2 a medical termination. The rest followed an extremely premature birth, or, in 3 cases, foetal death *in utero*. Among the recurrent cases, this mother[448] had two episodes after short gestation, the first of which followed severe pre-eclamptic toxaemia and had much evidence of an organic psychosis, so that a Donkin psychosis was possible:

> A woman, who had a mentally ill sister, developed kidney disease and swollen feet during her 1st pregnancy. At six months gestation she gave birth to a dead child. Within two weeks she developed trembling of her whole body, and began to fantasize, saying that God was calling her and she would be punished for her sins. She attacked her step-mother and husband, and tore her clothing. Admitted to hospital, her urine contained much albumin and casts, and she had a fever of 39°. She was strikingly immobile and almost mute, giving a dazed, perplexed impression, and had to be

fed. Three months later she was removed against medical advice, still not improved. For months she remained confused, did not remember her admission, and mistook evening for morning. A year after the birth she suddenly recovered, though still depressed. After two years she was again delivered at five months gestation. On day 9 she began to fantasize, gave odd answers and talked to the cat as if it were a child. On admission nearly a year later she always sat on the same stool in the same position. She was transferred to an asylum, where she eventually recovered.

The occurrence of non-organic puerperal psychosis in these circumstances is of interest because, in mid-pregnancy, the levels of oestrogen and progesterone are about half those at full term[449]. If (as some believe) a 'cascade' of reproductive hormones is involved in triggering episodes, the fall is much less.

Parturition

Section 3 discussed the onset of various organic and non-organic psychoses during labour.

Day 1 Onset

This term covers episodes that start explicitly within 24 hours of the birth. Three of Esquirol's[84,103,104] cases started on day 1, and Burrows[23] also drew attention to these very early postpartum onsets. He wrote,

> Delirium sometimes immediately succeeds a natural labour or as early as the following day. I have seen all the symptoms of genuine mania or melancholia thus early displayed.

Organic Psychoses

Section 3 described a number of cases of delirium and stupor starting *immediately* after the birth. In addition, eight eclamptic, two epileptic and four infective psychoses, one hyperammonaemic psychosis and one case of Sheehan's syndrome (with confusion on day 1 and death from necrosis of the anterior pituitary within 27 hours) all started at this time. A mother in my series developed an organic psychosis, associated with gestosis, starting on day 1.

Non-Organic Psychoses

In the literature 29 prolonged episodes began within 24 hours of the birth. This is a rate/trimester of 2,639, about half that of early postpartum onset.

Three started on recovery from an anaesthetic, with the alternative diagnosis of a postoperative psychosis[450–452], as in this example[451]:

> A 24-year old was delivered of her 1st child by Caesarean section. When she came round, she was excited and expressed the idea that her child had been kidnapped because he was too beautiful. The obstetricians were impostors acting on the orders of the person pretending to be her husband, who had been killed trying to prevent the kidnapping. Her admission to hospital was an imprisonment, to prevent her getting to the bottom of the plot, and giving the impostors time to establish their identities. She refused to see her husband and child. She recovered, relapsed two months later, again recovered in 15 days, and remained well.

Widerøe[250] mentioned a mother who had recurrent onsets on the first day:

> A 32-year old gave birth to five children. After each delivery she became mentally ill, starting the very day of the birth: she was restless, talkative, shouting, leaping, hopping and dancing. On each occasion this lasted 2–3 months.

In my series there were 17 episodes that undoubtedly started within 24 hours of parturition, including one that started on recovery from an anaesthetic given for caesarean section. Six had typical bipolar disorder with many episodes, followed for 15–36 years. With one exception (a mother who was murdered on day 11) the duration was at least six weeks, including, in three cases, at least one relapse. This is an example of a mother with recurrent cycloid psychosis, including a day 1 onset:

> A 20-year old gave birth to her 1st child. Five hours later she seemed drowsy and slow and did not understand what was being said to her; her abnormal behaviour came to the attention of the obstetricians. Admitted to hospital, she heard the voices of God and her parents. Her affect was distant, vacant, overexcited, perplexed and labile. She believed she had extra-sensory perception, could communicate without speaking, could speak any language and type in Braille. She was two people, one of whom was dead and was using her voice. She saw things plainer and more vividly. She wanted to dance, laugh, sing and play the piano. She wandered into other patients' rooms and took their possessions. She was talkative, disinhibited and distractible. She tried to feed her baby with rose hip syrup and jam. After a rapid response to neuroleptics and ECT, she was discharged, but relapsed eleven weeks after the birth. A deceased aunt was trying to take over her body and was speaking through her. Voices discussed her and answered each other, reprimanding her, and commanding her to put her hand through a window. She was being poisoned; her husband was dead and she was blind. She finally recovered five months after the birth. Eighteen months later she gave birth to her 2nd child. For the first week she felt 'on top of the world', but on day 8 became puzzled, perplexed and bewildered ('living in a dream world'). Her dead aunt had taken her over again. Auditory hallucinations, coming from outer space, commenting on her actions, were the main symptom. She again recovered quickly and had one relapse.

The 29 cases in the literature, and my own 17 cases, establish beyond reasonable doubt that bipolar/cycloid episodes can begin within 24 hours of labour.

Early Postpartum Onset

This is defined as onset within the first three weeks after childbirth. It is the time when most organic and non-organic psychoses begin. This is what most practitioners mean by 'puerperal psychosis'.

Organic Psychoses

Table 20.3 (on the next page) shows the numbers of organic and non-organic cases reported in the literature in each generation. Apart from infective delirium and eclamptic psychosis, whose numbers are shown in columns 2 and 3, the other organic psychoses were vascular disorders (19); Wernicke–Korsakow syndrome (15); urea cycle disorders (11); chorea psychosis, ethanol and sedative withdrawal syndromes and Sheehan's syndrome (4 each); water intoxication (1); plus nineteenth century brief psychoses (see page 26) and 40 of unknown cause. In the nineteenth century organic psychoses outnumbered the non-organic; equality was reached in the first 25 years of the twentieth century.

Non-Organic Psychoses

These are the 'puerperal psychoses' now most commonly seen in high-income nations. They are so familiar that no illustrative cases are required; but their number (1,211 including short gestation, intrapartum and day 1 onsets) is only 30 per cent of the cases published in the literature. In my series, 235 mothers had at least one early onset episode,

Table 20.3 Organic and non-organic psychoses with early postpartum onset in the literature

Epoch	Organic				Non-organic		
	Infective	Eclamptic	Other	Total	Single episodes	Multiple episodes	Total
Before 1850	22	22	16	**60**	52	13	**65**
1851–1875	41	25	31	**97**	55	8	**63**
1876–1900	95	31	24	**150**	96	24	**120**
1901–1925	91	70	18	**179**	147	33	**180**
1926–1950	88	23	22	**133**	244	16	**260**
1951–1975	12	9	10	**31**	201	33	**234**
After 1975	1	2	23	**26**	131	38	**169**
Total	**350**	**182**	**144**	**676**	**926**	**165**	**1,091**[a]

[a] This excludes short gestation, intrapartum and day 1 onsets.

with a total of 340 episodes. The episode diagnoses are compared with those of other onset groups in Tables 20.7 and 20.8 on page 207.

Day-by-Day Onset

The onset of psychoses is important in the search for causes. Unfortunately the data, both in the literature and in my own series, are poor: there were many cases with vague statements, such as 'immediately after the birth', 'in a few days', 'in the first week', 'in the second week' *et cetera*. But there are at present no better data. Focusing on those with more precise information, the day-to-day onset in 804 cases from the literature and 155 of my series is shown in Table 20.4 (on the next page).

The findings are similar: in the literature the median is day 8, with the highest totals on days 3, 8 and 10; a fall on day 11 and a steep fall after day 15. In my series, the median is day 5, with the highest totals on days 3 and 6, a fall on day 11 and hardly any cases after day 14. Thus, although the period is sometimes defined arbitrarily as the first three weeks (or in DSM 5 four weeks) post partum, there were few onsets in the third week, and a more precise delimitation would be from parturition to the 15th day.

Serial Early Postpartum Onset

In the literature there are 165 cases with multiple onsets, in which at least one episode had early postpartum onset. In 74, all onsets were early postpartum; most of these had two episodes, but eight had three and two had brief details of four episodes[453,454]. There were some impressive examples of mothers who suffered only from early postpartum onsets, with long periods of normal mental health. For example, this mother had three early psychoses after four births and five unrelated episodes in 23 years ($p < .0001$)[109].

A woman, whose brother suffered from manic episodes, became depressed at the age of 15, coincident with 'diminished menses'. At the next menses she was worse, and believed the police were after her. Admitted to hospital, she was perplexed, and complained that everything seemed strange and threatening. At 20 she gave birth to her 1st child. On day 3 she became febrile, restless and irritable. She seemed depressed and said she felt anxious 'as in war'. She noticed strange smells

Table 20.4 Day-to-day onset

Day	Literature	My series
1	28	14
2	68	17
3	89	19
4	65	15
5	71	14
6	56	19
7	39	15
8	96	5
9	41	8
10	88	11
11	20	2
12	27	6
13	21	2
14	31	4
15	43	1
16	3	1
17	4	Nil
18	6	Nil
19	3	1
20	5	Nil
21	Nil	1
Total	**804**	**155**

and expressed ideas of persecution and poisoning. Her speech was incoherent with flight of ideas, and she may have had auditory hallucinations. She recovered after four weeks in hospital. Two years later she gave birth to her 2nd child. Within 2–3 days she became overactive with elevated mood and incoherent speech and behaviour; she was running about at night, and making senseless purchases. After two months she switched to depression and thought her husband should shoot her. Four months after the birth she recovered. Eighteen months later she gave birth to her 3rd child, who died some hours later; there was no recurrence, but in the next year she suffered an episode unrelated to childbearing, with depression, mutism, a suicide attempt and hypomania. At 26 she gave birth to her 4th child. On day 18 another episode began with depression swinging to hypomania, for which she was hospitalized for six months. In the next 12 years she had three more unrelated bipolar episodes (case 5).

Gödtel[455] described a mother with two episodes after three births and no unrelated episodes in 17 years ($p = .007$), and Boutet[456] described a mother who had two day 8 onsets, three unaffected births and only one further episode 39 years after the first ($p = .003$). Fallgatter's[369] third patient had three pregnancies in 15 years, with four episodes (days 11 and 7 post partum, at 24 weeks gestation and day 9 after completion of the same pregnancy); she remained well for 15 years ($p < .0001$). Robertson–Blackmore's[106] series of women with post-menopausal episodes included two who suffered early postpartum episodes after both their births and no other episodes for 20 years. I can add 41 mothers with two early onset episodes and three who had three episodes. There were four mothers, each of whom had two early onset postpartum psychoses and no other episodes in the span of 26–33 years ($p = < .0001$).

Complex recurrent cases are discussed under Matrix of Associations on page 209.

4–13 Week Onset

Hoffmann[262] gave the first description of a psychosis starting in this time frame:

> Four weeks after childbirth a 20-year old, rather melancholy and anxious by temperament, had a severe fright – she 'saw' the ghost of her long-dead mother. Three days later she became confused and started to rave. She was restless, talked day and night (mainly in rhyme), and ate and drank little, but had no fever. The infant was given to a wet-nurse, leeches were applied to her feet, and medicines given to bring on the menses; but her raving increased more and more, and she had to be restrained. It was two months before she calmed down. She immediately became pregnant again and remained well.

Burns[457] was the first to assert that some cases of puerperal insanity had onset several weeks after delivery. Marcé[203] believed that it could start either immediately after the birth or several weeks later at the first menses; among his cases that meet my definition of psychosis, his figures were 10/29. It is remarkable how little attention has been paid to this, perhaps his most important contribution, by those who venerate him. Fürstner[274] also commented that puerperal psychosis broke out either at days 10–12 or at 4–6 weeks, with a free period between; two of his patients with *hallucinatorische Irresein* began late in the puerperium. Few other authors have mentioned this.

Surveys

Some provided data on the vague concept of 'lactational psychosis'. The ratio of 'lactational' to puerperal cases, calculated in 72 surveys, shows a huge range. For example, an American survey had only one lactational among 118 cases[458], while an asylum survey from Halle had 50 puerperal and 103 lactational[433]. The median figure is 30 lactational to 58 puerperal. 'Lactational' psychoses included those that begin as early as the 4th week, and as late as the 11th month. In the present work I shall make an arbitrary distinction between those starting within three months of the birth and those starting later in the first postpartum year.

A number of surveys have reported that a considerable proportion of postpartum psychoses are admitted after the first month. For example, the ratio of second and third month to first month admissions was 19/33[153], 48/164[156], 11/61[459], 16/80[405] and 8/30[460] (all at 1/5 or above), while Trixler[445] reported that 33/102 were admitted in weeks 4–6. The recent surveys of Kendell[41] and Munk-Olsen[355] give more detail. Kendell[41] quantified admissions with psychosis for each trimester: the mean before conception and during pregnancy was 6, in the first postpartum month 51 (153/trimester), in the next two months

38 (57/trimester, almost 10 times the base line) and in the rest of the first postpartum year 16/trimester. Munk-Olsen[355] reported 239 admissions in the first two postpartum weeks, 48 in the third week (a sharp fall), 145 in the fourth week and 222 in the second and third months (almost as many as in the first two weeks); the risk factor for late postpartum admission was above 2.0. These surveys reported hospital admissions, not onset.

Week-by-Week Onset

Table 20.4 listed the day-to-day onsets of non-organic psychotic episodes during the first three weeks after the birth. Table 20.5 extends this to two months, enumerating onsets on a weekly basis. The totals are higher than in Table 20.4 because cases with more approximate onset were included.

Table 20.5 Week-by-week onset of non-organic postpartum psychoses

Week	Literature		My series			
			All cases		Bipolar/cycloids	
	Episodes	Fall, %	Episodes	Fall, %	Episodes	Fall, %
1	610		159		139	
2	405	34	59	63	45	68
3	92	77	11	81	6	87
4	106		6		4	
5	26		11		3	
6	73		10		4	
7	14		4		4	
8	82		5		1	

In both series, there is a steep fall from week 2 to week 3; if this rate of fall were continued, one would expect only 21 onsets in the literature, and only 2 onsets in my series, in week 4. In the literature there are peaks in week 1, week 4, week 6 and week 8. In my series, which had relatively good data, there is a second mode at week 5–6, supporting Marcé's idea. But this does not survive the study of bipolar/cycloid patients, which shows a long tail, but no second mode; it does, however, show the same sharp fall from week 2 to week 3, and, if continued, there should be only one case in the fourth week, and none thereafter.

Case Lore

In the literature, 447 patients had onset 4–13 weeks after the birth. There were only 48 organic psychoses (11 per cent), fewer than after abortion (34 per cent), during pregnancy (32 per cent) or in the early puerperium (38 per cent). Almost all were infective (44), the others being chorea psychosis or an unusual recurrent delirium.

In this 10-week period, 399 mothers had episodes of non-organic psychosis, including 326 single and 73 recurrent cases (409 episodes). The rate/trimester (531/trimester) is one-tenth that of early postpartum onset (5,629/trimester), but much higher than the rate of those starting during pregnancy (146/trimester) or after abortion (108/trimester). The ratio of 4–13 week onsets to early postpartum onset is 1 to 3. In my series, there were only 41 episodes with 4–13 week onsets, and of these only 19 were bipolar/cycloid; the ratio of 4–13 week to early postpartum onset was 1 to 7, lower than in the literature or reported by Marcé, suggesting that some appeared to have late onset because they were hospitalized late.

Parity

Parity was as follows: *primiparae* 109, 2nd birth 65, 3rd birth 64, 4th birth 32, 5th birth 22, 6th birth 20, 7th birth 15, 8th birth 9, 9th–13th births 6; '*multiparae*' 12, with another 99 unknown. Thus 32 per cent were *primiparae*. Restricting the analysis to bipolar/cycloid patients, the mean for my series was 2.19, median 2, *primiparae* 38 per cent. Thus there are fewer first-time mothers than in the early onset group. There is some confirmation of this result from a Danish survey of 750,000 women: in *primiparae* the highest relative risk of psychiatric disorder (not just psychoses) occurred 10–19 days post partum (RR 8.7), but, when the first psychiatric episode followed the second birth, it was 60–89 days post partum (RR 2.7)[461].

Serial 4–13 Week Onsets

There are eight cases in the literature with two 4–13 week onsets and no other reproductive episodes. One mother had three episodes, but only a vague description – "She became insane some weeks later, each time with various delusions"[462]. In addition to those with multiple episodes limited to this time frame, one mother had seven postpartum episodes, including three late onsets – at four weeks, two months and three months, with the rest of unknown onset[463]. The following Danish patient[429] had three early and three 4–13 week postpartum onsets:

> A labourer's wife, aged 19, gave birth to her second child in 1834; on day 3 she became manic, and remained ill for seven months. In 1837 she gave birth for the 3rd time, and breast-fed for two months, at which point she became manic for eleven months. In 1839 she gave birth for the 4th time and breast-fed for one month, when she became manic for an entire year. In 1841 she had her 5th child, whom she breast-fed for 2½ months; when she weaned the child she became manic for 13 months. In 1844, after her 6th delivery, she failed to lactate, and immediately became manic, lasting eight months. In 1847 she gave birth to her 7th child, who died on the 8th day; she broke out into mania, less severe but chronic with remissions. In 34 years' observation, she also had four episodes unrelated to childbearing.

Her 6 postpartum episodes, all within the first trimester, cannot have been sporadic because she had only four unrelated episodes in 104 non-reproductive trimesters ($p = .0001$); but the postpartum episodes started in two separate time frames.

Recurrent episodes with other onsets are discussed under Matrix of Associations.

Marcé's interpretation that there are two distinct disorders is not the only explanation: it is possible that all non-organic postpartum psychoses are aspects of the same disorder, resulting from a single trigger associated with the birth itself, and that the late appearance of symptoms – the long tail in the onset distribution – is due to late presentation or the length of the pathogenetic process. But it seems unlikely that a trigger, which has its maximum effect within the first 15 days, can incubate a psychosis that breaks out a month later. Although there is no bimodal distribution of onsets, the steep fall from week 2 to week 3 supports Marcé's idea. It seems best provisionally to regard 4–13 week onset cases as a separate phenomenon. But psychoses with 4–13 week onset are not all of one kind. Indeed, in my series, they were significantly more common in non-bipolars (20/96 *versus* 22/218, $p = .018$). An important issue is whether, within this group, there are bipolar disorders triggered by a late postpartum event. The evidence for this will be discussed in Section 6 (page 360), as will Marcé's views on the menstrual origin of these cases.

Late Postpartum Onset

When a psychosis breaks out more than three months after an event, it begins to be incredible that there could be a causal relationship between the two. Onsets more than three months after childbirth are much less common than 4–13 week onsets. Very few surveys have provided figures for the two periods: they showed approximately equal numbers starting in the first month, the next two months and the last nine months, so that the rate/trimester was less than a third. Examining the case lore, the month-by-month onset in the literature and my series is shown in Table 20.6.

Table 20.6 Month-by-month onset

Month	Literature	My series
1	1,213	235
2	195	30
3	80	8
4	61	4
5	34	3
6	35	2
7	19	3
8	19	2
9	19	2
10	13	1
11	6	Nil

Of the 226 published cases, only 11 were organic psychoses (6 infective, 2 chorea psychoses, 1 uraemia, 1 *delirium tremens* and 1 of unknown cause). There were 157 single and 58 recurrent non-organic psychoses. In my series, 17 mothers had episodes with onset later than three months post partum (18 episodes). There were only three bipolar/cycloids after six months and none after eight months.

Recurrent Cases

Seven mothers had 2 or more episodes with onset later than three months, with a total of 24 episodes[345,374,464–468]. There are three interesting cases. Ménaché[466] described a mother who had 4 episodes of acute mania, with excitement, logorrhoea, clang associations and eroticism, with admission to hospital two months, five months, six months and six months after her four births; no other episodes were recorded in eight years ($p = .03$). Hurt[464] described this brief recurrent hallucinatory psychosis:

A French woman gave birth to six children. Five months after her 3rd birth she 'heard' people walking about in her bedroom – she opened the window and called for a ladder to make her escape. Admitted to hospital, she was in a state of terror with severe hallucinations, including left-sided hissing, barking, mewing and ticking clocks. She soon recovered and was discharged after 18 days. She gave birth again and, after 13 months lactation, developed a similar episode with terrifying auditory, visual, gustatory, olfactory and somatic hallucinations. Most of the time she was mute and stuporose, but she suddenly emerged to fight off a wild boar, and a man who was trying to push her into a stove. She rapidly recovered and was discharged after 28 days. Three months after the 6th child was born, she had a similar episode that lasted 15 days, and, one year later, long after weaning, she had the fourth episode that lasted three weeks, followed, seven months later by a 5th episode with mutism and visual hallucinations of intruders and flames, for one day only (case 9).

A Polish case[345] was similar:

A gentle, hard-working, and exemplary housewife had her first mental illness after 4–5 months of lactation. This took the form of confusion with disorientation, stupor and later excitement. She saw the judgment of God, the Virgin Mary and dead people everywhere – everyone had died, including her brothers, one of whom was buried as a woman wearing stockings, covered with a towel; she heard their voices. She gave birth eleven times, and had further episodes (with similar content) in the lactation phase after the 6th, 9th and 11th births, always with complete recovery (case 7).

The other five recurrent cases, with two to five episodes each, support the action of some unknown but specific late postpartum factor. Complex associations are discussed in the following, under Matrix of Associations.

Weaning Onset

This is a special instance of late postpartum onset; some cases have started more than 12 months after childbirth[92,203,443,469]. Excluding Williardts' case[470], in which 'manic fury' began eight weeks after the birth when 'the breasts were hanging and empty', the first (a recurrent) case was reported by Esquirol[104]:

A 30-year old was the mother of three infants. Two days after 'incautiously' weaning her 4th child, she suffered *délire général* with religious ideas, and recovered after four months. At 39 she gave birth to her 5th child: seven months later, the day after weaning, she developed a rash and *délire* and imaginary fears; she spent 20 months in the Salpêtrière in a state of hopeless melancholy with religious terrors.

She had only one other episode; in view of the infrequency of her depressions, the coincidence is striking. In his survey, he stated that 19/92 cases of puerperal insanity started a few days or immediately after weaning. Marcé[203] had eight patients with weaning onset, six of whom had suckled their infants for a long time (10–21 months).

Excluding cases with a birth interval less than three months (when other puerperal factors could compete), the literature consists of 32 cases – 18 single and 14 recurrent, including 4 with two or more weaning episodes. In most the interval between weaning and onset was not stated, or only in vague terms ('at the time of weaning', 'shortly after weaning'), and often there was little information: for example, Loiseau[471] gave this tantalizingly brief description of a mother with multiple episodes:

A woman always became mad in the third month of lactation. She had seven or eight children. With each new birth she insisted on breast-feeding her child, and every time, in the third month, her milk was suppressed and mania broke out.

Only four reports date the first postpartum menses.

The most convincing cases will be summarized: the first[87] describes a recurrent bipolar disorder, with 1st trimester prepartum and 4-month weaning episodes, and Cotard features:

> A 33-year old was mother of four children. When she became pregnant for the 5th time she started making ridiculous purchases, borrowing the money. She twice ran away, once to a distant destination reached by walking day and night, where she was found three days later covered with mud and bruises, her clothing in tatters. She improved after six weeks but remained feeble and had to be watched like a child. After the birth (during which she made not a single cry) there was an immediate and remarkable recovery, and she remained well until the 4th month of breast-feeding, when her milk supply failed. Five days later she became *gâteuse* [soft in the head] and lost her memory. Admitted to hospital, she was silent and sad, and refused to eat because she had no stomach, feet, arms or head. During her menses she became agitated, then lapsed into stupor. She could not walk without help, and became emaciated.

The second[471,472] describes a recurrent bipolar disorder, with first trimester prepartum, short gestation and 11-month weaning episodes:

> A young married woman had two children. During her third pregnancy, her character changed – she made obscene remarks, forgot her modesty and sought the company of men, reacting violently to criticism. At five months gestation, climbing out of a first floor window, she fell and provoked a miscarriage. She immediately returned to normal – calm, sweet and demure. Although sympathetic about the loss of the baby, everyone was happy that she had ceased to run wild. She then suddenly became manic – shouting, vociferating and assaultive – and had to be admitted to an asylum. After 48 hours she completely recovered – a good housewife and excellent mother. She became pregnant for the 4th time, and gave birth to a child, whom she breast-fed for eleven months. No sooner had she weaned the baby than she lost weight, became stranger to all tender affections and sank into a state of depression and inertia. Admitted to hospital, she was mute, completely immobile and ate nothing. While she was improving, she had her first haemoptysis and soon died of tuberculosis.

The next four patients were reported by Marcé[203]. The first had a brief manic episode 14 months after the birth, occurring three days after weaning and six days before the first postpartum menses:

> A 26-year old, an *enfant trouvée* who worked as a domestic at the Salpêtrière, breast-fed her 2nd child for 14 months. After an argument with her boss she abruptly weaned the child, and, three days later, became overactive, sleepless and incoherent. Admitted to the same hospital, she was excited and overtalkative. Three days later she menstruated for the 1st time since the birth. She recovered and was discharged well after only eight days (case 61).

The second had a brief manic episode six months after the birth, occurring 10 days after weaning with a menstrual exacerbation:

> A 25-year old developed acute mania ten days after she weaned her 6-month old child. She was agitated, sleepless and loquacious. Five days later there was an exacerbation, coincident with the return of her menses. After two days she recovered and remained well (case 65).

The third was a depressive psychosis, 16 months after the birth, starting three days after weaning:

> A 31-year old had to stop breast-feeding her 2nd child after 16 months. Three days later, she developed insomnia and *délire*. On admission to hospital she was melancholic, suicidal and

tormented by hallucinations including the crying of her infant; she thought she would be guillotined. She recovered a month later (case 70).

The fourth was a depressive psychosis that started nearly two years after the birth, a few days after weaning:

> A 20-year old weaned her 3rd child at twenty-one months. A few days later she developed *délire* and was admitted to hospital: she was melancholic and refused to eat or speak, tormented by imaginary fears. She remained ill for three months (case 72).

This is Révolat's[473] recurrent case:

> A 30-year old, while breast-feeding her 3rd child, had a scare that one of her children had been run over by a carriage; although this was not true, she immediately developed a *folie*, which lasted two years. The author did not know whether suppression of her milk came before, after or simultaneously with this event. Five years later, after breast-feeding her next child for a year, she weaned it abruptly and immediately became manic for four months. The same happened with the next pregnancy – the psychosis started at the moment of weaning, and lasted eighteen months. In the course of 8–9 years she had one other episode unrelated to childbearing.

Joyce[474] described this case from New Zealand:

> A 31-year old, whose father probably committed suicide, breast-fed her 1st child for twelve months; her milk had been drying up but the child appeared to initiate the weaning. Immediately afterwards, she developed a manic episode that lasted six weeks and was followed by depression lasting 4-5 months. Two years later, within a week of weaning her 2nd child, aged six months, she developed another psychosis, with perplexity, insomnia, restlessness, over-activity, over-talkativeness, pressure of speech and flight of ideas. She recovered within three weeks.

In my series, I had no convincing case of weaning onset. One mother had three late postpartum episodes: one, at five months, was perhaps coincident with weaning, but there was doubt about her reliability. It is curious that the majority of cases date from the nineteenth century, and it seems possible that, in Victorian times, mothers, with less access to safe supplementary feeding, breast-fed for longer. But in third world countries, breast-feeding rates are still high, and, if this is the explanation, one would expect to see weaning onsets.

The case for a weaning trigger of bipolar/cycloid episodes is further discussed in Section 6 (page 360).

Unknown Onset

In 259 cases (352 episodes) in the literature, and 15 of my own, the relationship between the onset of psychosis and the birth was not stated. This was also true of 51 recurrent cases.

Summary of Episode Diagnoses

Episode diagnoses, related to onset, are shown in Table 20.7 (the literature) and Table 20.8 (my series). Eighteen organic psychoses have been omitted from Table 20.8.

Comment

In the literature:

- In 66 per cent of cases the only possible diagnosis was unspecified psychosis.
- There are relatively few depressive psychoses in the early postpartum and post-abortion onset groups.

- There are surprisingly few bipolars in the early postpartum group, especially when compared with the post-abortion, prepartum and weaning onset groups; this is difficult to explain, but with data of this quality, it seems best to await further evidence.
- The last column shows the proportion of recurrent to single cases. The high proportion of recurrent cases among the weaning and post-abortion groups can be explained by failure to notice the association in single episodes.

Table 20.7 Non-organic psychosis in the literature episode diagnoses, related to onset

Onset	Psychosis unspecified	Depressive psychosis	Bipolar	Other	Total	Per semester	Recurrent/ single (%)
After abortion	52	9 (8%)	30 (27%)	17	**108**	108	40
Pregnancy	188	126 (29%)	99 (23%)	25	**438**	146	31
Early postpartum[a]	1,008	198 (15%)	76 (6%)	17	**1,299**	5,629	20
4–13 week onset	269	92 (22%)	40 (10%)	8	**409**	531	18
Late postpartum	133	50 (21%)	38 (16%)	13	**234**	78	27
Weaning	21	11 (28%)	8 (20%)	Nil	**40**		44
Unknown onset	243	83 (24%)	18 (5%)	8	**352**		20
Total	**1,914**	**569**	**309**	**88**	**2,880**		

[a] Includes short gestation with early postpartum onset, parturient and day 1 onsets

Table 20.8 Episode diagnoses in my series related to onset

Onset	Bipolar	Cycloid	Bipolar/ cycloids, %	Depressive psychosis	Other	Total	Per semester
Abortion	12	2	58	3 (10%)	7	**24**	24
Pregnancy	35	8	61	9 (28%)	18	**70**	23
Early postpartum	149	84	77	42 (14%)	27	**302**	1,308
4–13 week onset	12	7	46	12 (29%)	10	**41**	53
Late postpartum	5	1	35	10 (59%)	1	**17**	6
Unknown onset	7	Nil	46	1	7	**15**	
Total	**220**	**102**	**69**	**77 (16%)**	**70**	**469**	

The other diagnoses included psychogenic, cycloid and paranoid psychoses, and morbid jealousy as the sole symptom.

Comparing my series with the literature:

- The relative lack of depressive psychoses in the post-abortion and early onset groups is confirmed.
- There were no weaning onsets.
- There was a smaller proportion of 4–13 week onsets.
- The greater frequency of bipolar disorders in post-abortion and prepartum groups than in early onset group is not confirmed.
- The proportion of bipolar/cycloids is relatively low in the 4–13 week and late postpartum onset groups.

The other psychoses were psychosis unspecified (21), paranoid disorder (18), auditory hallucinations and disorders of the will and self as the sole symptom (10), non-psychotic disorders mistaken for psychoses (4), psychogenic episodes (3) and recurrent postpartum stupor (1).

Although depressive psychoses were more frequent in the 4–13 week onset group, they were still a small minority, so most mothers who become ill in this time frame are not suffering from depression, triggered by the birth but slow to develop or reach psychiatric care.

Matrix of Associations

History

Esquirol described, rather telegrammatically, a patient followed long term, who had four triggers – puerperal, seasonal, weaning (with a relapse) and abortion[104]:

> A 26-year old gave birth to her 1st child. On day 3 she developed furious mania that lasted for two months. Every spring she showed exaltation without psychosis. At 30, when weaning her second child aged one year, she developed mania, from which she recovered soon after hospitalisation; but, two days after her discharge, she relapsed, recovering after three months. At 34 she had a 2-month miscarriage; the next day she became loquacious and developed mania that lasted only a few days (case 6).

Among Marcé's cases were two with evidence of three triggers. The first[203] had post-abortion, recurrent prepartum and late postpartum (menstrual) onsets:

> A 34-year old suffered from a transient mental disorder after a miscarriage. She became ill in the last days of four pregnancies and remained ill until 8–10 days after weaning; after her 5th delivery, the psychosis began at the first menses (case 57).

The second was the description of a menstrual psychosis after weaning, with hints of a seasonal element, summarized on page 327[92].

Analysis of Cases with More than One Reproductive Episode

In the literature there were 397 recurrent childbearing psychoses, from which the following were omitted:

54 In which all episodes were of unknown onset

50 With only one episode of known onset

8 With the other episode(s) having no psychotic features

9 Involving weaning onsets

8 In which the other episode was an organic psychosis

3 In which the other episode was post-operative

This left 265 for analysis, of which 133 had onsets limited to one time frame, and 132 had onsets starting in different time frames. When constructing the matrix (Figure 20.1), cases were assigned to boxes when a mother had one or more episodes in both time frames. Thus, a mother with two early and three 4–13 week onsets scored just one in the box for associated early and 4–13 week onsets, but a mother with onsets three weeks, three months and four months after the birth counted one in each of three boxes – early and 4–13 week onsets, early and >3 month onsets and 4–13 week and >3 month onsets.

	Abortion	Prepartum	Early onset	4 – 13 week	> 3 months	Total cases
Abortion	4 (4%)	8	15	2	1	99
Prepartum		41 (10%)	51	8	12	407
Early onset			74 (6%)	19	20	1,211
4 – 13 week onset				8 (2%)	12	399
> 3 months					7 (3%)	215

Figure 20.1 Matrix of associations in the literature. The percentages refer to the proportion of all cases in that time frame.

	Abortion	Prepartum	Early onset	4 – 13 week	> 3 months	Total cases
Abortion	1 (5%)	3	11	3		21
Prepartum		9 (13%)	23	9	3	70
Early onset			57 (19%)	12	4	302
4 – 13 week onset				4 (10%)	3	41
> 3 months					1 (6%)	17

Figure 20.2 Matrix of associations in my series. The percentages refer to the proportion of all cases in that time frame.

In my series, there were 151 mothers with multiple episodes, of which 33 were excluded because there were data on only one psychotic episode, leaving 118 for the analysis.

Findings

- In the literature, all associations between onset groups had at least five examples, except the association between post-abortion and both groups of late postpartum onsets. In my series, all had at least three examples except post-abortion and >3 month postpartum onsets. There is, therefore, a *prima facie* case for a general factor underlying all these onsets, although it remains possible that the shared factor is the bipolar/cycloid diathesis
- The large number of recurrent prepartum onsets (proportionately more than for any other group, except, in my series, early postpartum onset) supports the case for a specific prepartum trigger
- The large number of cases with shared prepartum and early postpartum onset (more in both series than 4–13 week onset, which had a similar number of cases) suggests that the prepartum factor is closer to the early postpartum factor than is the 4–13 week factor.

When considering the possibility that the association between all onset groups is due to a shared bipolar/cycloid diathesis, the baseline frequency of episodes unrelated to reproduction, determined in mothers followed long term, is germane. To address this question, one needs mothers with different reproductive onsets and a relative lack of unrelated episodes, studied for many years. There are none in my series, but, in the literature, there were three informative cases. The first[419], followed for more than 10 years, had one post-abortion, one prepartum and no unrelated episodes:

> A 26-year old was first admitted in the 8th month of her 1st pregnancy, with eight days history of anxious confusion; she had made three suicide attempts. Her 2nd admission was seven years later, eight days after curettage for an incomplete abortion. She was confused with catatonic features (case 20).

The second, followed for 20 years, had episodes related to weaning, menstruation, childbirth, pregnancy and short gestation, as well as three unrelated episodes[109]:

> At the age of 28, a woman, with a strong family history of mental illness, gave birth to her 1st child, and breast-fed for four months. After weaning she developed insomnia and restlessness; her ideas were lively, she acted on a fear that the house was burning down and thought she was under surveillance because of her poor child-care. Admitted to hospital, she was perplexed and confused and had difficulty in distinguishing dream from reality; she misidentified people and had a persistent idea that she was pregnant. She improved, relapsed and then recovered, but had several premenstrual deteriorations. Three years later she gave birth to her 2nd child. On day 3 she was sleepless and anorexic, and believed the child was not getting enough milk. Admitted to hospital, she was perplexed, agitated and depressed with ideas of guilt and 'paranoid-hallucinatory elements'. Discharged after two months, she became hypomanic, spent a lot of money and gave presents to everybody. A year later she became pregnant for the 3rd time. In the 2nd trimester she became depressed, then manic. She heard voices – the neighbours were talking about her, but God and his angels were protecting her. Admitted to hospital, she was anxious and retarded and had difficulty with her memory; she was instructed by good and bad voices. She gave birth to a 5-month macerated foetus. Two weeks after improvement she relapsed with hypomania. She had three unrelated episodes (case 8).

The third, one of those comprehensively described by Van Steenbergen–van der Nordaa[96], and followed for 39 years, suffered an untimed postpartum episode, a possible eclamptic episode, one with onset 4–13 weeks after childbirth, one in the ninth month of pregnancy and only two unrelated episodes:

A 27-year old was admitted to an asylum for nine months following the birth of her 2nd child. Two years later she gave birth to her 4th child, after which she suffered a seizure, associated with albuminuria and oedema of the feet. The child soon died. She became disturbed - laughing, singing, restless and disorientated, with visual and auditory hallucinations, stereotypies and catalepsy. She recovered 18 months later. Nine weeks after her 5th delivery she started to sing and pray. Her speech was disturbed with flight of ideas and neologisms, and she was restless and excited. She wanted to visit her mother, dead these two years. She seemed to be in a dream-like state. She recovered in four months. At the age of 36 she became 'confused' at the end of her 7th pregnancy – she was praying, had dead people in her mind, and two days before admission ran away from home and took a carriage to a celebration. She was somewhat elevated in mood, cheered the doctor, and had fits of laughing. Five years later she again developed hyperactivity with pressure of speech, singing and dancing, preoccupied with religion, visions of the Virgin Mary and auditory hallucinations. On admission she was cataleptic. She recovered in two months, and remained well for eleven years, when she became overactive and excited, spoke nonsense and tried to jump from a 2nd floor balcony. From that time she remained in hospital, with bizarre ideas, laughing attacks and grimacing until her death from cancer at 66.

It would be a mistake to apply multivariate statistics to data of the quality so far available. But the number of mothers with complex associations suggests that there are shared elements in the triggering of reproductive episodes.

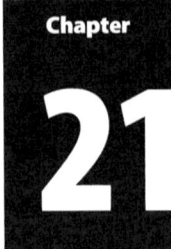

Chapter

21

The Bipolar/Cycloid Group

Introduction

One of the problems of research into 'puerperal psychosis' has been the heterogeneity of the samples studied. I had the opportunity to study a more homogeneous sample by focusing on 214 mothers (with 337 episodes), who suffered from bipolar/cycloid disorder, of which 115 were followed for at least ten years. This chapter will present some data on this group, referring to the literature, where appropriate.

Some Miscellaneous Data

Parity

This was known in 330 bipolar/cycloid episodes – 46 with prepartum onset, 252 early and 32 late postpartum onset. For prepartum the mean was 2.04, with 37% *primiparae*. For early postpartum the mean was 1.58, with 58% *primiparae*. For late postpartum the mean was 2.19, with 38% *primipara*. This accords with survey data on the association of early postpartum onset with the first birth, and greater parity in prepartum and late postpartum episodes. It agrees with the findings of Di Florio's[475] study of 934 women with 'bipolar I' that episodes with onset less than six weeks after the birth were associated with the first birth (odds ratio 2.0), but episodes starting in pregnancy or later in the postpartum period were not.

Secondary Sex Ratio

The child's sex was known in 317 pregnancies. Excluding a pair of dizygotic twins, 178 were boys and 138 girls, a ratio of 1.29. This could also be examined in 81 mothers who had both affected and unaffected pregnancies. In thirteen the child's sex was unknown; in the rest there were 60 boys and 58 girls, a ratio of 1.03, which is close to the usual figure for the general population (1.06). If the bipolar/cycloid group is subdivided into prepartum, early and late onsets, the ratios are 23/18 (1.28), 144/105 (1.37) and 11/15 (0.73). These findings require confirmation in a separate sample.

Treatment Response

Bipolar/cycloid mothers seem to be particularly susceptible to extra-pyramidal side effects of neuroleptic agents (see page 228).

Breastfeeding

Questions were asked about each birth in the Anne Roper interview (see Appendix), but the answers were often vague. I decided to omit such cases and focus on those who definitely did not breast-feed and those who continued for at least a week, or until the onset of the psychosis. On this basis, 79 mothers were breastfeeding or lactating (for example, expressing milk) and 36 were definitely not breast-feeding.

Evidence presented in chapter 5 above indicated that the onset of early postpartum episodes can (without doubt) occur on day 1, (probably) during labour and (possibly) shortly before labour. Breast-feeding can have little or no effect on hormone output for a few days after the birth. The early postpartum trigger, therefore, acts at an earlier stage. The same is not true of late postpartum episodes. It would be interesting to know whether their frequency and timing was affected by lactation.

Frequency in Different Onset Groups

Abortion

In my series, 139 abortions were recorded in mothers in the bipolar/cycloid group, including 90 miscarriages, 49 terminations and two mole pregnancies. Miscarriages were suffered by 48 mothers, affecting 22% of 435 pregnancies that were not terminated: this fails to confirm Kendell's[41] finding of a low miscarriage rate in mothers with postpartum psychosis; the figure is inflated by one mother who had 18 miscarriages, but, without her, 18% of pregnancies miscarried – about the same as the general population. All but two of the mothers with post-abortion psychosis, and 21/24 post-abortion episodes, belonged to the bipolar/cycloid group. The rates after termination and miscarriage were not significantly different.

Pregnancy

Twenty bipolar/cycloid mothers presented with prepartum episodes: two of them (after recovery) went on to suffer intrapartum or late postpartum episodes after the same pregnancy. Another 17 mothers presented with a postpartum episode, and later had a prepartum episode.

Short Gestation, Intra-Partum, Day 1 Onsets and Early Postpartum Onsets

Almost all mothers with short gestation episodes (5/6), intra-partum onsets (3/4) and day 1 onsets (15/17) were bipolar/cycloid. This is different from the main group of early postpartum onsets (between days 2–21), in whom 165/218 (76%) were bipolar/cycloid and 53 (24%) depressive, organic or paranoid.

Later Postpartum Onset

Only 20/43 mothers, who had 4–13 week onsets, were bipolar/cycloid. This was a surprisingly low figure, considering that there is no impediment to mother & baby units admitting mothers with psychoses that begin in this time frame.

Of those starting more than three months after the birth, only 7/17 were bipolar/cycloid and the rest suffered from depressive psychoses.

These longitudinal data confirm that bipolar/cycloid mothers can have a wide variety of reproductive onsets, not just early postpartum.

The Course

Duration of Episodes

In my bipolar/cycloid group, duration could be estimated for 288 episodes. The mean was 2.4 months (73 days); only 18 lasted less than two weeks. Recovery and resumption of normal life, with the care of children and grandchildren, was the rule. Only two mothers in my series were in hostel or residential care, and one of these suffered from multiple sclerosis.

Recurrences

There were 148 mothers with at least two full-term pregnancies. Of their 383 subsequent births, 105 were unaffected and 278 (73%) complicated by a reproductive episode. This is much higher than in the 'follow-up studies' reviewed in chapter 16 (pages 143–146). The onsets were prepartum (40), early postpartum (204), 4–13 weeks (20), >3 months (3) and unknown (11).

Table 21.1 (on the next page) compares recurrences in four onset groups. The first column gives the number of mothers who *first* presented with an episode in that onset group, and had a subsequent pregnancy.

All four onset groups had the same high recurrence rate (70–80%). The onset groups seem completely intermingled, almost as if they were interchangeable.

Mothers with Both Puerperal and Non-Puerperal Episodes

Reich & Winokur[131] reported a 100% relapse rate in six bipolar mothers with both reproductive and unrelated episodes. Bergink[476], as part of a prevention programme, followed eight bipolar women with both puerperal and non-puerperal episodes: only four (50%) had a 'peripartum' relapse during their next pregnancy. In my series there were 44 mothers who had a non-reproductive episode before the 'index episode', or between it and the next pregnancy; nine were not bipolar/cycloid, leaving 35 for the analysis. The onsets were early postpartum (25), post-abortion and prepartum (three each), and 4–13 week and 5–6 months (two each). There were 50 subsequent full-term pregnancies, 45 of which (90%) were complicated by a psychosis, although this was subclinical (hypomania) in three and considered to be psychogenic in one – a recurrence rate of 82% for undisputed major episodes. The recurrences were prepartum in 15, early postpartum in 24, 4–13 week onset in four and 7-month onset in one; two of those who remained well, and one with subclinical hypomania, were on lithium prophylaxis, and one was taking progesterone as a prophylactic. This gives some support to the claim that mothers with both reproductive and unrelated episodes are at higher risk. The recurrence was prepartum in one third.

Frequency of Episodes Unrelated to Reproduction

Those followed long term had 166 episodes unrelated to childbearing (3.8 each) in a mean of 23 years – an average of one non-reproductive episode every six years.

Table 21.1 Recurrences in Bipolar/Cycloid Mothers with Different Onsets

Onset group	Number of mothers	Number of subsequent pregnancies	Post-abortion recurrence	Prepartum recurrence	Early postpartum recurrence	Late postpartum Recurrence*	Unknown onset	Total
Post-abortion	11	22	2	1	11	3		17/22 (77%)
Prepartum	20	14		7	1	2¶		10/14 (71%)
Early postpartum	103	141	4	18	67	4¶	6	99/141 (70%)
4–13 week onset	11	5	1	1	3	1§		5/5 (100%)

* All 4–13 week onset unless otherwise stated

¶ This includes one with onset >3 months postpartum

§ This mother had a prepartum and 4–13 week onset episode in the same pregnancy

215

Relapses

These were noted in 74 mothers, of which 61 were in the bipolar/cycloid group and 13 among the others (p = .012). The high figure in the bipolar/cycloid group (28%) is underpinned by the higher rates found in three French studies[94,101,102]. Focusing on this group, the great majority followed an early postpartum episode with a frequency of 62/296 episodes (21%): there was one after a post-abortion episode, two after 4–13 week onsets, and two with unknown onset. Multiple relapses were noted in 24 mothers: twelve relapsed twice, eight thrice, and one each four, five and six times. Five had relapses after two separate postpartum episodes, including two with different onsets – one with a post-abortion and early postpartum onset, and one with a 4–13 week and early postpartum onset. Two had relapses after each of three early postpartum episodes.

The Menopause

There was one mother in my series with a single recurrence within a few months of the menopause:

> A 31-year old professional woman gave birth to her 1st child. On day 5 she became elated, sleepless and talkative, then unable to communicate (so that she had to write everything down). She could not make sense of what was happening, and was unsure whether she was dreaming, or had died. God was talking to her, and the psychiatrist was Jesus. Committed to hospital, she recovered within three weeks, but suffered from prolonged depression, aggravated by the death of her beloved father. She remained in good mental health for many years in spite of a second birth and Graves' disease, treated by radioactive iodine. At 47 she stopped oral contraceptives and was fitted with a Mirena coil, after which there were hardly any signs of menstrual bleeding (but no menopausal symptoms such as nocturnal sweating). Ten months later she developed a delusional bipolar illness that continued, almost without interruption, for 12 months, until arrested by valproate.

Even though 59 mothers were followed for more than 20 years, and 43 beyond the age of 50, my study has failed to find any convincing evidence of a menopausal effect.

Association with Medical and Surgical Disease

Since some postpartum psychoses are bipolar disorders, one might expect an association with other known bipolar triggers, such as seasonal changes, surgical operations and corticosteroid treatment. Data from the literature and my series are reported here.

Seasonal Affective Disorder

This was mentioned by Van Swieten[477] in this cryptic passage:

> In others, the footsteps of the old distemper have continued strong enough to cause recurrences about the time of the vernal or autumnal equinoxes . . . I have visited several who are accustomed to the raving madness during 3–4 weeks of the Spring season, remaining well for the rest of the year.

In the literature there are only four cases with even a hint of this association: Esquirol's 6th case[104] 'showed exaltation without *délire* every spring', Westphal's[478] had attacks of raving (when she was sleepless and unstoppably talkative for two weeks) in the autumn and spring, and regular episodes of melancholia in the summer, Raty-Vohsen's 3rd case[366] showed a tendency to depression in the spring and autumn, and Casiano's 2nd case[479] had exacerbations at least once/year, usually in the autumn.

In my series one mother's bipolar disorder worsened in the winter, and it was decided to provide her with a light machine. Another, who suffered six bipolar/cycloid episodes in 37 years, including two with onset within three weeks of childbirth, said that in the winter she lay in bed, and needed to increase her antidepressant medication. These published and personal cases offer scant evidence of an association of postpartum psychosis and seasonal affective disorder. Since many mothers in my series were followed long-term, it is fairly certain that there is no association.

Post-Operative Psychosis

In the literature there are eight instances of the association of postpartum and post-operative psychoses, three following sterilization[96,417,480], two after oöphorectomy[106] and three after other surgical operations[96,480,481]. In my series, only 46 surgical operations were known to have been performed during the study period. Five mothers had post-operative episodes. These are the details:

A 33-year old, with a bipolar/cycloid disorder, had one onset during labour, and one in the 3rd trimester in close temporal relationship to the surgical removal of an ovarian cyst. She had nine other episodes in the course of 15 years.

An 18-year old suffered a perforated duodenal ulcer, treated by partial gastrectomy. On the day of discharge, she developed 'acute schizophrenia' – up all night, talking incoherently, hearing voices and replying to messages from the radio saying that someone was trying to take over her brain. Admitted to hospital, she was unkempt and labile in mood, and was considered to have hallucinations, thought disorder and thought insertion. She later had three early postpartum schizo-affective or cycloid episodes as well as suicidal depressions.

A 29-year old suffered a postpartum episode with unknown onset, and later four other bipolar episodes. At 44, after a hysterectomy, she immediately became high and giggly, overtalkative, and required only two hours of sleep. She recovered, then, one month later, relapsed and was ill for another month.

A 25-year old became elated in the 3rd trimester of her only pregnancy, and, six weeks after the birth, depressed, with mutism. In the next 35 years she suffered 45 bipolar episodes. At 27 she was sterilized. After the operation she became elated, then depressed for 6–8 weeks.

The 5th mother had only three psychotic episodes in 39 years, one after one of her three births (but none after four abortions), and two after surgical operations:

A 25-year old developed a puerperal cycloid episode, with onset day 9, after her 1st birth. She had only two other episodes, both following surgery: after hysterectomy she was briefly hypomanic, and after a double knee replacement she suffered an acute psychosis, with pressure of speech, incoherence, violence and delusions of reference, poisoning and jealousy.

The frequency 5/46 (11%) is about the same as post-abortion episodes (14%).

It should be noted that many mothers were delivered by Caesarean section or forceps under general anaesthesia; in my bipolar/cycloid group, this was the mode of delivery in 30 episodes, only one of which was conducted under spinal anaesthesia. In addition, surgical evacuation of the uterus is sometimes necessary after miscarriage: one mother (summarized on pages 187 and 189) had two post-abortion episodes, both followed by dilatation and curettage under anaesthesia.

Corticosteroid Therapy

This was introduced into therapeutics about 1950. There is scattered evidence that adrenal corticosteroids can trigger psychotic episodes, as recently reviewed[482,483]. In the literature there are two instances of the association of puerperal and steroid psychoses[484,485], to which I can add six, which are briefly summarized below:

A 29-year old became pregnant for the 1st time. Because of foetal distress, she was delivered at 35 weeks gestation by emergency Caesarean section. She had two doses of dexamethasone at the time of delivery. On day 2 she became sleepless and began writing copious notes. By day 7 she became overactive and aggressive, and said the television and radio referred to her, and her husband was trying to infect her and the baby with AIDS, which he had contracted during an affair. She later had a second episode of postpartum mania, with onset six weeks after the birth.

A 35-year old, after six years of infertility, conceived with gamete intra-fallopian transfer, and became pregnant with twins. At 30 weeks gestation, she was given dexamethasone to increase the maturity of the foetal lungs. A week later she was admitted to the maternity hospital with antepartum bleeding. She became excited, elated and sleepless and expressed persecutory ideas. She was talking constantly, giving a running commentary on everything that was happening. At 32 weeks gestation, she gave birth; one of the twins had Down's syndrome. Three weeks later her psychosis recurred, with head-banging, restlessness, insomnia and racing thoughts. On admission to hospital she was depressed, and did not recover until five months later. She remained well during the next 20 years.

A 28-year old gave birth to her 1st child. For two weeks she was 'on a high', talking non-stop. Six weeks later she developed pityriasis rosea, treated with steroids. She became very high, 'brilliant', her mind racing. This lasted a week until she stopped the steroids. She then became depressed for a year. Her baby also became high on steroids.

A 35-year old, who for several years had suffered from poly-arthritis and Crohn's disease, developed pre-eclamptic toxaemia during her 1st pregnancy, and was delivered by Caesarean section. On day 12 she developed a cycloid psychosis – slow, confused and perplexed – from which she recovered within three weeks. When the baby was four months old, her arthritis recurred. Treated with ibuprofen, she developed a purpuric vasculitis with bullous lesions (Stevens-Johnson syndrome), together with laboratory evidence of systemic lupus erythematosus. She was treated with prednisolone 60 mg/day. Within four days she became withdrawn and mute, staring into the distance. She washed obsessively, complaining of sweating and halitosis. A CAT scan showed diffuse cerebral abnormalities, and an EEG low frequency activity. She was again treated with steroids, and recovered in three months. Her failure to respond to lithium prophylaxis is described on page 231, and her later psychogenic episode on page 171.

A 24-year old, whose mother suffered from puerperal psychosis after her own birth, became pregnant for the 1st time. Two days before the onset of labour she developed a rash, which was treated with prednisone 20mg/day. After the birth, on day 7, she became weepy, and disorientated, then elated and confused. She felt her brain was exploding. She thought her partner was trying to kill her and believed she was the Messiah. She telephoned a minister to say she had the solution to the Irish problem. She was writing reams of gibberish, which she believed was important to the future of humanity. After recovery she suffered severe bonding problems, which continued after the second baby was born. In 28 years she suffered one further manic episode.

A 28-year old, at 35 weeks gestation, was treated with prednisolone for idiopathic thrombocytopenia. At 39 weeks she was delivered by forceps, and steroids were discontinued.

On day 3 she became agitated, weepy and perplexed, with confusion and 'paranoid' ideation. On admission to hospital, prednisolone was started again. She remained retarded, vague and suspicious, staring into space, and speaking in a monotonous voice of being evil, hopeless and a failure. She denied the existence of her husband and the baby. She suddenly disrobed and started shouting, "Let me die!" After seven days she abruptly improved. Two weeks later steroids were stopped, but were soon started again because a diagnosis of systemic lupus erythematosus was made. She had no further episode in the course of nine years.

Only four other mothers were treated with steroids in any form. Furthermore, these six mothers, in a total of 88 years observation, had only one psychotic episode between them, apart from those associated with childbearing or steroid therapy. It seems best to regard these episodes as steroid psychoses not childbearing psychoses.

Thyroid Disease

In the literature there are 18 instances of an association with thyroid disease, to which I can add ten. Some of these seem obviously fortuitous: one had carcinoma of the thyroid[486] and one in my series had thyroglossal cysts . Two in the literature[101,487], and two in my series had non-toxic goiters. Two in the literature developed incidental hypothyroidism[97,488] (before the use of lithium to treat bipolar disorder), and two in my series developed hypothyroidism following lithium prophylaxis.

Recently an association with auto-immune thyroiditis has been claimed[58]. During pregnancy antibody titres decrease to protect the foetus[489], and, when they rebound after the birth, a destructive auto-immune thyroiditis can develop[490]; this is mainly due to anti-thyroid peroxidase antibodies, and can lead to transient or persistent hypo-thyroidism, hyper-thyroidism or both in sequence; its frequency is about 5%[491,492] and onset 1–3 months after the birth. There are also recent publications claiming that bipolar disorder is associated with auto-immune thyroiditis[493], although this was not confirmed by large American and Danish epidemiological studies[494,495]. Three relevant cases have been published[58,496,497]:

A 28-year old gave birth to her 1st child. On day 3 she became convinced that her husband would kill the baby. Over the next four days she became impulsive, irritable, violent and disorganized. With haloperidol and lithium therapy she recovered in three weeks. Three months postpartum a diagnosis of auto-immune thyroiditis was made.

Eleven weeks after her 3rd child was born, a 29-year old developed insomnia, weight loss and fatigue intolerance. She appeared confused and was disorientated in time and place. She heard Jesus talking to her, and had visual hallucinations. She believed she was pregnant with the Christ child, and would be killed by hospital staff. She had thyrotoxicosis, associated with thyroiditis. Her psychiatric symptoms improved concurrently with its treatment.

A 35-year old gave birth to twins. Seven months later she presented with increased energy, lack of the need for sleep and racing thoughts; she was preoccupied with bible reading, and the belief that God had fathered her babies. On admission she was found to have myxoedema due to postpartum thyroiditis. With thyroxin and risperidone she recovered within six days.

One of my series developed this disorder at the age of 52, nine years after her last child was born.

Auto-immune thyroid disease was first recognized in 1956, since when about 1,000 detailed cases of postpartum psychosis have been published. A rebound auto-immune phenomenon cannot account for early onset postpartum episodes (which can begin on day 1 or even earlier), but might be relevant to late postpartum episodes, such as those of Bokhari[496] and Stowell[497]; but the psychosis could be due to the thyroid dysfunction, not auto-immunity: Graves' disease is occasionally associated with acute psychosis, as shown by at least nine case reports and Brownlie's survey in New Zealand[498]: three patients have recovered after surgical treatment[499–501], and others after treatment with propylthiouracil[502] or propranolol[503].

The association of childbearing psychoses with thyrotoxicosis deserves consideration. Normal pregnancy may be associated with transient thyrotoxicosis[504,505]. The prevalence of thyrotoxicosis is 0.5–2%[506], so that at least 20 patients in the literature and up to six of my series would be expected to have this disease in their lifespan. One can therefore discount several cases in the literature with a history of Graves' disease not synchronous with postpartum episodes[90,507–509], together with a mother in my series who developed thyrotoxicosis four years before her postpartum episode, and two who became thyrotoxic some years later. Table 21.2 (on the next page) shows those with a closer temporal relationship:

In all there are eleven mothers with concurrent childbearing psychosis and thyrotoxicosis; one had prepartum, four late postpartum, five early postpartum and one unknown onset. Three had other episodes of postpartum psychosis that were not accompanied by thyrotoxicosis. One may have responded to thyroid treatment alone but there is no consistency in this evidence. It is possible that thyrotoxicosis acts as a trigger, or synergistically with the puerperal factor but more information is required.

Other Associations

Epilepsy was covered in section 2 (pages 56–58). Among the occasional associations are polycystic ovaries (two in my series), virilising disorder[418], galactorrhoea independent of lactation and treatment with neuroleptic agents[395] and systemic lupus erythematosus, closely related to postpartum episodes (two from my series). All these other associations were found in single cases and were presumably incidental. Several mothers in my series had a mild degree of learning disability, but this seems less common than in menstrual psychosis (see page 337).

Repetition of the Matrix of Associations

The last chapter reported a matrix of associations in 118 mothers from my series. After eliminating all non-bipolar/cycloid mothers, Figure 21.1 (on page 222) shows the revised matrix. The last column shows the number of mothers with an episode in this time frame.

When compared with the matrices reported in chapter 20, the associations between groups are upheld, except those between prepartum and 4–13 week and late postpartum onsets, and between 4–13 week and >3 months onset.

Affected and Unaffected Pregnancies

This strategy has the same aims as population-based epidemiology, but compares reproductive events in the lives of the mothers themselves. After excluding all those who suffered a psychotic episode after each full-term pregnancy, there were 76 bipolar/cycloid mothers with at least one unaffected pregnancy. It seemed best to exclude those in whom this was complicated by a subclinical episode (four episodes), hypomania (four episodes) or depression (in one case anxiety) severe enough to require treatment (eleven episodes in all). This

Table 21.2 Association with Thyrotoxicosis.
This omits the cases of Bokhari[496] and Stowell[497] summarized in the text.

1st author	Clinical features	Evidence of thyrotoxicosis	Comment
Johnstone (1884)[510]	Onset of psychosis six months after the birth of her 3rd child	Signs of exophthalmic goitre developed concurrently	Late postpartum onset
Knauer (1897)[69] Case 65	Onset of a chronic depressive psychosis after her 6th birth	She developed thyrotoxicosis	No data on timing
Sivadon (1933)[86] Case 15	Onset of psychosis on day 9 after her 1st birth	She had an enlarged thyroid and tremor. She also had a fever of 38°	She died on day 22, possibly due to infection
Schröder (1936)[110] case 38	She gave birth at 38, and on day 11 developed a psychosis	She had a goiter at the age of ten and puerperal psychosis at 38; seven months later, while still psychotic, she was noted to have slight exophthalmos and sweaty hands	Thyrotoxicosis was noticed seven months later
Abély (1947)[511]	Onset of psychosis shortly after the 2nd, 3rd, 4th & 5th births	During two episodes, thyroid enlargement was noted. During the 4th episode, tests showed transitory hyperthyroidism, whose disappearance coincided with clinical improvement	Only the 4th episode of postpartum psychosis was affected
Retzeanu (1960)[512]	Onset of psychosis in the 9th month of gestation	She had a large soft thyroid and tachycardia; she refused surgery on her goiter and was treated with psychotropic drugs and radioactive iodine. Improvement in mental state and reduction in goiter were concurrent	Prepartum psychosis, with a possible response to anti-thyroid treatment. She also had pleurisy and galactorrhoea
Butts (1968)[488]	Psychosis of unknown onset after 1st birth, and with onset day 7 after the second	During the second episode she had an enlarged thyroid, systolic murmur and tremor; but her protein-bound iodine was only 4.4μg/100ml and her basal metabolic rate minus 12%	Only the 2nd episode of postpartum psychosis was affected. Evidence of thyrotoxicosis was equivocal
My Series	Onset of depressive psychosis seven months after her 2nd birth	Goitre, loss of weight and tremor during the pregnancy	Late postpartum onset, response to ECT
	Psychosis on day 5 after both her 1st and 2nd births	During her 2nd postpartum episode she was noticed to have a goiter & clinical signs; the diagnosis was confirmed by laboratory tests. Treatment included radioactive iodine	Only the 2nd episode was affected.

221

Figure 21.1 Revised Matrix of Associations

	Abortion	Prepartum	Early onset	4 – 13 week	> 3 months	Number in onset group
Abortion	**1** (6%)	3	11	3		18
Prepartum		**6** (17%)	17	2	1	35
Early onset			**55** (33%)	8	3	165
4 – 13 week onset				**2** (5%)	1	20
> 3 months onset					**nil**	7

left a maximum of 66 for further study; there was much missing information, and only mothers in the Roper series had the full set. There were trends to more premature births among the affected pregnancies, and to a protective effect of progesterone prophylaxis, but only two statistically significant differences emerged: lithium prophylaxis was associated with unaffected births, and stress (such as domestic violence, imprisonment of the child's father and extreme poverty) with affected births; the latter finding conflicts with the systematic studies reported on page 146.

Correlation of Childbearing and Unrelated Episodes

Winokur[513] suggested that puerperal psychoses were 'a different illness', not just bipolar disorder, because some bipolars do not suffer puerperal episodes. At one extreme, there are mothers who had episodes after each birth and no other episodes in more than 25 years. At the other extreme, there are manic depressive women who give birth to many children, without suffering any postpartum episodes; for example a patient of mine had five manic episodes in 16 years, and gave birth to four children without complications.

Restating this hypothesis, the childbearing factors are distinct from the other triggers of bipolar/cycloid episodes. This can be tested by comparing the severity of childbearing and non-reproductive bipolar/cycloid disorder. Focusing on mothers followed for at least ten years, the non-reproductive severity was measured by counting the number of unrelated psychotic episodes, and dividing by the years between the first episode and the end of the observation, after subtracting one year for each birth and one trimester for each abortion. The severity of the childbearing trigger(s) was measured by the proportion of pregnancies affected.

After eliminating 23 mothers with only one pregnancy and four with inadequate data, there were 87 bipolar/cycloid mothers followed for a mean of 23.5 years. Subtracting the time spent in pregnancy and the puerperium left 21.5 non-reproductive years. During this time they had 338 episodes unrelated to childbearing, that is, 3.5 episodes each (.17/year, one every six years). Table 21.3 compares the non-reproductive frequency in various groups. The final column shows the mean number of non-reproductive episodes/year.

Table 21.3 Relation between Childbearing and Non-Reproductive episodes

Group	Pregnancies affected	Ratios of affected pregnancies	Number of mothers	Episodes/ year
All childbearing episodes	Less than half	1 of 3 and 1 of 4	9	.15
	Half	1 of 2	22	.11
	At least two, one spared	2 of 3, 3 of 4, 4 of 5	13	.18
	Both	2 of 2	35	.15
	Additional episodes	3 of 3, 4 of 4, 3 of 2, 4 of 3, 6 of 5*	8	.22
Any prepartum episodes			23	.24
Any late postpartum episodes			12	.27

* Six mothers had additional prepartum episodes.

There is a difference between onset groups: mothers with prepartum and late postpartum episodes had more non-reproductive episodes (about one every four years) than those who suffered only early postpartum episodes (about one every six years). Excluding them, and focusing on mothers whose episodes all started early in the puerperium, severity bore no relation to the frequency of non-reproductive episodes: exactly the same figure was obtained (.15 non-reproductive episodes/year) in nine mothers who had one puerperal episode in three or four births, and 35 mothers, who suffered bipolar/cycloid episodes after both their children were born. This, from a different and unique data set, confirms the genetic findings of Jones & Craddock[194] that the early puerperal trigger is independent of other triggers of bipolar disorder.

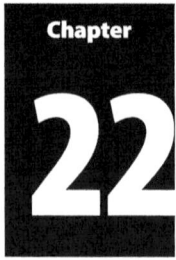

Management

This chapter will cover pre-conception planning, pre-birth planning, the setting of treatment, ECT, sedation, mood stabilizers and hormonal treatment. Because of the relative infrequency of postpartum psychosis, there is a dearth of prospective randomized, controlled double blind trials[514,515]. Reports on teratogenesis and other complications are voluminous, and this review covers only the best-established findings.

Pre-Conception Planning

Where possible, women with bipolar disorder (particularly those taking psychotropic medication), or a family history of puerperal psychosis, should be offered pre-conception counselling. The issues include the risks of pregnancy (to themselves, the child and future generations), the frequency of recurrence, and the risks and benefits of various treatment options during pregnancy and breast-feeding. In addition, education and advice should be readily available (for example, on-line) so that women can obtain the information at short notice.

Since there are potential effects on the infant, the decision whether or not to continue prophylactic medication is best shared with husbands, partners and family. Various adverse effects will be discussed below, but they must be evaluated against the risk of stopping long-standing prophylactic medication[516,517]. Viguera has found that stopping lithium or other mood stabilizers has the same effect in pregnancy as in women at other times. In 2007[140] she reported on various prophylactic agents (55 lithium, 15 valproic acid, and 13 with other agents) in over 80 bipolar patients: the recurrence rate was 53/62 (86%) in those who discontinued treatment compared with 10/27 (37%) in those who maintained the prophylaxis ($p < .001$). Lamotrigine also reduces the risk of relapse[518].

The balancing of risks involves a difficult judgment. As for teratogenesis, the period of organogenesis is days 18–55 of foetal life[519]. Congenital malformations are common in the general population, with 2.2% having lethal or severe malformations[520]. Bipolar disorder (whether treated or not) has increased risks of adverse pregnancy outcome: for example, 68/874 (7.7%) had a pre-term birth, compared with 15,785/331,263 (4.8%) in the Swedish population[521].

Planning During Pregnancy

If a mother with a history of psychosis becomes pregnant, a multidisciplinary planning meeting should be convened as soon as possible, to share information and coordinate management. The reason for urgency is that the interval between diagnosis of pregnancy (which may be delayed) and birth (which may be premature) can be short. The meeting should include all those involved in treatment, (in some countries) the general practitioner, a representative of the obstetric and mental health teams, (if appropriate) a social worker, and (if possible) the expectant mother and family members. There are many issues to be addressed – pharmaceutical treatment, antenatal care, early signs of a recurrence, the management of the puerperium, the care of the infant and sometimes action to protect the child. It is important that the mental health team be alerted as soon as the mother goes into labour.

The Setting of Treatment

Home Treatment

With a psychosis that is known to remit within weeks or months, this alternative should be considered. At home, the mother can maintain her roles and her relationship with the newborn. But there are risks, which were first mentioned in the 16th century[522]:

> A beautiful and fertile wife in Delft developed phrenitis, and then *furor* after every child was born. Through neglect she was left alone, and sprang cat-like from the couch on to a table and then climbed up into a chest and hid there. Attendants were unable to find her until she cried out from the hiding place to which she had miraculously ascended. She could only be brought down by ladder, with great danger. She accidentally sustained a head injury, and through brain damage remained delirious[a].

> In the Hague, a woman became phrenetic after childbirth, was not watched by the midwife, and still less by others; left alone, she got up from the couch and jumped out of the window, and came to a miserable end. From this example we learn that phrenitic patients should never be left alone, but diligently guarded.

In spite of the difficulties, Godding[523], concerned about the stigma of insanity, advised against hospital admission, and Conolly[524] gave directions on home nursing – securing windows and fires, removing anything that could be used for suicide, never leaving the patient unwatched. In Edinburgh, Clouston[434] treated a mother, who was sleepless, uncooperative and deluded, and refused food, for six weeks at home, seconding an experienced attendant from his team:

> The strain and responsibility on relations, attendants and nurses were no doubt most severe, and they were nearly exhausted, but she got through it (in six weeks) just as well as if she had been sent to an asylum.

Recently home treatment has been practised in Nottingham and Birmingham, where we treated a mother in Wednesbury (17 miles from the University) for six weeks, with daily visiting.

Since the building of public asylums about 200 years ago, many newly-delivered mothers have been admitted without their babies. Alienists were resourceful in managing these extremely severe disorders; for example, giving beef tea (with milk and eggs beaten in) by enema or stomach tube, under chloroform anaesthesia, to those with obstinate food refusal[525,526]. There were, however, risks from prolonged hospitalization, including infections, such as tuberculosis. Jolly's follow-up study[113] (see page 144) suggested that there were also risks for the infant.

Main[527] and Douglas[528] pioneered conjoint mother-and-infant hospitalization. This is widely practised in UK, Australia, New Zealand, France, Germany, the Netherlands,

---

[a] I thank Dr John Godwin, head of classics at Shrewsbury School, for translating this passage.

Belgium and India. Many believe, as I do, that it has advantages, but they have never been demonstrated objectively[529]. Its safety has not been established, and the risk of harm to the infants hangs like a sword of Damocles over the heads of those who work on these units. The risk was discussed in some detail in *Motherhood and Mental Health*[67] on pages 566–568. It is known that babies have been killed by their own mothers[530], but there are no systematic records. In 1978[531] the murder of a baby by another patient was reported:

> A 19-year old was admitted for the investigation of epilepsy. She was noticed to be in contact with a drug-user, and was told that drugs would not be tolerated on the ward. After abusing ethanol, she became angry and broke a bottle in the kitchen, then made a trivial assault on another mother. While staff were occupied with this complaint, she went into a bedroom and battered a baby, which died an hour later.

Margison[532], in an unpublished masters thesis, documented incidents by examining the medical, nursing and social work records of 245 mothers admitted in five years to the Withington mother & baby unit: there were 37 instances of threatened or actual non-accidental injury involving 21 babies. The most serious was a fractured skull:

> This mother had already made several impulsive attacks on staff, and three on the baby. While nurses were sitting on either side of her, she suddenly pushed her baby off her lap onto a hard floor; he suffered a parietal facture, from which he made a full recovery.

Is this risk acceptable? This is a complex question. There may be one answer for specialized units with experienced personnel and optimized surveillance, and another for admission to general psychiatric wards. Margison found that the risks were low when mothers were admitted with puerperal psychosis, and higher when they were admitted with depression, personality disorder or bonding disorders. There is a need for accurate figures for both types of unit and various disorders – data which are at present completely lacking. Babies are also at risk at home, in the care of their mentally ill mothers, or (if the mothers are in hospital) relatives or foster parents. Even if they are safer at home, there is the further question of their long term safety, after prolonged rupture of the mother–infant relationship. In 1996[67] I took the view that the risk was small and acceptable, provided that staffing levels and procedures were adequate, and the level of risk was fully researched; but, in the last 20 years, this research has not been funded.

Electroconvulsive Therapy

The beneficial effect of seizures was first noted by Worthington[533], whose patient suddenly recovered after a spontaneous fit. Convulsive therapy was developed by 1934, first with camphor then pentelenetetrazol; electroconvulsive therapy followed in 1937[534]. The first mention of the use of convulsive therapy in postpartum psychosis was in the theses of Gentis[535] and Haas[536], using pentelenetetrazol with apparent success. In the early 1940s, Van Steenbergen[96] used ECT in the Netherlands, Jacobs[537] in Britain, Mori[538] in Italy and von Hagen[539] in USA, with claims that it was effective. Ross[540] used ECT to treat seven mothers hospitalized with depression 1–14 months after delivery; all improved, while one mother not given this treatment was still in hospital after six months. Feldman[541] used ECT or metrazol convulsions in 24 patients: 15 were 'much improved'. Lafon[542] reported a negative result: ten patients treated before 1940 with sedatives, rest, baths and isolation had a mean duration of 48 days; 31 patients treated after 1940 by ECT had a mean duration of 135 days; but the groups were not matched. Twenty years after its introduction, Impastato[543] reviewed its use in the puerperium, assembling data on 57 mothers from the literature and 14 treated by themselves: they were sanguine about the lack of complications - two died, the cause of death being uncertain in both cases, though both had some evidence of thrombophlebitis; in their own series, only six completed the treatment (with definite improvement in three), the other eight being certified and sent to an asylum. Baker[544] compared ECT with chlorpromazine in 40 women, almost all of whom required it for full recovery. Over 20 years later, Sneddon[545] reported on her experience in Sheffield, where 55 mothers (36 with puerperal psychosis) with 59 episodes were treated: in her view, puerperal mental illness "is particularly sensitive to ECT; even the 1st treatment may change a mute catatonic mother into one that will eat, drink and communicate". Reed[546] made a retrospective case record study of 114 patients treated in Manchester, 58 of whom were puerperal: although the length of stay was the same, the 58 puerperal patients showed more improvement ($p<.001$), which was better maintained ($p = .001$); the largest difference was in 28/42 puerperal depressed patients, who showed substantial improvement, compared with only 9/33 non-puerperal depressed patients. Forray[547] reported its use in postpartum affective disorders: all five mothers recovered after seven treatments. Finally Babu[548] reported its effects in 34 mothers treated in Bangalore, of whom 16 had mania and eight a non-affective psychosis: there was no significant difference in the recovery of those who did and did not receive ECT.

In the last 70 years ECT has been used in a very large number of mothers based on the clinical impression that it is effective. Commenting on these reports:

- There have been no randomized, controlled, double-blind trials.
- Results reported for postpartum depression may not be relevant to postpartum psychosis.
- It is a clinical impression that manic and cycloid variants respond as well as depressive, but this has not been shown objectively. In my series, 61 mothers were treated with ECT for psychosis without depression, stupor or catatonia. In three it was given as an emergency treatment, and five others responded after pharmaceutical treatment had failed.
- Satisfactory results have been obtained without ECT: in the Netherlands, 64 mothers were treated in three phases – benzodiazepines for three days, neuroleptics for two weeks and (if this failed) the addition of lithium. ECT was recommended only after the failure of this regime for 12 weeks, and was required only once. Although there were relapses, all the other mothers recovered from their primary episode within six weeks[58].

Other evidence comes from historical data: Prothero[115] compared the outcome of 52 patients treated in 1927–1941 with 82 treated in 1942–1961 (by which time chlorpromazine was also available): there was not much difference in recovery rates (65% *versus* 79%), but the mortality rate was lower (13 *versus* one, $p = .0001$) and the mean duration was reduced from eight months to 2.5 months. In the present literature review, the effect on duration was less dramatic (as shown below).

1875–1940	6.8 months	
1941–1953	5.3 months	Treated by ECT
1953–1975	2.3 months	After the introduction of chlorpromazine.

The benefits of ECT have not been established beyond doubt.

The Safety of ECT During Pregnancy

When a mother becomes dangerously depressed during pregnancy, ECT has the advantage of avoiding pharmaceutical effects on the unborn child. The use of ECT in pregnant patients has been the subject of two authoritative reviews. Miller[549] reviewed 300 cases and listed 28 reported complications. Anderson[550] reviewed 309 cases: 78% improved, but there were 25 foetal or neonatal complications, including two deaths, one through maternal *status epilepticus* and the other through an 8-week miscarriage. The maternal complications included uterine contractions or preterm labour (nine mothers). Induction of uterine contractions is a definite risk: Sherer[551] gave ECT repeatedly to one mother, and each time it caused uterine contractions, controlled by subcutaneous terbutaline; after delivery by Caesarean section, a large retroperitoneal clot was found.

Sedation

It was not until the second half of the 19th century that sedation by bromides (1857), chloral (1869) and paraldehyde (1882) was introduced, while the barbiturates did not replace them until 1912. Chlorpromazine, the first of the neuroleptic (anti-psychotic) agents, was introduced to psychiatry in 1953. Haloperidol, a butyrophenone, was also discovered in the 1950s. Clozapine, the first of a 'second generation' of 'atypical' anti-psychotic drugs, with fewer anti-parkinsonian side effects, was introduced in 1971. In the 1990s risperidone, quetiapine and olanzapine followed. In this century, ziprasidone and aripiprazole have been added, but it is too early to assess their effects. This review will not cover effects in laboratory animals, but only teratogenic effects in man, and toxic effects on the newborn and breast-fed infants.

Adverse Effects on the Mother

Treatment of the acute episode now almost always involves the use of neuroleptic agents. Their harmful effects have perhaps been under-emphasized. Hypotension[552] and parkinsonian side effects are common. Extrapyramidal side effects were recorded in 54 of my series, of whom 49 were bipolar/cycloids ($p<.001$). There have been two published cases of neuroleptic malignant syndrome[553,554], and one fatal 'idiosyncratic reaction to neuroleptics'[75]; a fourth case occurred on my unit when trainees, using haloperidol for sedation, misdiagnosed a mother's symptoms as catatonic schizophrenia and added more haloperidol, until she had to be transferred to a neurological unit. Another in my series, who suffered four episodes related to childbearing, developed a neuroleptic malignant syndrome during a later non-reproductive episode. It is possible that pregnant women are themselves more vulnerable, because neuroleptic syndrome occurred in a woman given haloperidol 'for agitation'[555], and a mother given haloperidol as an anti-emetic developed torticollis and oculogyric crisis in labour[556]. To avoid these effects, other neuroleptics have been suggested – perfenazine[557], pimozide[558,559], clozapine[560,561], chlomethiazole[562], aripiprazole[563] and olanzapine[516], but there has been no systematic study.

Teratogenic Risk

Depot neuroleptic agents are widely used in the prophylaxis of chronic psychoses, and there is a great deal of information on their teratogenesis, using large data bases to examine the risk. Since they are seldom used in the prophylaxis of bipolar disorders, it is only necessary to touch on this literature. As early as 1977, Slone[564] used the American Collaborative Perinatal cohort (50,282 pregnancies) to examine the frequency of congenital malformations in 1,309 children exposed to phenothiazines during the first four months of pregnancy: the RR was 1.16 overall, and 1.68 for cardiovascular malformations. For haloperidol, the European Network of Teratology Information Services[565], comparing 188 infants exposed with over 500 controls, found congenital anomalies in 3.4% (slightly raised). As for the second generation anti-psychotic drugs, the Lilly Worldwide Pharmacovigilance Safety Database[566] found no major malformations in 23 prospective olanzapine pregnancies. Gentile[567], reviewing literature, found that clozapine (176 pregnancies) and olanzapine (96 pregnancies) did not increase the teratogenic risk. Databases from Canada, Israel and UK[568] found no adverse effects from olanzapine (60 pregnancies), risperidone (49 pregnancies) or quetiapine (36 pregnancies). The Swedish Medical Birth Register[569] covering 77 pregnancies on haloperidol, 98 on flupenthixol, 79 on olanzapine and 51 on risperidone, compared with 958,729 women in the general community reported a small collective increase in congenital malformations (odds ratio 1.52). A review of literature on 1,090 pregnancies with 1st trimester exposure to quetiapine (443), risperidone (432) and aripiprazole (100) found the teratogenic risk only slightly raised for risperidone (RR 1.5) and aripiprazole (RR 1.4)[570]. A search of the Benefit Risk Management Worldwide Safety database found 713 pregnancies in women taking risperidone: there were 12 retrospectively reported major malformations (1.7%)[571]. A German study[572] of 561 mothers taking second generation anti-psychotic agents found an increased major malformation rate (5.2% versus 2.5%) due mainly to an increase in cardiovascular anomalies (2.8% versus 0.6%). The teratogenic risk of neuroleptic agents is small.

Gestation Period and Birth Weight

The European Network of Teratology Information Services[565] reported that pre-term birth was more frequent (13.9% versus 6.9%, p = .006) in infants born to mothers on butyrophenones (mainly haloperidol); birth weights were accordingly lower (mean 3.16 kg versus 3.42 kg, p = .004). This was confirmed by a German group[572], who reported 15.7% preterm births (versus 9% in controls) in 284 mothers taking first generation anti-psychotic agents (64 of whom took haloperidol). The effect of second generation anti-psychotic agents is disputed: in a prospective study of over 50 mother-infant pairs, 4/14 infants born to mothers taking olanzapine had a birth weight less than 2.5kg and were admitted to intensive care[573]. But the British Neonatal Teratology Information Service, reporting on 45 infants exposed to typical and 22 to atypical anti-psychotic drugs, found that 13 exposed to olanzapine were heavier than a reference group[574]. Data from the Swedish National Health Register found that olanzapine and clozapine (N = 169 versus 357,696 other Swedish mothers) led to heavier infants due to their increased risk of gestational diabetes (odds ratio 1.94)[521]; this was also true of other anti-psychotic drugs (N = 338, odds ratio 1.77). Other Swedish findings were similar[569]. But a German study[572], comparing 561 second generation anti-psychotic agents (including 187 olanzapine, 185 quetiapine, 73 clozapine, 64 risperidone and 60 aripiprazole) with 1,122 controls, reported that gestation was normal (9.2% preterm versus 8.7%) and the median birth weight was 3.35kg (versus 3.38kg); there was no mention of gestational diabetes.

Effects on the Neonate

Phenothiazines, such as chlorpromazine and fluphenazine, given late in pregnancy, have caused somnolence and apathy[575,576] and neonatal icterus[577,578]. They have also caused lasting extrapyramidal symptoms, including hypertonicity, jitteriness, tremor, choreiform or dystonic movements, hand-flapping, tardive dyskinesia, nystagmus, jerky irregular breathing and/or arching of the back[579-583], still detectable six months later. As for butyrophenones, exposed infants have suffered from similar movement disorders[584,585] as well as hypothermia (35°)[586], hypotonia and nephrogenic diabetes insipidus[587]. These may be withdrawal symptoms not toxic effects[584]. As for second generation anti-psychotic agents, 21/197 infants born to mothers taking risperidone had tremor, irritability, feeding problems and somnolence, suggesting drug withdrawal[571], and a German study reported jitteriness, somnolence and seizures, especially in mothers taking quetiapine (26%) or aripiprazole (24%)[572]; but in both studies the mothers were taking other drugs as well.

Effects on the Breast-Fed Infant

Clozapine is lipophilic and notoriously associated with agranulocytosis – a contra-indication to its use in lactating mothers. Gardiner[588] studied seven mother–infant pairs under treatment with olanzapine: it was not detected in the plasma of six infants.

Lithium

Therapeutic Effects

As soon as the link between postpartum psychosis and bipolar disorder was recognized, the beneficial effect of lithium therapy was reported[557,589]; but its therapeutic effect has never been established in these patients by a double-blind, randomized controlled trial. Nevertheless, Bergink's findings[58] support its effect: of the 64 mothers in her prospective study, 48 failed to respond within two weeks to benzodiazepines and neuroleptics and proceeded to the addition of lithium, with remission in a median of 44 days; 63 recovered completely[98]. In Manchester, McKenzie[590] studied the effect of continued lithium treatment after recovery: in 69 mothers discharged from a mother & baby unit, the relapse rate was 0/9 in those discharged on lithium, and 27/60 in the others ($p < .01$). This needs replication.

Prophylactic Effects

Stewart[591] reported a prophylactic effect in four mothers, only one of whom had a mild recurrence. In collaboration with Dutch colleagues and Kendell, she collected 21 mothers[592]: with lithium prophylaxis, only two had a recurrence, both mild. Klompenhouwer[75] described a mother with two episodes of puerperal mania, who remained well with lithium after three more births. Austin[593] studied nine mothers: 6/8 patients not on lithium suffered a recurrence, as did 2/9 patients on lithium, but the illness was milder than in previous episodes ($p = .023$). Van Gent[594,595] reported a postpartum recurrence in 3/5 without lithium *versus* 3/11 on lithium ($p = .38$). Cohen[596] found that only one of 14 manic depressive women treated with lithium, carbamazepine or both had a recurrence within three months of childbirth, compared with 8/13 who did not receive these 'mood stabilisers' ($p = .004$). In Birmingham we planned a study involving

18 other units, but, in the event, only one non-Birmingham case participated (from Adelaide): Abou-Bakar collected 18 cases, divided into three groups – lithium (seven mothers), haloperidol (four mothers) and placebo (seven mothers): there was one severe relapse on lithium, two on haloperidol and three on placebo (comparing lithium with the other groups, $p = .15$). Most recently and cogently, Bergink[58,476] studied 70 patients in Rotterdam with the following results:

- Of 29 with a history of postpartum episodes, all 17 who accepted lithium prophylaxis remained well, while 3/9 who refused it developed a manic, hypomanic or mixed psychosis ($p = .03$).
- Of 41 with a history of bipolar episodes, 31 had prophylactic medication throughout pregnancy and ten did not. Prepartum recurrences occurred in 6/31 and 4/10 ($p = .22$), and postpartum episodes in 9/41.
- These 41 bipolar women included eight who also had a history of postpartum episodes (though one had depression not psychosis): three suffered manic or mixed psychoses during pregnancy and two postpartum episodes; these frequencies did not differ from bipolar women without postpartum episodes.

Bergink's thesis[58] did not provide a summary of all cases, and the tabulation of data left some uncertainties, for example which were 'bipolar I' and which 'bipolar II', but this extensive study provided the best available evidence for the benefit of lithium prophylaxis. In pregnancy, however, it is not very effective. Lithium prophylaxis can fail, as in this case:

A Birmingham woman suffered from Crohn's disease and systemic lupus. On day 13 after her first birth, she developed puerperal psychosis, from which she recovered within three weeks. Six months after the birth she had a recurrence, associated with steroid therapy. Five years later she became pregnant again, and entered the lithium trial. On day 11 she developed severe mania, and was, with difficulty, controlled by two police officers, two social workers, her general practitioner and her husband. Her serum lithium was 1.0 mE/l.

Teratogenicity

In 1974 Nora[597] briefly reported, in the infants of mothers taking lithium in early pregnancy, two cases of Ebstein's anomaly; this is malposition of the tricuspid valve, so that the right ventricle is 'atrialised', with a frequency is about 1/20,000 infants. Schou in Denmark and Weinstein & Goldfield in San Francisco set up an International Register of Lithium Babies. At the time of its closure (after the death of Weinstein) in 1979, 225 lithium babies had been registered, of whom 25 (11%) were malformed. There is a tendency for such a register to include excessive numbers of abnormal infants, and there are other methodological problems, including the lack of a control series of manic depressive women, and the prescription of additional medication; but there were 18 malformations involving the heart. In 1973, reporting the first 13 of these, Weinstein & Goldfield[598] listed six cases of Ebstein's[a]. Since then, ten additional cases have been reported[600–608]; including three Israeli cases[607], this is a total of sixteen. Another infant had tricuspid valve regurgitation without Ebstein's[609]. There is some contrary evidence: Edmunds & Oakley[610] found no mothers with manic depression or

---

[a] Weinstein's[599] article is sometime cited as showing six cases of Ebstein's, but the number is not specified. Schou[437] stated that there were six Ebstein's, but they may include Nora's[597].

lithium use among 34 infants with Ebstein's. A review of four case control studies of Ebstein's anomaly, with a total of 207 cases, found that none of the mothers had taken lithium[611]. Most recently a literature search found 385 relevant studies, including seven cohort studies, seven case-control studies and 48 case reports: the six case-control studies with a total of 264 lithium babies showed no excess of Ebstein's anomaly[612]; the authors quoted a Hungarian study of major abnormalities: 6/10,698 with a major congenital abnormality had been exposed to lithium, compared with 5/21,546 controls ($p = .13$). The risk may have been exaggerated, but with 16 reported cases, there is not much doubt about the association with Ebstein's. This disorder can be diagnosed by ultrasound and is surgically correctable.

Toxicity During Labour

In pregnancy the increase in body fluid and glomerular filtration rate raises lithium clearance, and higher doses may be required to maintain a therapeutic level. At parturition, this is suddenly reversed and serum lithium can reach dangerous levels. In *Motherhood and Mental Health*[67] I gave details of six cases of severe toxicity developing in mothers taking a dose of lithium they normally tolerated; in the last 20 years, eight more have been described. Since this phenomenon seems not to be widely known, Table 22.1 on pages 233 and 234 gives details of fourteen cases[614-628]. The last of these publications offered an explanation: this mother had obstruction of the right ureter by a urinoma, resulting in hydronephrosis. In normal pregnancy, the pressure of the gravid uterus can cause asymptomatic ureteric obstruction, even occasionally renal failure[613]. It seems likely that labour itself, as the foetal head is forced through the pelvis, aggravates this obstruction.

Toxic Effects on the Infant

The foetus, exposed to lithium, is highly susceptible to adverse effects. In a prospective study Newport[629] studied ten mothers who took lithium throughout labour, and combined their results with 32 from the literature: even when the mother's blood level was not abnormally high, babies exposed in the womb have been lethargic, hypotonic, hypothermic and cyanosed[630-633]; 12 infants with a serum level above 0.64 mE/l had lower Apgar scores, more CNS and neuromuscular complications and longer hospital stay. Källén & Tandberg[634] found by record linkage that 6/59 infants of mothers taking lithium died as neonates. A review of 241 lithium babies reported that 36% were born before 38 weeks gestation, and 37% had macrosomia (body weight above the 90th centile)[635]; the perinatal mortality was 8.3% including eight stillbirths. A prospective multicenter study confirmed the higher birth weight (3.48 kg *versus* 3.38 kg at the same gestational age), but had only one stillbirth among 138[604]. Some infants had transient effects on the heart[609,621,632,636,638-641], such as bradycardia[638], atrial flutter[621,632], supraventricular tachycardia[640] or pulmonary hypertension[641]. Several have developed goiters[642-646]. Five developed nephrogenic diabetes insipidus, which could be a reason for polyhydramnios, since the foetal kidney contributes to the formation of amniotic fluid[641,645,647,648]; one infant was unable to concentrate urine for two months, and was resistant to vasopressin. Hypothyroidism, hypoglycaemia and hyperbilirubinaemia have also been described[632,645,685]. Although most of these effects are transient, lithium prophylaxis in pregnancy is not fully effective[140], and there is a need to find a safer form of prevention.

Table 22.1 Toxicity of Lithium during Parturition

Vacaflor (1970)[614]	This mother received 1.2g daily during pregnancy and developed ankle oedema; she was treated with salt restriction and diuretics. She developed tremor and diarrhea. Lithium was discontinued the day before the birth, but she obtained a supply from a friend. Three days after the birth the serum level reached 5 mMl/l. She became confused and incontinent, had seizures and sank into coma. Her serum lithium fell to normal in ten days, but she remained confused for three weeks.
Wilbanks (1970)[615] Woody (1971)[617]	A 30-year old, with a history of three episodes of puerperal and one of prepartum psychosis, was maintained at or below a serum level of 1.0 mM/l during pregnancy; she was well at the beginning of labour, with a serum lithium of 0.9 mM/l. It rose to 3.4 mM/l on the day of the birth, and then, even though the drug was stopped, to 4.4 mM/l. She developed clonic twitching, and by day 3 was in coma, with diarrhea and incontinence of faeces. With a massive diuresis she recovered after nine days. The infant, whose serum lithium on the second day was 2.4 mM/l, was cyanosed and flaccid with poor grasp and absent Moro and sucking reflexes; although lithium was detected for 13 days, it recovered by the 8th day.
Aoki (1971)[616]	A 30-year old with a 14-year history of recurrent mania was taking 1.8g daily until the day of the birth of her 4th child, and was treated with diuretics and salt restriction because of oedema. She developed diarrhea and neuromuscular irritability before labour, then three seizures, with impaired consciousness. Her serum lithium reached 5 mM/l. She recovered in ten days, but developed puerperal mania. The infant had multiple congenital abnormalities, an Apgar score of 4 and serum lithium of 2.05 mM/l.
Piton (1973)[618]	A 33-year old was receiving 1.5 g daily during pregnancy, with a blood level of only 0.4 mM/l; for some unexplained reason she was on a salt-free diet. On day 1 she became confused and disorientated and her serum lithium was found to be 3.6 mM/l. It fell to normal in nine days. The child's serum lithium was 1.6 mM/l; it had hypotonia, hyperbilirubinaemia, tachycardia and cardiomegaly, and required exchange transfusion.
Schou (1973)[619]	A manic depressive woman, whose renal lithium clearance was normally 30 ml/min, sustained a rise to 48 ml/min during pregnancy, and the dose had to be raised to maintain serum lithium at a level of 1.0 mM/l. After the birth it rose to 1.5 mM/l, and she experienced 'slight intoxication symptoms' (few details).
Casparie (1974)[620]	A 29-year old was receiving 2 grams of lithium carbonate daily during pregnancy, and had a blood level of only 0.4 mM/l. At 35 weeks gestation, a low salt diet was started, and the serum lithium rose to 5.4 mM/l. She was delivered by emergency Caesarean section and sodium infusion, but the infant, whose serum lithium rose to 4.9 mM/l, died two days later from respiratory failure.
Karlsson (1975)[621]	A woman in the 8th month of pregnancy developed lithium toxicity (no details) with a serum level of 2.5 mM/l. Sixteen days later, after the maternal lithium had fallen to 0.9 mM/l, an infant was born with transient muscular hypotonia.

Table 22.1 (*cont.*)

Morrell (1983)[622]	A manic depressive woman had been treated with lithium for seven years, and was maintained on 1.2 g lithium carbonate throughout her 4th pregnancy. At 35 weeks she developed hydramnios. At 37 weeks she developed lithium toxicity with a serum level of 2.6 mM/L. The following day she went into labour. The infant, weighing 2.8 kg, was apneic for 15 minutes, then again three hours later, with signs of myocardial failure; its serum lithium was 2.8 mM/L. It was profoundly hypotonic and suffered from polyuria and paralytic ileus, required exchange transfusion, and showed delayed motor development at 12 months of age
Jenniskens-Bruins (1992)[623]	A mother took 800–1,200 mg lithium throughout her 1st pregnancy, developing diabetes insipidis and hypertension; her serum lithium level was never more than 0.8 mM/l. At 36 weeks she gave birth to a cyanotic and hypotonic infant weighing 3 kg. For five days it needed assistance with breathing, and on the 4th day had seizures. Its serum lithium was 0.64 mM/l 24 hours after the birth. The mother's lithium level was not stated. The infant recovered with exchange transfusion.
Nishiwaki (1996)[624]	A 29-year old was admitted in coma at 31 weeks gestation. She was in labour. It was not known what drugs she had been taking. She was treated with frusemide and tocolysis with ritrodine. Because of a grossly abnormal foetal heart rhythm, she was delivered by emergency Caesarean section of a 1.5 kg infant. The mother was treated with haemodialysis. The laboratory then reported a serum lithium level of over 4.0 mM/l in mother and baby. She recovered and the baby survived.
Flaherty (1997)[625]	A 17-year old with pre-eclampsia and a history of manic depression gave birth to an infant at 37 weeks gestation. Her serum lithium, several hours before the birth, was 2.6 mM/l, and the infant was born with a level of 2.1 mM/l, falling to 1.4 mM/l on day 3; it was lethargic and had to be fed by naso-gastric tube for six days.
Pinelli (2002)[626]	A 28-year old, who required 1.6g/day lithium carbonate during pregnancy gave birth at 34 weeks gestation. Labour was induced because of hypertension. The infant, with birth weight 2.3 kg, had poor respiratory effort, hypoglycaemia, hyperbilirubinaemia and nephrogenic diabetes insipidus; it had a serum lithium of 1.7 mM/l. The mother's serum lithium was not stated.
Malzache (2003)[627]	A 36-year old, during her 2nd full pregnancy, developed lithium toxicity (nausea and diarrhea) at 35 weeks gestation. Her serum lithium was 1.25 mM/l. She gave birth to an infant weighing 2.7 kg that was lethargic with marked hypopnea; its serum lithium was 3.6 mM/l. It was flaccid with poor reflexes for several days, but its serum lithium fell to normal in a few days.
Blake (2008)[628]	A 39-year old mother of six was admitted to hospital at 34 weeks gestation in a state of agitation, restlessness and confusion with disorientation. She was receiving 1.7 g lithium/day, with the last lithium level 0.6 mM/l, but it rose to 1.7 mM/l. Twins were delivered by emergency Caesarean section; they were said to have signs of lithium toxicity but their serum lithium levels were not stated. After the operation the mother was slow to recover consciousness. Her serum lithium was 3.3 mM/l; with haemodialysis she recovered in 14 days.

Lithium and Breast-Feeding

Lithium passes readily into the milk. In a prospective study of ten breast-feeding mothers, Viguera[637] found that the mean breast milk concentration (0.35 mEq/l) was half the maternal serum level (0.76 mEq/l), and the infant serum level was half the milk level (0.16 mEq/l); four infants had mild thyroid or renal abnormalities. They recommended vigilance rather than prohibition of breast-feeding. There is one published case of lithium toxicity: the infant caught a cold and developed nystagmus, fasciculation and paresis; its blood level was 1.4 mM/l, twice that of its mother[649]. Fever, gastro-intestinal illness or other causes of fluid and electrolyte loss could result in lithium toxicity; the resulting lethargy, hypotonia and poor feeding would require intravenous hydration. This may be a greater problem in countries where these infant disorders are common.

Conclusion

It would be wise for a woman on lithium prophylaxis to use contraception, and to withhold lithium during the first trimester of a planned pregnancy. If the parents decide that the balance of risk favours resuming lithium prophylaxis, it should be given in divided doses to avoid transient peaks and the blood level checked frequently. Sodium depletion, salt restriction and diuretic medication should be avoided. The drug should be stopped 24–48 hours before the birth. Afterwards, it should immediately be started again. Breast-feeding is permitted, with close monitoring.

Anti-Epileptic Agents

These paragraphs will discuss carbamazepine and valproate. Lamotrigine may be used more in future, because of its lower teratogenic risk[650,651], but at present little is known about its effects.

Carbamazepine

This has been used to treat epilepsy and trigeminal neuralgia since 1962 and a great deal was already known about its teratogenicity before, in 1973, it began to be used in bipolar disorder. An Israeli study[652] found various major abnormalities in 12/160 infants exposed, compared with 18/560 controls (RR 2.24). A meta-analysis of 16 prospective studies, with a total of 1,255 cases, reported a malformation rate of 5.3–6.8 (depending on definition), compared with 2.3 normal and 2.8 epileptic controls; the most frequent were cardiovascular anomalies[653]. The Eurocat Anti-epileptic Study Database[654] together with eight cohort studies of carbamazepine monotherapy (2,680 pregnancies) reported only 3.3% major congenital malformations, with one statistically significant increase – spina bifida (odds ratio 2.6). The EURAP epilepsy and pregnancy register[651] reported on 1,402 carbamazepine pregnancies, and found a dose effect, with 7.7% abnormalities in those taking over 1,000 mg/day, and only 3% in those below. In Australia[655] a study of 1,733 infants found an association with renal tract anomalies. In Norway, the Mother & Child Cohort Study compared 333 born to mothers taking anti-epileptic agents with over 60,000 other children: those taking carbamazepine alone had impaired fine-motor and social skills at 18 months and were more aggressive at 36 months[656]. These results are inconsistent, but suggest a modest teratogenic risk.

Valproate

This was introduced for the control of epilepsy in the 1960s. By 1981 a link with microcephaly in exposed neonates was noticed: in the Rhône-Alpes region of France, 9/72 infants with lumbo-sacral neural tube defects had been exposed to it[606,657]. By 1988 pooled French and Italian data obtained a figure of 14/334 children with spina bifida (RR 36)[658]. In a joint European prospective study[659], a dose effect was established, and replicated[677]: offspring of mothers taking >1,000 mg/day were at high risk (RR 6.8); but even those taking less than 700 mg/day had a malformation rate of 4.2%[651]. This effect has been confirmed many times – in Finland[660], Australia[661,662], Italy[663], UK & Ireland[664,665], Canada & Japan[666] and the European epilepsy and pregnancy register[651]. Folic acid may be preventive: mothers taking valproate are advised to take 4–5 mg/day[667] supplement, after excluding vitamin B_{12} deficiency; but it does not eliminate the risk[668]. Apart from spina bifida, valproate has also been associated with malformations of the heart and great vessels[655], facial cleft and genito-urinary malformations[665] and limb defects[669]. The most recent study from the EURAP registry reported that 105/1,224 (8.6%) pregnancies on valproate monotherapy resulted in major congenital malformations. In addition, there is also a 'foetal valproate syndrome' with developmental delay, speech disability and dysmorphic faces[670]. In Britain 44/57 had learning difficulties, and in Finland 4/21 exposed children had an IQ less than 80[671]. At least 16 cases of Asperger's syndrome or early childhood autism have been reported[672–674]. Other effects include withdrawal symptoms in 9/17 infants[675]; a Danish study found that 13/22 newborn infants became hypoglycaemic, and developed jitteriness, irritability, hypertonia and vomiting[676]. Valproate may be essential in the control of epilepsy, but there are alternatives for the prophylaxis of bipolar disorder, and it is contra-indicated in women contemplating pregnancy.

Hormonal Treatment and Prophylaxis

Some believe that hormonal treatment is therapeutic or preventive. This was suggested by three American studies:

In an account of 39 mothers with postpartum mental illness, including 16 with psychosis, progesterone was given as initial treatment, or additional treatment, to mothers who failed to remain well when treated with ECT. One recovered with progesterone alone as initial treatment, and five as the only treatment after 1–4 relapses[99].

In a study of 44 mothers, progesterone was given, usually in addition to ECT, medication or psychotherapy. It was claimed that schizo-affective patients, who responded well to ECT but tended to relapse in the premenstrual phase, responded to progesterone[678].

A third study treated eight patients with mestranol and norethynodrel (a combined oral contraceptive). Five recovered, and two did not; one recovered with no other treatment[679].

This mother reported her own experience:

Within a week of her first birth she became depressed and at six weeks developed various delusions. She was admitted to hospital and within five days menstruated. She improved and was discharged after 12 days. Three weeks later she relapsed. Readmitted, she again recovered rapidly with the menses and was discharged within 14 days. She relapsed again and this time recovery was gradual. Treated with progesterone, she remained well for 18 months[680].

These results can all be explained by the natural history of the disease, which often involves a brief series of relapses. Other anecdotal reports have not confirmed the efficacy of progesterone, either in treatment of the acute episode[681] or prophylaxis[286].

A beneficial effect of oestrogen therapy has also been claimed, originally in an early account of treatment by whole ovarian gland[682]. In another study, seven patients with a history of puerperal psychosis were treated prophylactically with oestrogen, starting with an intravenous dose, and continuing with oral treatment for four weeks: only one relapsed[683]. Finnish papers claimed a beneficial effect[287,684]: Ahokas reported a series of ten patients, who suffered an early onset puerperal episode; ten weeks after the onset of symptoms, all mothers, who were given sublingual oestrogen until their serum concentration reached 400 mg/day, recovered within two weeks. At the Institute of Psychiatry, its prophylactic effect was studied in 29 women with a history of bipolar or schizoaffective disorder (not puerperal psychosis); they were given transdermal oestrogen from day 1 after the birth: 12/29 (41%) relapsed within three months, including 6/13 of those who received the top dose of 800 µg/day[188].

Chapter

Risks

Suicide Attempts

There is a remarkable description of survival from determined suicide attempts, written by the husband[686] (see Clinical Gem 23.1):

Clinical Gem 23.1   Survival of Several Determined Suicide Attempts

At the age of 30, the author's wife developed typhus, complicated by delirium, which changed to melancholy: she tried to drown herself. During the next two years, her parents were ruined, her father became mentally ill and died, a much loved brother died and two other siblings were ill, all of whom she nursed. She was a good wife, although she only submitted to sexual intercourse for the sake of having children. She became pregnant, and after a long labour, a child was extracted with difficulty, only just alive. On day 3 she became febrile; this lasted six weeks and was followed by thrombophlebitis. She slowly recovered, but was troubled by the constant crying of the child, who suffered from a skin disease. There was a further family dispute, and she became depressed: she was sleepless, crying all night, and lacked any feeling for the baby. She had various delusions – they had no food, the king would be murdered, and the town had been destroyed by an earthquake. Using her husband's scalpel, she cut her cubital artery and stabbed herself 13 times, sinking the knife to the handle and breaking the blade against a rib. With determined medical efforts she survived, and was absolved by a priest for the crime of suicide. She tried to strangle her husband in the night. Visiting a friend, she seized a knife and stabbed herself to the hilt, wounding her liver and stomach; she obstructed efforts to stem the bleeding, cursing, biting, hitting out, and tearing off the bandage. With inconceivable strength she tried to tear open the window, to throw herself out. She had to be restrained, but refused food, drink and medicine, clamping her mouth and arching her back. The wound suppurated; she had a rigor and became delirious, howling like a dog, trying to destroy everything, and almost sleepless for 14 days. After six months she recovered, with an incoherent memory of events. Two years later she gave birth to a healthy son.

Babu[19] found, in Bangalore, that 10/56 postpartum mothers with mania or acute psychosis had suicidal ideas. Several mothers in my series made determined, but unsuccessful, suicide attempts. One, suffering from day 9 with depressive stupor and delusions, jumped into a canal and was rescued by a bystander. Another, who suffered an early onset cycloid episode with disorientation and catatonia, threw herself from a first-floor window, sustaining a 15- to 20-cm laceration of her scalp, through which skull was showing; she said, "Something compelled me to do it; I wasn't trying to kill myself". The following two mothers made determined suicidal attempts during later episodes unrelated to childbearing:

A woman, with over 20 admissions for recurrent bipolar/cycloid psychosis, including three postpartum episodes, made several suicide attempts. At the age of 21, she smashed her way through a window and jumped off a balcony, resulting in a wedge fracture of a lumbar vertebra, fractures of both heels, a mid-tarsal dislocation, and permanent nerve damage to her left leg. At the age of 44 she poisoned herself with lithium: her blood level reached 7 mM/l, resulting in dementia.

A woman, who suffered 12 episodes of bipolar disorder, made multiple suicide attempts, but not during her only pregnancy. At 18, in the context of a violent relationship, she took an overdose, set fire and tried to hang herself. The following year she drove to the coast and threw herself off a 250 ft cliff, suffering fractures of her skull, pelvis and limbs, and leaving her with retrograde amnesia; she was bitter to have survived – "I could not even get that right". At 33 she became pregnant, and developed her 11th episode in the third trimester, with a postpartum recurrence starting on the maternity ward, from which she made a full recovery.

Completed Suicide in Follow-Up Studies

Fifteen studies provided data on suicide. Most had a mixed sample, including depression without psychotic features. Collectively they reported 46 suicides in about 15,000 person/years – about 3/1,000 person/years. This figure is much influenced by Schöpf's study[118]: he found 13 cases among his 119 mothers, with a mean survival of 13 years after the index episode. Klompenhouwer's study[75] is unique in calculating a precise suicide rate (1.13/1,000 person/years), which was 17 times the rate for Dutch women (.065/1,000 person/years).

Case Lore

Excluding parturient suicide, whose cause is not psychosis, but the ordeal of labour, there are two relevant cases of completed suicide, reported in detail. One, mentioned only briefly, was a post-abortion psychosis occurring two months after an extra-uterine pregnancy[687]. The other[688] probably occurred during an infective delirium:

A doctor's wife, herself a doctor, gave birth to a stillborn child. She had rigors and developed a fever of 39.5°, which reached a peak of 40.6°. She became restless, and expressed persecutory ideas. On day 11, in an unguarded moment, she jumped from the window to her death.

In my legal work I encountered two postpartum suicides. Both were suffering from depression. One, accompanied by filicide and with no psychotic features, is summarized on page 245. This is the other:

A 25-year old soldier's wife was delivered of her 1st child by emergency Caesarean section, because of foetal distress. The baby received phototherapy for jaundice, and the mother developed a fever, which soon settled with metronidazole. A week later she became depressed, and on day 16 was hearing voices instructing her to commit suicide. She drank toilet disinfectant, filled a bath to drown herself and tried to strangle herself with the flex from her iron. She told a psychiatrist, "I've got to do it". In letters discovered after her death, it was clear that she thought she had cancer. "You don't know how happy it would have made me (if I killed myself), because my brain was full of it. People like me they put in a padded cell, where you just lay there until you die. I pray you are reading this, and know that I am at peace". There were words of love, and a remark about how lovely the baby was. To her mother, she wrote: "I don't want to die and love you all, but I am going mad". On day 22 she disappeared. Three days later she was found hanging from a tree.

In the literature five suicides occurred later in the mother's life, after recovery from the postpartum episode[111,280,362,689,690]. In Schöpf's study[118] the earliest suicide was two years after the index episode. Rhode[691] stated that one mother died from suicide during the index episode, but her series was mixed, and she gave no details of the psychopathology. A mother in my series, who suffered two early postpartum depressive psychoses in the context of bipolar disorder, threw herself from a bridge some years later.

Suicide in First Degree Relatives

Many mothers lost close relatives by suicide: 18 lost fathers, 8 lost mothers (one after her own birth), 6 lost brothers and 3 lost sisters, one of whom lost a twin sister who had just given birth to twins. One lost both father and brother, and one lost father, mother and a brother. In my series, 13 lost 1° relatives – 4 a father, 3 a brother, 4 a sister, one a 'sibling' and one her mother after her own birth. All except one had a lifetime diagnosis of bipolar/cycloid disorder; the exception had six episodes of a recurrent brief psychosis, two episodes with premenstrual onsets (possibly a bipolar/cycloid variant).

Conclusion

The suicide rate is high in the families of mothers with postpartum psychosis, and in subsequent psychotic episodes, but no one has reported suicide during a puerperal manic/cycloid episode.

Filicide

Frequency

As part of another study, I have compiled 800 published cases of filicide. I excluded 65 due to depression or psychosis within a year of the birth. Eleven were depressed without psychotic features. One had a chronic psychosis and 12 had insufficient evidence either of depression or of psychosis. The literature contains this tragic South African case, remarkable for the killing of five infants[692]:

> A 25-year old gave birth to twins, who were admitted for phototherapy to treat neonatal jaundice. The mother was a lodger, and was noticed collecting shoes and placing them in lines. One evening she went into the neonatal intensive care ward, grabbed her twins and threw them against the wall, and killed three other babies. She later had further children without mental illness.

After these exclusions, only 48 had evidence of psychosis[a] – just above 1 per cent of the 4,029 cases reviewed. Recent American papers have given the much higher figure of 4 per cent[693,694]. This error can be traced to a misreading of a Scottish study[367], in which 82 patients were followed for a mean of 16 years: only 29 were suffering from bipolar, paranoid or schizophrenic psychoses, the rest from depression; one definite and one probable filicide were committed by depressed mothers, and a mother probably suffering from a chronic psychosis killed two children. None of the filicides was committed by a mother suffering from an acute puerperal psychosis without depression.

Filicides in the Literature

Six cases occurred during organic psychoses – 6/1,368 organic psychoses is 1/228. This is an example of filicide during an infective psychosis[696]

> A 26-year old single woman concealed her pregnancy and gave birth alone. She developed puerperal fever, and on day 13 became disturbed, singing and shouting. In this state she strangled her child, said so, and immediately began singing and roving around again. Peritonitis set in, but she recovered with no memory for the deed.

Two filicides that occurred during epileptic psychoses were summarized on page 57.

Most of the non-organic filicides occurred during depressive psychoses – 3 with pre-partum onset, 10 with early postpartum onset and 11 with late postpartum onset. This is a famous case of early onset melancholia, leading to filicide a fortnight after the birth:

> A 37-year old showed signs of derangement – she was going to die and would go to hell. She was 'prostrated of strength', her eyes vacant and wild, her countenance haggard. The doctor gave instructions that she should not be left alone, and should not be given the child. But, thirteen days after the birth, she angrily demanded that her teenage daughter bring it to her. She nearly decapitated the baby with a razor[697].

In the following cases, filicide was an issue after two births:

> A 24-year old gave birth to her 1st child. Within the first three weeks she became depressed and had impulses to kill the child although she loved it very much [obsessions of infanticide]. Two years later she gave birth to her 2nd child. On day 20 she became depressed, said her brain was gone, she could not concentrate or remember anything and thought she was going to hurt the child. During a failure of supervision, she cut its throat, then her own. On admission to hospital she was confused; she could not remember killing the baby, only seeing herself in the mirror with her throat cut (case 1)[698].

> A 29-year old woman from Kazakhstan, whose father hanged himself, gave birth to a child, and within a month became depressed. She tried to suffocate the infant, but was prevented by the family. Ten years later they came to Germany. She gave birth again. On day 5 she became ill, with a staring expression. On day 10 the baby was found drowned in the bath. Admitted to hospital she was in a perplexed and sub-stuporose state with ideas of guilt and punishment, and auditory hallucinations; she heard the baby cry; it had a bad mother and a bad future (case 1)[369].

In the next case, four children were killed:

> A 32-year old, whose husband had a severe pulmonary infection, became depressed and asked him to kill her – she was a great sinner. She cut the throats of all four children, tucked them up in bed,

---

[a] All 48 cases have been tabulated in *What Is Worth Knowing about, 'Puerperal Psychosis'*,[695].

lit candles so that they would not be in darkness, and disappeared. She was found wandering three days later. In prison, she lay on the floor, sleepless, without the strength to kill herself. She had no sympathy for others' grief, having no love left in her heart[699].

Melancholic filicides, often accompanied by suicidal actions, are a notorious risk in severely depressed mothers. Twenty-four cases among 535 depressive psychoses is 1/22 (4.5 per cent).

The remaining cases occurred during postpartum psychoses without overt depression. There were three with late postpartum onset and five with unknown postpartum onset. Ten cases with early onset psychoses will now briefly be summarized. In one there were no details of the psychopathology, which may have been depressive; suppression of an unwanted child is an alternative diagnosis[700]:

In 1756, Agnes Crockat, an unmarried woman, called for help with her delivery, but a week later became strange in speech and behaviour, and strangled the child. She kept it beside her on the bed, and, when visitors came, said 'the Devil had tempted her'. She was sentenced to death, but pardoned by Royal Mercy.

In five of the remaining nine, there may have been no *mens rea* – no intention to kill, and the baby's death was accidental:

A 25-year old, whose mother suffered from depression, gave birth to her 1st child. From that time she became excited. She left home at 2 am, naked, and made her way to a river, where the infant was carried away. After her arrest she was sleepless and anorexic and completely indifferent to people and her own injuries[701].

A 23-year old, with a history of two psychotic episodes, gave birth to her 1st child: afterwards she became sleepless, talking and gesticulating. On day 4 she became violently agitated and suffocated her infant by forcing a thimble into its mouth. Admitted to hospital, she did not know where she was and appeared not to recognize anyone. She was terrified by visual and auditory hallucinations, fought and tried to escape, colliding with doors, walls and furniture that she appeared not to see. She lapsed into stupor, mute, cataleptic and resistant to all approaches. From time to time she took on an ecstatic attitude, as if in prayer. Mysticism gave place to eroticism. Three months later she recovered, with amnesia for her illness, which seemed like a dream (case 5)[363].

A 20-year old, whose father suffered two 'affective episodes', gave birth to her 1st child. On day 9 she developed a confused and dream-like episode. Six hours later she covered her daughter with talcum powder, inhalation of which caused her death. She spoke of the end of the world and said she covered the child with powder to prevent its freezing or to reanimate it after death. She danced with the child, not realising it was dead. She told her husband they could have other children, or adopt them. She was in hospital for 15 days but showed little sign of illness[702].

Two days before giving birth, a woman began to have lacunae in her memory, which persisted until the explosion of a postpartum psychosis with illusions and hallucinations. She drowned her infant while bathing it, then seized the dead baby and showed it to a neighbour in a state of morbid exaltation[703].

A woman gave birth to her 1st child: 17 days later, she became agitated and sleepless. For four days she walked about her apartment, breast-feeding the infant, although she had no milk. On the 4th day the child died, apparently of neglect. Admitted to hospital, she was in a state of manic agitation, confused with auditory and visual hallucinations and illusions. She believed her husband had died, God had told her the baby would be resuscitated, she was still pregnant and would give birth at the end of the year (case 3)[95].

In these remaining four, filicide seemed deliberate:

14 days after childbirth, a woman began to have ideas of sin, then became more disturbed with swearing, violence, seeing the Devil, dancing with raised skirts, saying obscene things, and singing

in a crazy tone. In the night she stabbed her three children, and was about to stab her husband when he woke and overpowered her[704].

At the age of 17, a woman developed auditory hallucinations and persecutory delusions. At 24 she gave birth to her 1st child. Three weeks later she became agitated, saying that her child was controlled by the Devil. She strangled it and took an overdose (case 2)[705].

A woman became depressed after giving birth to her 1st child. After her 2nd birth, on day 4, she developed an acute psychosis with exaltation, hallucinations and themes of guilt and religiosity. She killed the child (no details)[706].

A 34-year old suffered from a periodic disorder with three days of jocularity, creativity and high energy alternating with tearfulness and withdrawal. She gave birth to her 2nd child: on day 2 she became sleepless and suspicious that her husband would harm the baby. She had thoughts of throwing him out of the window, believing he had gas inside him. She became agitated and confused, and could not think straight. On day 20 she felt as if she was being taken over by 'a force': she did not feel connected to her hands. In a dazed, trance-like state, she strangled her baby with a telephone cord, then attempted to cut her wrists[693].

The frequency in early onset psychoses, including accidental filicides, is 9/1,115 (less than 1 per cent).

Filicide in My Series

As mentioned in Section 1 (page 5), my interest in menstrual psychosis was aroused by a mother who nearly killed her infant accidentally during a relapse of puerperal mania occurring at the first postpartum menses.

There were five minor or half-hearted attempts to suffocate the infant, and five mothers made deliberate and dangerous assaults on their babies. In the first, the only evidence of psychosis was a delusion (possibly subcultural) about the infant:

An Indian woman came to UK at the age of five. As a child she was happy, jokey and energetic. After an arranged marriage, her in-laws enslaved, scapegoated and ill-treated her. Her husband would punch and kick her, pull her hair and threaten to 'smash her head in'. She gave birth to a child and then, as a result of marital rape, became pregnant again. She tried to induce a miscarriage, and felt like punching her stomach. The birth of a girl was more like a death in the family. "It's going to be hell for me now. I did not want her, and have no love for her". The family accused her of adultery and prostitution. "Where did you get this piece of rubbish from? It's not my son's child". There were more beatings. She became depressed and attempted suicide several times. She abused the infant, put toilet water or bleach in the feeding bottle, shook her, swung her by her legs, put ice in her bath and left her outside in the cold. After yet another beating (because she was seen talking to an aunt), she purchased a knife and some petrol. She stabbed her sister-in-law 46 times, and, when her 4-year old nephew intervened, stabbed him eleven times. She then stabbed her mother-in-law 16 times, put her body in a bag, dragged it across the road to her sister-in-law's house and set fire to the bodies. After her arrest she suddenly grabbed her 4-month old daughter by the legs and smashed her against the wall, fracturing her skull. She believed the baby was the Devil.

The second took a knife to her 18-month old son in a recurrence of a cycloid episode:

A 28-year old gave birth to her 1st and only child; this was followed by a cycloid episode, starting on day 1. Eighteen months later she became depressed, withdrawn and preoccupied, 'on a downward spiral'. One night she was restless; at dawn she saw vapour trails in the sky, which she thought were angels. She said, "It's the end of the world. Look at the clouds". She appeared confused, preoccupied and distressed, holding her head and screaming. She was afraid devils would take her son away. At 5.30 am she attempted to sacrifice him, stabbing him in the chest five times with a large kitchen knife, penetrating the skin, but causing little damage. She was shouting, "I've got to kill the Devil's baby and free the world". Her husband disarmed her, suffering wounds to his hands. She telephoned a friend and said, "I've done it. I've killed the Devil's baby, like you told me to". As the baby was being taken to hospital, she grabbed the ambulance doors and said, "Don't let them take him. They will kill him"; she had to be wrenched away from the door. While waiting for a doctor, she asked her husband to kill her. During the next 20 years she suffered several more episodes, all of which were thought to be premenstrual.

The next mother stabbed her 13-year old, and attempted to immolate herself and her 6-week old baby, when in the grip of a paranoid psychosis:

A 37 year old, in an unstable relationship, was delivered of her 4th child by Caesarean section at 36 weeks gestation. After the birth she was sleepless and anorexic. She took St John's Wort for depressive symptoms, and smoked an unknown amount of cannabis. At five weeks postpartum she confided in her aunt that she believed the child's father was trying to abduct the baby and take it to Spain. She expressed the idea that he had been tape-recording her, to gather evidence about her mothering. A week later, after two sleepless nights, she made incoherent, rambling telephone calls to her aunt and the police, implying that others were involved (organized crime, 'a sick and perverted syndicate'), not just her partner, and naming individuals: the children would be introduced to an internet paedophile ring and, before death, would suffer horrific sexual abuse and torture. She had a knife ready to protect her family, and a bucket of bleach to throw at an intruder. When the police arrived, she waved them away, believing they were imposters. After gazing at her sleeping 13-year old for half-an-hour, she stabbed her in the chest with a 5-inch knife. Her intention was to kill her, but when she woke and cried out, she came to her senses. She then cut her own wrists and neck. At 5.30 am the terrified children were running into the garden in the freezing cold. There was smoke coming from a window in a top room, where she had set light to the duvet to kill herself and the baby. Her daughter had two quarter-inch wounds on her left nipple and sternum, a punctured lung and pneumothorax. At the police station, the mother said, "I wanted to kill them, so that they would not suffer the pain I have suffered".

The following mother attacked her 4-month-old child in the context of a postpartum depressive psychosis with a menstrual relapse, which had manic features:

A 24-year old gave birth to her 2nd child @ 38 weeks gestation. Within two weeks she became depressed, and lost two stones in weight. She developed ideas that people were talking about her, and the family was plotting against her. Four months after the birth she perceived that her son's eyes were green, like the Devil's eyes, and his voice had changed. She believed the Devil was trying to take him. She shook him, "tried to poke the Devil out of his eyes" and banged his head against the refrigerator, shouting for the Devil to leave him. "When I attacked my son, I was actually protecting him. I thought I was one of God's messengers, and was getting a message from God, saying that everybody was evil except the angels". The baby suffered severe injuries, including swollen eyes and mouth, lacerations to his gums and an eye, leaving scarring. Admitted to hospital the mother was high, irritable and suspicious, and showed pressure of speech and flight of ideas. She attacked the doctor and nursing staff. She thought she could fly, and attempted to baptise other patients. She washed repetitively and ritualistically, gargling to the point of choking. The next day she lay in bed and refused to speak, then hit her head on a brick wall and had to be prevented from jumping from a 3rd floor window. Her menses started and, within two days, she improved, apologised, full of remorse, and was soon discharged well.

The last mother was the only one who attacked the baby when in the grip of a psychosis of early postpartum onset:

A 26-year old was delivered of her 1st child, by ventouse under epidural anaesthesia; this was followed by a renal infection. During labour she experienced auditory hallucinations. During the next two weeks she developed a system of persecutory ideas involving her sister, who had bugged her home, and wanted to kill her and the baby. She taped the letter-box to prevent her sister passing a letter bomb. She asked for more locks and closed circuit television, in case her sister broke in at night. She misidentified pedestrians as her sister in disguise. She became tirelessly overactive, starting a new business, organizing holidays and spending £1,000 on mail-order goods. She believed she was destined to become an amazing artist. After four weeks she came to believe her sister was living in the garage, or in a cupboard under the stairs. Early one morning she telephoned her father to warn him that her sister wanted to kill their mother too; she used a public phone booth because she believed the police had bugged her telephones as well as the baby monitor, and were watching the house. A voice told her to kill the dog and cat, her sister and herself, so that they would all go to Heaven. That evening she telephoned for an ambulance, saying, "It is suicide . . . My sister tried to kill me. I am afraid I have had to kill her in self defence, because I have got a young baby here." When the paramedics arrived, they heard screams and inarticulate rantings. She was kneeling on the floor over the infant, compressing its chest with an 8-inch knife, rocking forward and pressing down. When a paramedic seized the knife, she said, "Kill me quickly". The baby sustained two one-inch wounds in the chest, with no damage to underlying organs. The patient was in hospital for several months, made a complete recovery, had another child and remained well for 13 years.

One mother suffered from 4-13 week onset delusional depression; her attempt at combined suicide and filicide was frustrated by the fortuitous intervention of a stranger.

A 34-year old gave birth to her 2nd child, and, five weeks later, developed a depressive psychosis, with delusional ideas about the infant. After four months she deliberately dropped her baby on the floor. She was admitted to the Mother & Baby unit, where she dissimulated her suicidal intentions. Six months after the birth, she drove for an hour, bought a hose-pipe, looked for a deserted place, drove into a field, attached the hose pipe to the exhaust, and locked the windows, leaving the engine on. A farm worker saw her, and rescued them.

There were three completed filicides. The first mother suffered from bipolar disorder, but there were no psychotic features in the postpartum episode (so she has not been included in my series). Filicide and suicide occurred three months after the birth.

At the age of 34, a doctor, with a history of eight bipolar episodes in 15 years, was delivered by Caesarean section of her 1st child. She became depressed, and, 14 weeks later, killed her baby ('to protect her') with multiple stab wounds using a kitchen knife, then set fire to herself and her baby. She suffered 25% burns and died from pneumonia.

The second mother also suffered from bipolar disorder, and had several episodes related to subsequent pregnancies. At the time of the filicide, she was depressed, without psychotic features:

A 23-year old gave birth to her 1st child. She was discharged from the maternity hospital after ten days. She was attached to the baby, but felt 'really low' and would cry, cry and cry and bang her head against the wall. The baby took two hours to feed and required another feed 1½ hours later. She was "so tired" and had no family to help. She ate nothing and her weight went down from 10 to 7½ stones. "I felt like pulling out my hair, I was that bad". After seven days at home she 'just smothered the baby'. "I must have thought, 'for Christ's sake shut up' and put a pillow over him". Her husband found the baby dead, and his wife gone. She did not remember the act, and could not believe she had done it.

The third mother killed her 4½-month old baby in the context of a postpartum depressive psychosis.

> After a pregnancy complicated by pre-eclamptic toxaemia, a 31-year old was delivered of her 2nd child by emergency Caesarean section @ 34 weeks gestation. She became depressed, losing one stone in weight. Two months later she started to worry about her baby's health. She asked for blood tests and a brain scan. He was very cold and in danger of hypothermia. She became obsessed with these ideas and was continually checking on him. A letter from a physiotherapist about a minor hip problem was interpreted as removing him because of maltreatment, causing brain damage. She could not be reassured, and "unbearable pressure" built up in her head. When the baby was 4½ months old, she drowned him in the sink, and cut her neck and wrists. She was ill for a year but recovered after ECT and successfully mothered another child.

Thus, in my experience, all the attempted and completed filicides occurred in the context of depressive psychoses, but two major assaults (one accidental) occurred during early onset postpartum psychosis.

Summary

The literature of only 2,452 works includes:

- A total of 419 reviews, only one of which covered more than 10 per cent of published work. Attention is drawn to the pernicious effect of incomplete reviews.
- A total of 352 surveys, which show the prevalence of these psychoses worldwide:
  - They agree on an incidence of about 1/1,000 births.
  - There is evidence of a fall in frequency at the end of the nineteenth century.
  - There is an increased rate of non-organic psychoses with early postpartum onset in *primiparae*.
  - There is an association with manic-depressive (bipolar) disorder, but postpartum episodes are more severe.
  - After 1940 the mean duration fell from seven months to 10 weeks.
  - There is a tendency to relapse.

- There are 50 'follow up studies', but only 194 detailed cases have been followed for at least 10 years. The risk of a recurrence is at least 30 per cent in mothers who have already suffered one childbearing episode, and is also raised in bipolar women.
- Investigations of obstetric variables and laboratory tests have drawn blank, with no replicated findings.
- There is no doubt that genetic factors are important, but molecular genetics has not yet found a replicated locus for the genes responsible. The inheritance of the puerperal disorder may be distinct from that of bipolar disorder.
- More than 4,000 cases have been described, the majority by French and German authors; In spite of the great opportunity presented by mother & baby units, their number has declined since 1950.
- A citation analysis of more than 2,000 articles showed abysmal standards of scholarship, especially by Anglo-Saxon authors. Many excellent contributions have received few citations, and some none at all.

The symptoms cover the whole range found in psychoses.

Classification by the *International Classification of Diseases* and American *Diagnostic and Statistical Manual* has not facilitated epidemiological research or clinical practice.

In a review of the clinical forms observed in the literature and my series, the main findings were:

- The literature includes descriptions of 1,368 cases of organic psychosis, including:
  - Several hundred infective psychoses, which can present with mania
  - Nearly 300 eclamptic and Donkin psychoses
  - More than 130 with Wernicke–Korsakow syndrome, which has returned as a result of the treatment of pernicious vomiting by dextrose infusion without thiamine
  - At least a dozen less common neuropsychiatric disorders

- The non-organic psychoses in the literature include more than 500 depressive psychoses, as well as psychogenic psychoses, Fürstner's postpartum hallucinatory disorder, amentia, unusual cyclical disorders and bromocriptine psychoses.
- The lifetime diagnoses in my series included:
  - A total of 130 mothers with manic-depressive or manic episodes (40 per cent).
  - A total of 86 mothers with cycloid episodes (27 per cent).

Long-term observation showed that bipolar and cycloid elements were inextricably mixed, and a combined 'bipolar/cycloid' group is proposed. This amounted to only two-thirds of the series. The other mothers suffered from depressive psychoses (with or without minimal bipolar features), paranoid and schizo-phreniform psychoses, and some rarer disorders.

Cases in the literature and my series have been divided into nine onset groups – post-abortion, prepartum, short gestation, parturient, day 1, early postpartum, weeks 4–13, later postpartum and weaning onsets. Analysis showed:

- Organic psychoses are common after abortion, during pregnancy and parturition, and in the early puerperium, but are less common later in the postpartum period.
- Non-organic psychoses most frequently start soon after the birth (within the first 15 days). The onset is as early as day 1 or even during parturition.
- There is evidence for reproductive triggers following abortion, during pregnancy, several weeks after the birth and after weaning.

Combining the literature and my series, there are more than 450 recurrent cases. A matrix of their associations shows a general association among abortion, prepartum, early postpartum and late postpartum onset groups, suggesting shared elements in causation or pathogenesis.

A study of 214 bipolar/cycloid mothers showed:

- The recurrence rate after later pregnancies was 73 per cent overall, and this high rate was also found in mothers with prepartum, late postpartum and post-abortion onsets.
- A total of 28 per cent had at least one relapse.
- Surgical operations and steroid treatment have the same potency to provoke episodes as do abortions.
- There was no correlation between the frequency of reproductive and non-reproductive bipolar disorder.

Management should include pre-conception and pre-birth planning. The efficacy and safety of conjoint mother and baby in-patient care have not been researched. There is a dearth of randomised, controlled treatment trials, but experience suggests:

- The value of ECT may have been exaggerated.
- Neuroleptic agents, prescribed during pregnancy, can occasionally cause extra-pyramidal symptoms in infants. Bipolar/cycloid mothers are particularly susceptible to adverse effects.
- Lithium is teratogenic and, when taken during pregnancy, has various toxic effects on the infant. There are 14 reported cases of dangerous toxicity during parturition. There is much evidence of its prophylactic effect when given post partum. Adverse effects on the breast-fed infant have been exaggerated.
- Valproate is contraindicated during pregnancy because of teratogenicity.
- There is no satisfactory evidence for the efficacy of oestrogens or progesterone in treatment or prophylaxis.

The suicide rate is high in the families of mothers with postpartum psychosis, and in subsequent psychotic episodes.

The filicide rate is 1 per cent overall.

References

1   Anton G. Über Geistes- und Nervenkrankheiten in der Schwangerschaft, im Wochenbett und in der Säugungszeit. In: Anton G et al., editors, *Handbuch der Gynäkologie*. Wiesbaden: Bergmann; 1910. p. 1–41.

2   Sit D, Rothschild AJ, Wisner KL. A review of postpartum psychosis. *Journal of Women's Health.* 2006;15:352–368.

3   Lewis T. Observations on research in medicine, its position and its needs. *British Medical Journal.* 1930;i:679–683.

4   Hill AH, Keedy DM. Psychoses related to childbirth. *Texas Journal of Medicine.* 1951;47:635–638.

5   Victoroff VM. Dynamics and management of parapartum neuropathic reactions. *Diseases of the Nervous System.* 1952;13: 291–298.

6   Gautam S, Nijhawan M, Gehlot PS. Postpartum psychiatric syndromes – an analysis of 100 consecutive cases. *Indian Journal of Psychiatry.* 1982;24:383–386.

7   Trixler M, Ferenc J. Genetikai és szociális tényzók szerepe a terhességhez társuló pszichés megbetedésekben. *Ideeggyógyászati Szemie.* 1982;35:433–440.

8   Howard LM, Goss C, Leese M, Appleby L, Thornicroft G. The psychosocial outcome of pregnancy in women with psychotic disorders. *Schizophrenia Research.* 2004; 71:49–60.

9   Davenport YB, Adland ML. Postpartum psychoses in female and male bipolar manic-depressive patients. *American Journal of Orthopsychiatry.* 1982;52: 288–297.

10 Brewer C. The incidence of post-abortion psychosis: a prospective study. *British Medical Journal.* 1977;i:476–477.

11 Somers RL. *Risk of admission to psychiatric institutions among Danish women who experience induced abortion: an analysis based on national record linkage.* PhD Thesis, University of California at Los Angeles; 1979.

12 Gilchrist AC, Hannaford PC, Frank P, Kay CR. Termination of pregnancy and psychiatric morbidity. *British Journal of Psychiatry.* 1995;167:243–248.

13 Shearer ML, Davidson RT, Finch SM. The sex ratio of offspring born to state hospitalised schizophrenic women. *Journal of Psychiatric Research.* 1967;5:349–350.

14 Loudon I. Puerperal insanity in the 19th century. *Journal of the Royal Society of Medicine.* 1988;81:76–79.

15 Austin MP, Kildea S, Sullivan E. Maternal mortality and psychiatric morbidity in the perinatal period: challenges and opportunities for prevention in the Australian setting. *Medical Journal of Australia.* 2007;186:364–367.

16 Blehar MC, DePaulo JR Jr, Gershon ES, Reich T, Simpson SG, Nurnberger JI Jr. Women with bipolar disorder: findings from the NIMH genetics initiative sample. *Psychopharmacology Bulletin.* 1998;34: 239–243.

17 Harlow BL, Vitonis AF, Sparen P, Cnattingius S, Joffe H, Hultman CM. Incidence of hospitalization for postpartum psychotic and bipolar episodes in women with and without prior prepregnancy or prenatal psychiatric hospitalizations. *Archives of General Psychiatry.* 2007;64: 42–48.

18 Reardon DC, Ney PG, Scheuren F, Cougle J, Coleman PK, Strahan TW. Deaths associated with pregnancy outcome: a record linkage study of low-income women. *Southern Medical Journal.* 2002;95:834–840.

19 Babu GN, Subbakrishna DKS, Chandra PS. Prevalence and correlates of suicidality among Indian women with post-partum psychosis in an inpatient setting.

Australian & New Zealand Journal of Psychiatry. 2008;42:976–980.

20 Borri C, Mauri M, Oppo A, Banti S, Rambelli C, Ramacciotti D, et al. Axis 1 psychopathology and functional impairment at the third month of pregnancy: results from the perinatal depression-research and screening unit (PND-ReScU) study. *Journal of Clinical Psychiatry.* 2008;69:1617–1624.

21 Haslam J. *Observations on Insanity, with Practical Remarks on the Disease, and an Account of the Morbid Appearences on Dissection.* London: Rivington; 1798. p. 51–53.

22 Rush B. (18th century) quoted by Esquirol (1816, reference 84).

23 Burrows GM. *Commentaries on the Causes, Forms, Symptoms and Treatment, Moral and Medical of Insanity.* London: Underwood; 1828.

24 Macdonald J. Observations on puerperal mania. *New York Medical Journal.* 1831;1:268–280.

25 Macdonald J. Puerperal insanity. *American Journal of Insanity.* 1847;4:113–163.

26 Reid J. On the causes, symptoms and treatment of puerperal insanity. *Journal of Psychological Medicine.* 1848;1:128–151 and 284–294.

27 Gundry R. Observations upon puerperal insanity. *American Journal of Insanity.* 1859: 294–320.

28 Anderson EW. A study of the sexual life in psychoses associated with childbirth. *Journal of Mental Science.* 1933;79:137–149.

29 Brush EN. Does sepsis play a prominent causative role in the production of puerperal insanity? *American Medical Quarterly.* 1899;1:141–144.

30 Poulsen A. Nogle Bemaerkninger om Puerperalpsychoser. *Hospitals-Tidende.* 4th series. 1899;7:251–260.

31 Ostrander H. Puerperal insanity. *Journal of Michigan State Medical Society.* 1931; 6:49–54.

32 McCarthy DJ. Psychoses and neuroses of pregnancy and the puerperium. *American Journal of Obstetrics.* 1915;72:269–280.

33 Oltman JE, Friedman S. Trends in postpartum illnesses. *American Journal of Psychiatry.* 1965;122:328–329.

34 Ličina M, Mlakar J. *Poporodne i Laktacijske Psihoze Zdravstveni Vestnik.* 1984;53: 3099–3012.

35 Elsässer. Bericht über die Ereignisse in der Gebäranstalt des Catharinen-Hospitals in Stuttgart vom 1 Juli 1842 bis zum 30 Juni 1844. *Medicinisches Correspondenz-Blatt des Würtembürgischen Ärztlichen Vereins.* 1844;14:17–32 and 281–299.

36 Weebers WT. *Over puerperaal-psychosen.* Thesis, Leiden; 1893.

37 Engelhard JLB. Über Generationspsychosen und den Einflus des Gestationsperiode auf schon bestehende psychische und neurologische Krankheiten. *Zeitschrift für Geburtshülfe und Gynäkologie.* 1912;70: 727–812.

38 Guzman A. Trastornos psicóticos vinculados a la función reproductora de la mujer (las psicosis puerperales). *Revista de Obstetricia y Ginecologia de Venezuela.* 1986;46:7–18.

39 Ndosi NK, Mtawali ML. The nature of puerperal psychosis at Muhimbili National Hospital: its physical co-morbidity, associated main obstetric and social factors. *African Journal of Reproductive Health.* 2002;6:41–49.

40 MacLeod MD. An address on puerperal insanity. *British Medical Journal.* 1886; ii:239–242.

41 Kendell RE, Chalmers JC, Platz C. Epidemiology of puerperal psychoses. *British Journal of Psychiatry.* 1987;150: 662–673.

42 Spitzer R, Endicott J, Robins E. *Research diagnostic criteria.* Instrument no. 58, New York: New York State Psychiatric Institute; 1975.

43 Terp IM, Mortensen PB. Postpartum psychoses: clinical diagnoses and relative risk of admission after parturition. *British Journal of Psychiatry.* 1998;172:521–526.

44 Nager A. Johansson LM, Sundquist K. Are sociodemographic factors and year of delivery associated with hospital admission

for postpartum psychosis? A study of 500,000 first-time mothers. *Acta Psychiatrica Scandinavica.* 2005;112:47–53.

45 Munk-Olsen T, Laursen TM, Mendelson T, Pedersen CB, Mors O, Mortensen PB. Risks and predictors of readmission for a mental disorder during the postpartum period. *Archives of General Psychiatry.* 2009; 66:189–195.

46 Friedreich JB. *Systematisches Handbuch der gerichtlichen Psychologie für Medicinalbeamte, Richter und Vertheidiger.* Leipzig: Wigand; 1835. p. 682 and 694–722.

47 Leopold JH. Eigenthümlicher Fall von Melancholie in der Schwangerschaft und im Wochenbette. *Neue Zeitschrift für Geburtskunde.* 1851;29:67–68.

48 Marcé LV. De l'influence de la grossesse et de l'accouchement sur la guérison de l'aliénation mentale. *Annales Médico-psychologiques.* 3rd series. 1857;3: 317–360.

49 Hammouda AA. Selective gestational psychosis: a case report. *Practitioner.* 1966;196:281–282.

50 Taylor MA, Levine R. Puerperal schizophrenia: a physiological interaction between mother and fetus. *Biological Psychiatry.* 1969;1:97–101.

51 Melges FT. Postpartum psychiatric reactions: time of onset and sex ratio of newborns. *Science.* 1969;166:1026–1027.

52 McNeil TF, Kaij L, Persson-Blennow I. Offspring sex and degree of maternal mental disturbance near reproduction among female patients. *Comprehensive Psychiatry.* 1975;16:69–76.

53 Robertson Blackmore E, Jones I, Doshi M, Haque S, Holder R, Brockington IF, et al. Obstetric variables associated with bipolar affective puerperal psychosis. *British Journal of Psychiatry.* 2006;188:32–36.

54 Nager A, Sundquist K, Ramirez-León V, Johansson LM. Obstetric complications and postpartum psychosis: a follow-up study of 1.1 million first-time mothers between 1975 and 2003 in Sweden. *Acta Psychiatrica Scandinavica.* 2007;117: 12–19.

55 Bartholomaeo de Battista a St Georgio. Von der Tollsucht den Kindbetterinnen. In: *Abhandlung von den Krankheiten des schönen Geschlechtes.* Vienna: Sonnleithner; 1784. p. 113–114 in the 1819 edition.

56 Abrahamson M. Von dem Wahnsinn bey Kindbetterinnen. *Meckels Neues Archiv der Praktischen Arzneykunst für Ärzte, Leipzig.* 1789;1:47–49.

57 Weber F. Über *mania puerperalis. Allgemeine Medizinsche Central-Zeitung.* 1870;39:1037–1039 and 1049–1051.

58 Bergink V. *First-onset postpartum psychosis.* Thesis, Rotterdam; 2013.

59 Böszörmenyi Z, Villeneuve A. A comparative study of psychoses following childbirth in Hungary and Quebec. *Confinia Psychiatrica.* 1974;17:111–121.

60 Kadrmas A, Winokur G, Crowe R. Postpartum mania. *British Journal of Psychiatry.* 1979;135:551–554.

61 Brockington IF, Cernik KF, Schofield EM, Downing AR, Francis AF, Keelan C. Puerperal psychosis: phenomena and diagnosis. *Archives of General Psychiatry.* 1981;38:829–833.

62 Katona CLE. Puerperal mental illness: comparisons with non-puerperal controls. *British Journal of Psychiatry.* 1982;141: 447–452.

63 Wisner KL, Pindl K, Hanusa BH. Symptomatology of affective and psychotic illnesses related to childbearing. *Journal of Affective Disorders.* 1994;30:77–87.

64 Hays P. Taxonomic map of the schizophrenias, with special reference to puerperal psychosis. *British Medical Journal.* 1978;ii:755–757.

65 Hays P, Douglass A. A comparison of puerperal psychosis and the schizophreniform variant of manic-depression. *Acta Psychiatrica Scandinavica.* 1984;69:177–181.

66 Brockington IF, Margison F, Schofield E, Knight RJE. The clinical picture of the depressed form of puerperal psychosis. *Journal of Affective Disorders.* 1988; 15:29–37.

67 Brockington IF. *Motherhood and Mental Health*. Oxford: Oxford University Press; 1996.

68 Robertson A. Cases of puerperal insanity. *Glasgow Medical Journal*. new series. 1969;2:125–128.

69 Knauer O. *Über Puerperale Psychosen, für practische Ärzte*. Berlin: Karger; 1897.

70 Paris G. *Des psychoses puerpérales envisagéees au pointe de vue du prognostic*. Thèse, Paris; 1923.

71 Balduzzi E. La psychose puerpérale: essai d'interprétation pathogénique. *Encéphale*. 1951;40:11–43.

72 Dean C, Kendell RE. The symptomatology of puerperal illness. *British Journal of Psychiatry*. 1981;139:128–133.

73 Schöpf J, Bryois C, Jonquiere M, Le PK. On the nosology of severe psychiatric post-partum disorders. *European Archives of Psychiatry and Neurological Sciences*. 1984;234:54–63.

74 Meltzer ES, Kumar R. Puerperal mental illness, clinical features and classification: a study of 142 mother-and-baby admissions. *British Journal of Psychiatry*. 1985;147: 647–654.

75 Klompenhouwer JL. *Puerperal psychosis*. Thesis, Rotterdam; 1992.

76 McNeil TF. A prospective study of postpartum psychoses in a high-risk group. 1. Clinical characteristics of the current postpartum episodes. *Acta Psychiatrica Scandinavica*. 1986;74:205–216.

77 Brockington IF, Kendell RE, Leff JP. Definitions of schizophrenia: concordance and prediction of outcome. *Psychological Medicine*. 1978;8:387–398.

78 Brockington IF, Leff JP. Schizoaffective psychosis: definitions and incidence. *Psychological Medicine*. 1979;9:91–99.

79 Clayton PJ, Rodin L, Winokur G. Family history studies. III. schizoaffective disorder, clinical and genetic factors, including a one to two year follow-up. *Comprehensive Psychiatry*. 1968;9:31–39.

80 Brockington IF, Hillier VF, Francis AF, Helzer JE, Wainwright S. Definitions of

mania: concordance and prediction of outcome. *American Journal of Psychiatry*. 1983;140:435–439.

81 Brockington IF, Winokur G, Dean C. Puerperal psychosis. In: Brockington IF, Kumar R, editors, *Motherhood and Mental Illness*. London: Academic Press; 1982. p. 37–69.

82 Oosthizen P, Russow H, Roberts M. Is puerperal psychosis bipolar mood disorder? A phenomenological comparison. *Comprehensive Psychiatry*. 1995;36:77–81.

83 Robertson Blackmore E, Rubinow DR, O'Connor TG, Liu X, Tang W, Craddock N, et al. Reproductive outcomes and risk of subsequent illness in women diagnosed with postpartum psychosis. *Bipolar Disorders*. 2013;15:394–404.

84 Esquirol JED. Folies. In: Panckoucke CLF, editor, *Dictionaire des Sciences Médicales*. Paris: Panckoucke; 1816. p. 192–193.

85 Clauser F. Contributo allo studio delle psicosi puerperali. *Rivista Italiana di Ginecologia*. 1922;2:379–401.

86 Sivadon P. *Les psychoses puerpérales et leurs séquelles*. Thèse, Paris: 1933.

87 Dubrisay J. Délire extatique éclatant tout à coup dans le cours de la grossesse à la suite d'une émotion morale. *Annales Médico-psychologiques*. 3rd series. 1858;4:428–430.

88 Mares J, Barre R. Quelques aspects des accidents psychiatriques de la puerpéralité en milieu musulman Algérien. *Annales Médico-psychologiques*. 1962;1:31–49.

89 Wise MG, Ward SC, Townsend-Parchman W, Gilstrap LC II, Hauth JC. Case report of ECT during high-risk pregnancy. *American Journal of Psychiatry*. 1984;141:99–101.

90 Luauté JP, Sanabria E, Bidault E, Lusset P, Meunier P. Psychose puerpérale récidivante et calcifications des noyaux gris centraux. *Annales Médico-psychologiques*. 1991;149:257–261.

91 Lértora A. En torno a una psicosis gravido-puerperal curada con cortone. *Obstetricia y Ginecologia Latino-Americanas*. 1955;13:20–30.

92 Marcé LV. Manie hystérique intermittente à la suite de sevrage; accès revenant à chaque époque menstruelle: traitement infructueux par les toniques; guérison par la diète lactée. *Gazette des Hôpitaux.* 1856;29:526.

93 Warburg B. *Über die im Jahre 1909 in der Kieler psychiatrichen und Nervenklinik beobachteten Fälle von Generationspsychosen.* Inaugural-Dissertation, Kiel: 1915.

94 Fauré-Amiel P. *Les états psychotiques et névrotiques de la puerpéralité.* Thèse, Toulouse: 1962. Case 73.

95 Moisan M. *Psychoses puerpérales: approche psychodynamique.* Thèse, Nantes: 1982.

96 Van Steenbergen-van der Noordaa MC. *Generatie-psychosen.* Amsterdam: Academisch Proefschrift; 1941.

97 Visscher GRA. *Generatie-psychoses en hersenstam: een katamnestisch onderzoek.* Thesis, Groningen; 1949.

98 Bergink V, Burgerhout KM, Koorengevel KM, Kamperman AM, Hoogendijk WJ, Lambregtse-van den Berg MP, et al. Treatment of psychosis and mania in the postpartum period. *American Journal of Psychiatry.* 2015;1–9.

99 Bower WH, Altschule MD. Use of progesterone in the treatment of postpartum psychosis. *New England Journal of Medicine.* 1956;254:157–160.

100 Bourson Y. *Contribution à l'étude des psychoses puerpérales.* Thèse, Strasbourg; 1958.

101 Delay J, Boitelle G, Corteel A. Les psychoses du postpartum: étude cyto-hormonale. *Semaines d'Hôpitaux de Paris.* 1948;24:2891–2901.

102 Cain J, Serment M, de Verville M. Les psychoses du post-partum. *Annales Médico-psychologiques.* 1959;117:229–253.

103 Esquirol JED. Observations sur l'aliénation mentale à la suite de couches. *Journal Général de Médecine, de Chirurgie et de Pharmacie Françaises et Étrangères.* 1818;62:629–648.

104 Esquirol JED. De l'aliénation mentale des nouvelles accouchées et des nourrices.

Annuaires Médicales-chirurgiques des Hôpitaux de Paris. 1819;1:600–632.

105 Dupouy R. *Les psychoses puerpérales et les processus d'auto-intoxication.* Thèse, Paris; 1904.

106 Robertson Blackmore E, Craddock N, Walters J, Jones I. Is the perimenopause a time of increased risk of occurrence in women with a history of bipolar affective postpartum psychosis? A case series. *Archives of Women's Mental Health.* 2008;11:75–78.

107 Hesso Norico J. (16th century) Quoted by Schenck (1609, reference 114).

108 Daseking JGW. *Verlauf und Prognose der im Puerperium entstandenen Schizophrenien und schizophrenieartigen Erkrankungen; eine katamnestische Untersuchung.* Inaugural-Dissertation, Berlin; 1931.

109 Bonse M. *Puerperaler Syndromwandel endogener Psychosen.* Inaugural-Dissertation, Münster; 1989.

110 Schröder P. Über Wochenbettpsychosen und unsere heutige Diagnostik. *Allgemeine Zeitschrift für Psychiatrie.* 1936;104: 177–207.

111 Beckmann E. Über Zustandsbilder und Verläufe von Puerperal-Psychosen. *Allgemeine Zeitschrift für Psychiatrie.* 1939;113:239–293.

112 Karnosh LJ, Hope JM. Puerperal psychoses and their sequelae. *American Journal of Psychiatry.* 1937;94:537–550.

113 Jolly P. Zur Prognose der Puerperalpsychosen. *Münchener Medizinische Wochenschrift* 1911;58: 130–133.

114 Schenck of Grafenberg J. *Observationum medicarum, rararum, novarum, admirabilum, et monstrosarum.* Published by his son JG Schenck after his death, 1609.

115 Protheroe C. Puerperal psychoses: a long-term study 1927–1961. *British Journal of Psychiatry.*; 1969;115:9–30.

116 Platz C, Kendell RE. A matched follow-up and family study of 'puerperal psychoses'. *British Journal of Psychiatry.* 1988;153: 90–94.

117 Dean C, Williams RJ, Brockington IF. Is puerperal psychosis the same as bipolar manic depressive disorder? A family study. *Psychological Medicine.* 1989;19:637–647.

118 Schöpf J. *Postpartum-Psychosen: Beitrag zur Nosologie.* Thesis, Zürich; 1992.

119 Pfuhlmann B, Stöber G, Franzek E, Beckmann H. Cycloid psychoses predominate in severe postpartum psychiatric disorders. *Journal of Affective Disorders.* 1998;50:125–134.

120 Pfuhlmann B, Franzek E, Beckmann H, Stöber G. Long-term course and outcome of severe postpartum psychiatric disorders. *Psychopathology.* 1999;32:192–202.

121 Pfuhlman B, Stöber G, Franzek E, Beckmann H. Differenzierte Diagnostik, Verlauf und Ausgang postpartaler Psychosen: eine katamnestische Untersuchung. *Nervenarzt.* 2000;71: 386–392.

122 Lanczik MH. *Entstehungsbedingungen und Verlauf postpartal auftretender psychischer Erkrankungen und Störungen.* Würzburg: Habilitationsschrift; 1994.

123 Terp IM, Engholm G, Møller H, Mortensen PB. A follow-up study of postpartum psychoses: prognosis and risk factors for readmission. *Acta Psychiatrica Scandinavica.* 1999;100:40–46.

124 Robling SA, Paykel ES, Dunn VJ, Abbott R, Katona C. Long-term outcome of severe puerperal psychiatric illness: a 23-year follow-up study. *Psychological Medicine.* 2000;30:1263–1271.

125 Garfield P, Kent A, Paykel ES, Creighton FJ, Jacobson RR. Outcome of postpartum disorders: a 10-year follow-up of hospital admissions. *Acta Psychiatrica Scandinavica.* 2004;109:434–439.

126 Robertson MMA, Jones I, Haque S. Holder R, Craddock N. Risk of puerperal and non-puerperal recurrence of illnesss following bipolar affective puerperal (post-partum) psychosis. *British Journal of Psychiatry.* 2005;186:258–259.

127 Bratfos O, Haug JO. Puerperal mental disorders in manic-depressive females. *Acta Psychiatrica Scandinavica.* 1966; 42:285–294.

128 Freeman MP, Smith KW, Freeman SA, McElroy SL, Kmetz GF, Wright R, et al. The impact of reproductive events on the course of bipolar disorder in women. *Journal of Clinical Psychiatry.* 2002;63: 284–287.

129 Ghaemi SN, Hsu DJ, Ko JY, Baldassano CF, Kontos NJ, Goodwin FK. Bipolar spectrum disorder: a pilot study. *Psychopathology.* 2004;37:222–226.

130 Rybakowski JK, Suwalska A, Lojko D, Rymaszewska J, Kiejna A. Bipolar mood disorders among Polish psychiatric outpatients treated for major depression. *Journal of Affective Disorders.* 2005;84: 141–147.

131 Reich T, Winokur G. Postpartum psychoses in patients with manic depressive disease. *Journal of Nervous and Mental Disease.* 1970;70:60–68.

132 Akiskal HS, Walker P, Puzantian VR, King D, Rosenthal TL, Dranon M. Bipolar outcome in the course of depressive illness: phenomenologic, familial and pharmacologic predictors. *Journal of Affective Disorders.* 1983;5:115–128.

133 McNeil T. Women with nonorganic psychosis: psychiatric and demographic characteristics of cases with *versus* without postpartum psychotic episodes. *Acta Psychiatrica Scandinavica.* 1988;78: 603–609.

134 Wehr TA, Sack DA, Rosenthal NE, Cowdry RW. Rapid cycling affective disorder: contributing factors and treatment responses in 51 patients. *American Journal of Psychiatry.* 1988;145:179–184.

135 Grof P, Robbins W, Alda M, Berghöfer A, Vojtechovsky M, Nilsson A, et al. Protective effect of pregnancy in women with lithium-responsive bipolar disorder. *Journal of Affective Disorders.* 2000; 61:31–39.

136 Jones I, Craddock N. Familiality of the puerperal trigger in bipolar disorder: results of a family study. *American Journal of Psychiatry.* 2001;158:913–917.

137 Akdeniz F, Vahip S, Pirildar S, Vahip I, Doganer I, Bulut I. Risk factors associated with childbearing-related episodes in

women with bipolar disorder. *Psychopathology.* 2003;36:234–238.

138 Di Florio A, Forty L, Gordon-Smith K, Heron J, Jones L, Craddock N, et al. Perinatal episodes across the mood disorder spectrum. *Journal of the American Medical Association Psychiatry.* 2013;70:168–175.

139 Viguera AC, Cohen LS. The course and management of bipolar disorder during pregnancy. *Psychopharmacology Bulletin.* 1998;34:339–346.

140 Viguera AC, Nonacs R, Cohen LS, Tondo L, Murray A, Baldessarini RJ. Risk of recurrence of bipolar disorder in pregnant and nonpregnant women after discontinuing lithium maintenance. *American Journal of Psychiatry.* 2000;157:179–184.

141 Viguera A, Whitfield T, Baldessarini RJ, Newport DJ, Stowe Z, Reminick A, et al. Risk of recurrence of women with bipolar disorder during pregnancy: prospective study of mood stabilizer discontinuation. *American Journal of Psychiatry.* 2007;164:1817–1824.

142 Viguera AC, Tondo L, Koukopoulos AE, Reginaldi D, Lepri B, Baldessarini RJ. Episodes of mood disorders in 2,252 pregnancies and postpartum periods. *American Journal of Psychiatry.* 2011;168:1179–1185.

143 Brockington IF, Martin C, Brown GW, Goldberg P, Margison F. Stress and puerperal psychosis. *British Journal of Psychiatry.* 1990;157:331–334.

144 Dowlatshahi D, Paykel ES. Life events and social stress in puerperal psychoses: absence of effect. *Psychological Medicine.* 1990;20:655–662.

145 Marks MN, Wieck A, Checkley SA, Kumar R. Life stress and post-partum psychosis: a preliminary report. *British Journal of Psychiatry.* 1991;158:45–49.

146 Marks MN, Wieck A, Checkley SA, Kumar R. Contribution of psychological and social factors to psychotic and non-psychotic childbirth in women with previous histories of affective disorder. *Journal of Affective Disorders.* 1992;24:253–263.

147 Tetlow C. Psychoses of childbearing. *Journal of Mental Science.* 1955;101:629–639.

148 Kendell RE, Rennie D, Clarke JA, Dean C. The social and obstetric correlates of psychiatric admission in the puerperium. *Psychological Medicine.* 1981;11:341–350.

149 Ostermann E. Des états psychopathologiques du postpartum: la fréquence, le développement et le pronostic de ces états. *Encéphale.* 1963;52:365–420.

150 Lange P. *Über psychische Erkrangungen in Schwangerschaft und Wochenbett: eine retrospektive Studie.* Inaugural-Dissertation, Münster; 1994.

151 Serretti A, Olgiati P, Colombo C. Influence of postpartum onset on the course of mood disorders. *BioMed Central Psychiatry.* 2006;26:4–12.

152 Paffenbarger RS. The picture puzzle of the postpartum psychoses. *Journal of Chronic Diseases.* 1961;13:161–173.

153 Jansson B. Psychic insufficiencies associated with childbearing. *Acta Psychiatrica Scandinavica.* 1963;39: supplement 172.

154 Paffenbarger RS Jr, McCabe LJ Jr. The effect of obstetric and perinatal events on risk of mental illness in women of childbearing age. *American Journal of Public Health.* 1966;56:400–407.

155 Hellerstedt WL, Phelan SM, Cnattingius S, Hultman CM, Harlow BL. Are prenatal, obstetric, and infant complications associated with postpartum psychosis among women with pre-conception psychiatric hospitalisations? *British Journal of Obstetrics & Gynaecology.* 2012;120:446–455.

156 Paffenbarger RS. Epidemiological aspects of parapartum mental illness. *British Journal of Preventive & Social Medicine.* 1964;18:189–195.

157 Yogananda BH. *A Study of the Phenomenology and Quality of Marital life in Major Postpartum Psychiatric Disorders.* MD Thesis, Bangalore; 1997.

158 Lewis, WB. *Insanity at the Puerperal, Climacteric and Lactational Periods.* New York: Wood; 1890. p. 295–347.

159 Parfitt DN. The blood urea in psychotics. *Journal of Mental Science.* 1933;79:501–507.

160 Haworth NA. Malnutrition and debility in puerperal psychoses. *Lancet.* 1939;ii: 417–418.

161 Jansson B, Selldén U. EEG investigation of women with psychic insufficiencies associated with childbearing. *Acta Psychiatrica Scandinavica.* 1966;42:89–96.

162 Enomoto S. [Pathophysiological studies of mental disorders in puerperium] *Journal of Kyushu Neuropsychiatry.* 1978;23:190–212.

163 Goode DJ, Meltzer HY, Fang VS. Increased prolactin levels during phenothiazine and butyrophenone treatment of six postpartum women. *Psychoneuroendocrinology.* 1980;5:545–551.

164 Whalley LJ, Robinson ICAF, Fink G. Oxytocin and neurophysin in postpartum mania. *Lancet.* 1982;ii:387–388.

165 Lindström LH, Nyberg F, Terenius L, Bauer K, Besev G, Gunne LM, et al. CSF and plasma β-casomorphin-like opioid peptides in postpartum psychosis. *American Journal of Psychiatry.* 1984; 141:1059–1065.

166 Lindström L, Nyberg F, Terenius L. Postpartumpsykos – nya rön om en gammal sjukdom. *Läkartidningen.* 1987;84:755–758.

167 Terenius L, Lyrenas S, Lutsch H, Lindstrom L, Nyberg F, Lindberg B. Opioid peptides at term pregnancy in the early puerperium and in postpartum psychosis. *Advances in Biochemical Psychopharmacology.* 1987;43:201–209.

168 Nyberg F, Lindstrom EH, Terenius L. Reduced beta-casein levels in milk samples from patients with postpartum psychosis. *Biological Psychiatry.* 1988;23:115–122.

169 Renlund S, Erlandsson I, Hellman U, Silberring J, Wernstedt C, Lindström L, et al. Micropurification and amino acid sequence of β-casomorphin in milk from a woman with postpartum psychosis. *Peptides.* 1993;14:1125–1132.

170 Mampunza M, Dechef G, Kinsala Y, M'Pania PM, Mbanzulu PN, Ntudulu N. Les psychoses post-gravidiques à Kinshasa. *Acta Psychiatrica Belgica.* 1984;84: 284–293.

171 Riley DM, Watt DC. Hypercalcaemia in the etiology of puerperal psychosis. *Biological Psychiatry.* 1985;20:479–488.

172 Sane AS, Pandya AK, Patel MJ, Vaishnav MD. Serum cholesterol and triglycerides in post-partum psychosis. *Panminerva Med.* 1985;27:143–146.

173 Frank E, Kupfer DJ, Jacob M, Blumenthal SJ, Jarrett DB. Pregnancy-related affective episodes among women with recurrent depression. *American Journal of Psychiatry.* 1987;144:288–293.

174 Urdén G, Thornwall M, Lyrenäs S, Lindström L, Nyberg F. Classification of CSF samples from normal and post-partum psychotic chromatographic profiles with bilinear projections: a multivariate approach. *Biomedical Chromatography.* 1996;10:149–154.

175 Becker T, Hofmann E, Knoche M, Lanczik M. Neuroradiological findings in postpartum psychiatric disorder. *European Psychiatry.* 1993;8:105–107.

176 Lanczik M, Fritz J, Hofmann E, Knoche M, Schulz C, Becker T. Neuroradiologische Befunde bei postpartalen Psychosen. In: Moeller HJ, Mueller-Spahn F, Kurtz G, editors, *Aktuelle Perspectiven der Biologischen Psychiatrie.* Vienna: Springer; 1996. p. 705–707.

177 Schulz C. *CT-MRT-Veränderungen bei Puerperalpsychosen.* Inaugural-Dissertation, Würzburg; 1996.

178 Bilszta JL, Meyer D, Buist AE. Bipolar affective disorder in the postnatal period: investigating the role of sleep. *Bipolar Disorders.* 2010;12:568–578.

179 Singh B, Gilhotra M, Smith R, Brinsmead M, Lewin T, Hall C. Postpartum psychoses and the dexamethasone suppression test. *Journal of Affective Disorders.* 1986;11: 173–177.

180 Eberl BM. *Verlauf und Klinik der Puerperal psychose: pro- und retrospektive Untersuchungen an der Psychiatrischen Universitätsklinik Würzburg.* Inaugural-Dissertation, Würzburg; 1989.

181 Paykel ES, Martin del Campo A, White W, Horton R. Neuroendocrine challenge studies in puerperal psychosis: dexamethasone suppression and TRH stimulation. *British Journal of Psychiatry.* 1991;159:262–266.

182 Nomura J, Hatotani N, Yamaguchi T, Inoue K, Kitayama I, Higashimura T. Endocrine studies on recurrent type of schizophreniform psychoses. In: Namba M, Kaiya, H, editors, *Psychobiology of Schizophrenia.* Oxford: Pergamon; 1982. p. 303–308.

183 Nomura J, Okano T, Komori T, Harada M, Kitayama I, Inoue K, et al. Clinico-endocrine studies of postpartum psychosis, In: Shagass C et al., editors, *Biological Psychiatry.* Amsterdam: Elsevier; 1986. p. 228–230.

184 Stewart DE, Addison AM, Robinson GE, Joffe R, Burrow GN, Olmsted MP. Thyroid function in psychosis following childbirth. *American Journal of Psychiatry.* 1988; 145:1579–1581.

185 Meakin CJ, Brockington IF, Lynch SE, Jones SR. Dopamine supersensitivity and hormonal status in puerperal psychosis. *British Journal of Psychiatry.* 1995; 166:73–79.

186 Wieck A, Kumar R, Hirst AD, Marks MN, Campbell IC, Checkley SA. Increased sensitivity of dopamine receptors and recurrence of puerperal psychosis. *British Medical Journal.* 1991;303:613–616.

187 Brockington IF, Meakin CJ. Increased sensitivity of dopamine receptors in puerperal psychosis, (followed by a reply). *British Medical Journal.* 1991;303:1334.

188 Kumar C, McIvor RJ, Davies T, Brown N, Papadopoulos A, Wieck A, et al. Estrogen administration does not reduce the rate of recurrence of affective psychosis after childbirth. *Journal of Clinical Psychiatry.* 2003;64:112–118.

189 Kaij L. Atypical endogenous psychosis: report on a family. *British Journal of Psychiatry.* 1967;113:415–422.

190 Wålinder J. Recurrent familial psychosis of the schizo-affective type. *Acta Psychiatrica Scandinavica.* 1971;48:274–283.

191 Craddock N, Brockington IF, Mant R, Parfitt E, McGuffin P, Owen M. Bipolar affective puerperal psychosis associated with consanguinity. *British Journal of Psychiatry.* 1994;164:359–364.

192 Sivagamasundari U, Fernando H, Jardine P, Rao JM, Lunt P, Jayewardene SLW. The association between Coffin-Lowry syndrome and psychosis: a family study. *Journal of Intellectual Disability.* 1994;38:469–473.

193 Thuwe I. Genetic factors in puerperal psychosis. *British Journal of Psychiatry.* 1974;125:378–385.

194 Jones I, Craddock N. Do puerperal psychotic episodes identify a more familial subtype of bipolar disorder? Results of a family history study. *Psychiatric Genetics.* 2002;12:177–180.

195 Arentsen K. Postpartum psychoses with particular reference to the prognosis. *Danish Medical Bulletin.* 1968;15:97–100.

196 Coyle N, Jones I, Robertson E, Lendon C, Craddock N. Variation in the serotonin transporter gene influences susceptibility to bipolar affective puerperal psychosis. *Lancet.* 2000;356:1490–1491.

197 Jones I, Middle F, McCandless F, Coyle N, Robertson E, Brockington I, et al. Molecular genetic studies of bipolar disorder and puerperal psychosis at two polymorphisms in estrogen receptor α gene (ESR 1). *American Journal of Medical Genetics (Neuropsychiatric Genetics.)* 2000;96:850–853.

198 Middle F, Jones I, Robertson E, Morey J, Lendon C, Craddock N. Variation at the coding sequence and flanking splice junctions of the estrogen receptor alpha (Erα) gene does not play an important role in genetic susceptibility to bipolar disorder or bipolar affective puerperal psychosis. *American Journal of Medical Genetics.* 2003;118B:72–75.

199 Middle F, Jones I, Robertson E, Lendon C, Craddock N. Tumour necrosis factor α and bipolar affective puerperal psychosis. *Psychiatric Genetics.* 2000;10:195–198.

200 Robertson E, Jones I, Middle F, Morey J, Lendon C, Craddock N. No association

between two polymorphisms at the 5HT2A gene and bipolar affective puerperal psychosis. *Acta Psychiatrica Scandinavica.* 2003;108:387–391.

201 Jones I, Hamshere M, Nangle JM, Bennett P, Green E, Heron J, et al. Bipolar affective puerperal psychosis: genome-wide significant evidence for linkage to chromosome 16. *American Journal of Psychiatry.* 2007;164:1099–1104.

202 Berkson J. Limitation of the application of 4-fold tables in hospital data. *Biometrical Bulletin. 1946;* 1946;2:47–53.

203 Marcé LV. *Traité de la Folie des Femmes Enceintes, des Nouvelles Accouchées et des Nourrices, et Considérations Médico-légales qui se rattachent à ce Sujet.* Paris: Baillière; 1858.

204 Rocher G. *Étude sur la folie puerpérale.* Thèse, Paris; 1877.

205 Lallier A. *De la folie puerpérale dans ses rapports avec l'éclampsie et les accidents infectieux suites de couches.* Thèse, Paris; 1892.

206 Senlecq F. *Du délire post-éclamptique.* Thèse, Paris; 1896.

207 Meyer E. Die Puerperalpsychosen. *Archiv für Psychiatrie und Nervenkrankheiten.* 1911;48:459–522.

208 Zilboorg G. Malignant psychoses related to childbirth. *American Journal of Obstetrics & Gynecology.* 1928;15:145–158.

209 Duval RAE. *Les psychoses puerpérales.* Thèse, Lille; 1934.

210 Vayssiere D. *Contribution à l'étude des psychoses du post-partum; étude cyto-hormonale.* Thèse, Paris; 1949.

211 Dazzi P. Le psicosi puerperali. *Rivista di Neuropsichiatria e Scienze Affini.* 1957; 3:1–162.

212 Berthier P. *Les Névroses Menstruelles ou la Menstruation dans ses Rapports avec les Maladies Nerveuses et Mentales.* Paris: Delahaye; 1874.

213 Powers EF. *Beitrag zur Kenntniss der menstrualen Psychosen.* Inaugural-Dissertation, Zürich; 1883.

214 Icard S. *La Femme pendant la Période Menstruelle.* Paris: Alcan; 1890.

215 Schwob A. *Contribution à l'étude des psychoses menstruelles, considérées surtout au point de vue médico-légal.* Thèse, Lyon; 1893.

216 Kowalewski PJ. Der Menstruationszustand und die Menstruations-psychosen. *St. Petersburg Medizinische Wochenschrift.* 1894;19:216–218, 227–229, 238–241, 247–250, 258–260.

217 Epstein L. A menstrualis elmezavarrol. Translated in *Pest Médico-chirurgical Presse.* 1897;33:744–750; 768–772; 803–810; 829–835.

218 v. Krafft-Ebing R. *Psychosis Menstrualis: eine klinisch-forensische Studie.* Stuttgart: Enke; 1902.

219 Häffner R. Beziehungen zwischen Menstruation und Nerven- und Geisteskrankheiten auf Grund der Literatur und klinischer Studien. *Zeitschrift für die gesamte Neurologie und Psychiatrie.* 1912;9:154–223.

220 Jolly P. Menstruation und Psychosen. *Archiv für Psychiatrie und Nervenkrankheiten.* 1914;55:637–686.

221 Splett T. *Die wissenschaftliche Erforschung der Menstruationspsychosen in der deutschen Psychiatrie bis 1945.* Inaugural-Dissertation, Würzburg; 1996.

222 Boyd DA Jr. Mental disorders associated with childbearing. *American Journal of Obstetrics & Gynecology.* 1942;43:148–163 and 43:335–349.

223 Kunst AH. Puerperal insanity. *Transactions of the Medical Society of West Virginia.* 1878;355–370.

224 Lee CP. Puerperal mania. *Kansas Medical Index.* 1881;2:200–208.

225 Hirst BC. A case of pregnancy complicated by anemia, chorea, insanity and pyelitis. *University Medical Magazine.* 1888;1: 151–152.

226 Castin P. *Des psychoses puerpérales dans leur rapports avec la dégénerescence mentale.* Thèse, Paris; 1899.

227 Esquirol JED. *Des Maladies Mentales considérées sous les Rapports Médicals, Hygiéniques et Médico-Légals.* Paris: Baillière; 1838. Translated into English in 1845.

228 Campbell Clark A. Aetiology, pathology and treatment of puerperal insanity. *Journal of Mental Science*. 1887;33:169–189, 372–379 and 487–496.

229 Donkin AS. On the pathological relation between albuminuria and puerperal mania. *Edinburgh Medical Journal*. 1863;8: 994–1004.

230 Schneider E. Zur Therapie der 'Menstrualpsychosen'. *Allgemeine Zeitschrift für Psychiatrie und Psychisch-gerichtliche Medizin*. 81:368–373.

231 Hirschmann-Wertheimer I. Wechselseitige Beziehungen von Menstruation und Psyche. *Monatsschrift für Psychiatrie und Neurologie*. 1927;66:215–254.

232 Aschner B. Neurosen und Psychosen bei Menstruations-störungen (Körperliche Behandlung von Geisteskrankheiten). *Wiener Klinische Wochenschrift*. 1931;44:1132–1135.

233 Goldschmidt E. Ursachen und Behandlung prämenstruell-menstruell psychisch nervöser Störungen. *Wiener Medizinische Wochenschrift*. 1935;85:612–615.

234 Martinius J. Periodic psychosis in adolescence. *Zeitschrift für Kinder und Jugendpsychiatrie*. 1992;20:121–125.

235 Kirkland T. *A treatise on childbed fevers and on the methods of preventing them*. London: Baldwin & Dawson; 1774; 56–63, 72–73 and 92–95.

236 Barth. Ein Fall von plötzlich nach der Entbindung entstandener *Mania transitoria*. *Henke's Zeitschrift für der Staatsarzneikunde*. 1828;16: 108–110.

237 Kelso J. Nervous exhaustion dependent on and complicating the puerperal state with cases. *Lancet* 1840;i:945–948.

238 Tott CA. Fälle von *melancholia attonita* bei Neuentbundenen. *Neue Zeitschrift für Geburtskunde*. 1844;16:187–190.

239 Imbert-Gourbeyer A. Des paralyses puerpérales. *Mémoirs de l'Académie Impériale de Médecine*. 1861;25:46–53.

240 Kutzinski A. Über eklamptische Psychosen. *Charité-Annalen*. 1909;33: 216–260.

241 Kirchberg P. Psychische Störungen während der Geburt. *Archiv für Psychiatrie*. 1913;52:1153–1163.

242 Kleinknecht F. *Die posteklamptischen psychosen*. Inaugural-Dissertation, Leipzig; 1914.

243 Sioli F. Eklamptische und post-eklamptische Psychosen. In: Hinselmann H, editor, *Die Eklampsie*. Bonn: Cohen; 1924. p. 597–524.

244 Herrmann E. *Die Eklampsie und ihre Prophylaxie*. Berlin and Vienna: Urban & Schwarzenberg; 1929. p. 150–159.

245 Kalbag RM, Woolf AL. *Cerebral Venous Thrombosis*. London: Oxford University Press; 1967.

246 Yamada N, Fukui M, Ishii K, Shibata H, Okabe H, Ohomiya H, et al. [Adult hypercitrullinaemia with consciousness disturbance and marked hypertransaminasemia after delivery]. *Nihon Shokakibyo Gakkai Zasshi*. 1980;77:1655–1660.

247 Breton A. *État mental dans la chorée*. Thèse, Paris; 1893.

248 Collet MJ. *l'Accouchement spontané rapide*. Thèse, Paris; 1904.

249 Osiander FB. *Neue Denkwürdigkeiten für Ärzte und Geburtshelfer*. Volume 1. Göttingen: Rosenbusch; 1797. p. 52–89 and 90–128.

250 Widerøe J. Puerperale Psykoser. *Saertryk av Tidschrift f Nordisk Retsmedesin og Psykiatri*. 1903: 1–103.

251 Mendel E. *Die Manie*. Leipzig and Vienna: Urban & Warzenberg; 1881. p. 80–83 and 90–93.

252 Wollenberg R. Drei Fälle von periodisch auftretender Geistesstörung. *Charité-Annalen*. 1891;16:427–476.

253 Ewald G. Fraktionerte Kastration mittels Röntgenstrahlen und Operation bei einer menstruell rezidivierenden Psychose. *Münchener Medizinische Wochenschrift*. 1924;71:336–338.

254 Brockington IF, Kelly A, Hall P, Deakin W. Premenstrual relapse of puerperal psychosis. *Journal of Affective Disorders*. 1988;14:287–292.

255 Horwitz WA, Harris MM. Study of a case of cyclic psychic disturbances associated with menstruation. *American Journal of Psychiatry*. 1935;92:1403–1412.

256 Brière de Boismont A. Recherches bibliographiques et cliniques sur la folie puerpérale, précédées d'un aperçu sur les rapports de la menstruation et de l'aliénation mentale. *Annales Médico-psychologiques*. 2nd series. 1851;3:574–610.

257 Yamashita I. *Periodic psychosis of adolescence*. Sapporo: Hokkaido University Press; 1993.

258 Siemerling E. Graviditäts- und Puerperalpsychosen. In: Schultz E et al., editors, *Lehrbuch der Psychiatrie*. Jena: Fischer; 1920. p. 220–236.

259 Delay J, Boitelle G, Corteel A. Explorations cyto-hormonales au cours des psychoses du post-partum. *Annales Médico-psychologiques*. 1948;106:62–68.

260 Thomas CL, Gordon TJE. Psychosis after childbirth: ecological aspects of a single impact stress. *American Journal of the Medical Sciences*. 1959;238:363–388.

261 Kendell RE. Emotional and physical factors in the genesis of puerperal mental disorders. *Journal of Psychosomatic Research*. 1985;29:3–11.

262 Hoffmann F. *De primipara ex terrore facta maniaca et feliciter restituta*, In: *Medicinae Rationalis Systematicae*. Dec. III, casus III. Venice: Coltei; 1721. p. 125–127.

263 Müller-Fahlbusch H, Ichikawa J. Zur Frage de Rezidive von Wochenbettpsychose. *Nervenarzt*. 1969;40:481–485.

264 Reichard. Eine heftige Raseren von zurückgetretener Milch, vorzüglich durch den Hurhamschen Spiessglas-Wein geheilt. *J Ch Starks Neues Archiv für die Geburtshülfe, Frauenzimmer und Neugebohrner Kinder-Krankheiten*. 1787;1:78–89.

265 Scott DH. Puerperal mania, beneficial effects of belladonna. *Dublin Medical Journal*. 1838;13:442–446.

266 Arnold AB. Insanity occurring in the puerperal state. *Maryland Medical Journal*. 1880;7:73–76.

267 Brooke H. Puerperal mania. *Journal of Nervous & Mental Disease*. 1887;14: 361–382.

268 Anderson EW. A clinical study of states of 'ecstasy' occurring in affective disorders. *Journal of Neurology, Neurosurgery and Psychiatry*. 1937;1:80–99.

269 Wessel J. *Die nicht wahrgenomme (verdrängte) Schwangerschaft*. Berlin: Habilitationsschrift; 1998.

270 Morel BA. Mémoire sur la manie des femmes en couche. *Bullétin des Travaux de la Société Médico-pratique de Paris*. 1842;35:52–67 and 36:5–56.

271 Worthington JH. On puerperal insanity. *American Journal of Insanity*. 1861;18: 42–60.

272 Perretti J. Über die Beeinflussung der Geistesstörung durch Schwangerschaft. *Archiv für Psychiatrie*. 1885;16:442–463.

273 Bruas FM. *Grossesse dans les névroses, les psychoses et en particulier la paralysie générale*. Thèse, Bordeaux; 1902.

274 Fürstner C. Über Schwangerschafts- und Puerperalpsychosen. *Archiv für Psychiatrie und Nervenkrankheiten*. 1875;5:505–543.

275 Underhill AS. Notes from my midwifery casebook. *Birmingham Medical Review*. 1874;3:112–116.

276 Bamford CB. An analytical review of a series of cases of insanity with pregnancy. *Journal of Mental Science*. 1934;80:58–63.

277 Berthier P. Délire mélancolique déterminé par une grossesse, passée inaperçue de tous, même de la malade, et jugé par un accouchement et une délivrance simultanés, également accomplis à l'insu de la malade. *Gazette Médicale de Lyon*. 1859;11:116–117.

278 Amann J. *Klinik der Wochenbettkrankheiten*. Stuttgart: Enke; 1876, p. 288–297.

279 Wu PL. *Psychosen nach Entbindungen und gynäkologischen Operationen*. Inaugural-Dissertation, Berlin; 1933.

280 Callieri B. Il problema nosologico delle psicosi puerperali. *Rassegna degli Studi Psichiatrici*. 1955;44:769–800.

281 Galletti L, Niccolo M, Rambelli L. Considerazioni sulle psicosi puerperali. *Rivista di Neuropsichiatrica e Scienze Affini.* 1962;2:92–110.

282 Nilsson R, Perris C. The Capgras syndrome: a case report. *Acta Psychiatrica Scandinavica.* 1971;221, supplement:53–58.

283 Scherrer P. Névroses et psychoses de la grossesse. *Revue Médicale de Dijon.* 1971;6:241–267.

284 Cohn CK, Rosenblatt S, Faillace LA. Capgras' syndrome presenting as postpartum psychosis. *Southern Medical Journal.* 1977;70:8.

285 Silva JA, Leong GB, Longhitano M, Botello TE. Delusion of fetal duplication in a Capgras patient. *Canadian Journal of Psychiatry.* 1991;36:46–47.

286 Murray D. Recurrence of puerperal psychosis not prevented by prophylactic progesterone administration. *Journal of Nervous and Mental Disease.* 1990;178: 537–538.

287 Ahokas A, Aito M, Rimon R. Positive treatment effect of estradiol in postpartum psychosis: a pilot study. *Journal of Clinical Psychiatry.* 2000;61:166–169.

288 Pazzagli A, Benvenuti P, Rossi Monti M. Psicosi puerperali: personalità, stati-limite e maternità. *Rassegna di Studi Psichiatrici.* 1979;68:1–18.

289 Ripping LH. *Die Geistesstörungen der Schwangeren, Wöchnerinnen und Säugenden.* Stüttgart: Enke; 1877.

290 Ferdière G, Daumézon G. Syndrome catatonique puerpérale avec aréflexie. *Annales Médico-psychologiques.* 1937;95:82–85.

291 Morison A. *Cases of Mental Disease with Practical Observations on the Medical Treatment.* London: Longman & Highley; 1828, p. 28–53 and 159–161.

292 Churchill F. *On the Diseases of Women Including Diseases of Pregnancy and Childbed.* 3rd ed. Dublin: Fannin; 1850, p. 424–429, 526–528 and 733–742.

293 Scherrer P. Névroses et psychoses de la grossesse. *Revue Médicale de Dijon.* 1971;6:241–267.

294 Hermes J. *Über die im Jahre 1907 in der Psych- und Nervenklinik behandelten Puerperalpsychosen.* Inaugural-Dissertation, Kiel; 1908.

295 Gooch R. *An Account of Some of the Most Important Diseases Peculiar to Women.* London: Murray; 1829, p. 108–175.

296 Capelle J. *Puerpéralité et psychoses.* Thèse, Bordeaux; 1929.

297 Weill. *Considérations générales sur la folie puerpérale.* Thèse, Strasbourg; 1851.

298 Bürgi S. Puerperalpsychose oder Diencephalosis puerperalis? *Schweizerische Medizinische Wochenschrift.* 1954;84: 1222–1225.

299 World Health Organization. *The ICD-7 Classification of Mental and Behavioural Disorders.* 7th revision. Geneva: WHO; 1957.

300 World Health Organization. *The ICD-8 Classification of Mental and Behavioural Disorders.* 8th revision. Geneva: WHO; 1967.

301 World Health Organization. *The ICD-9 Classification of Mental and Behavioural Disorders.* 9th revision. Geneva: WHO; 1975.

302 World Health Organization. *The ICD-10 Classification of Mental and Behavioural Disorders.* 10th revision. Geneva: WHO; 1992.

303 World Health Organization. *The ICD-10 Classification of Mental and Behavioural Disorders: Clinical Descriptions and Diagnostic Guidelines.* Geneva, WHO; 1992.

304 American Psychiatric Association. *Diagnostic and Statistical Manual of Mental Disorders.* Washington DC: APA; 1952.

305 American Psychiatric Association. *Diagnostic and Statistical Manual of Mental Disorders.* 2nd ed. Washington DC: APA; 1968.

306 American Psychiatric Association. *Diagnostic and Statistical Manual of Mental Disorders.* 3rd ed. Washington DC: APA; 1980.

307 American Psychiatric Association. *Diagnostic and Statistical Manual of Mental Disorders*. 3rd ed. revised. Washington DC: APA; 1987.

308 American Psychiatric Association. *Diagnostic and Statistical Manual of Mental Disorders*. 4th ed. Washington DC: APA; 1994.

309 American Psychiatric Association. *Diagnostic and Statistical Manual of Mental Disorders*. 5th ed. Washington DC: APA; 2013.

310 Brockington IF. Letter to the editor. *Archives of Women's Mental Health*. 2011;14:361.

311 Essen Möller E. On classification of mental disorders. *Acta Psychiatrica Scandinavica*. 1961;37:119–126.

312 Bydlowski M, Raoul-Duval A. Un avatar psychique méconnu de la puerpéralité: la névrose traumatique post-obstétricale. *Perspectives Psychiatriques*. 1978;4:321–328.

313 Brown WA, Shereshefsky P. Seven women: a prospective study of postpartum psychiatric disorders. *Psychiatry*. 1972;35:139–159.

314 De Armond M. A type of postpartum anxiety reaction. *Diseases of the Nervous System*. 1954;15:26–29.

315 Weightman H, Dalal BM, Brockington IF. Pathological fear of cot death. *Psychopathology*. 1998;31:246–249.

316 Zilboorg G. The dynamics of schizophrenic reactions related to pregnancy and childbirth. *American Journal of Psychiatry*. 1929;85:733–767.

317 Wimmer A. *Psykogene Sindssygdomsformer*. St. Hans Hospital 1816–1916: Jubilee; 1916.

318 Faergeman PM. *Psychogenic Psychoses: A Description and Follow-Up of Psychoses Following Psychological Stress*. London: Butterworths; 1963.

319 Strömgren E. The development of the concept of reactive psychoses. *Psychopathology*. 1986;20:62–67.

320 Melges FT. Postpartum psychiatric syndromes. *Psychosomatic Medicine*. 1968;30:95–108.

321 Asch SS, Rubin LJ. Postpartum reactions: some unrecognised variations. *American Journal of Psychiatry*. 1974;131:870–874.

322 Durand VJ, Vaneecloo P, Aurières M. À propos de deux cas de psychoses puerpérales. *Annales Médico-psychologiques*. 1978;136:630–638.

323 Trixler M, Jádi F, Wágner M. Adoptáció utáni 'post partum' pszichózisok. *Orvosi Hetilap*. 1981;122:3071–3074.

324 Remington GJ, Rosenblatt H. Spousal allegations of incest during transient psychotic episodes. *British Journal of Psychiatry*. 1991;159:287–288.

325 Van Putten R, LaWall J. Postpartum psychosis in an adoptive mother and in a father. *Psychosomatics*. 1991;22:1087–1089.

326 Privat de Fortunié J. *Étude sur le délire post-partum*. Thèse, Paris; 1904.

327 Cremer D. *Zur Klinik der Puerperalpsychosen*. Inaugural-Dissertation, Kiel; 1914.

328 Andersen HA. *Über Puerperalpsychosen*. Inaugural-Dissertation, Kiel; 1919.

329 Edelberg H, Galant S. Über psychotische Zustände nach künstlichem Abort. *Zeitschrift für die Gesamte Neurologie und Psychiatrie*. 1925;97:106–128.

330 Hilpert P. Zur Symptomatologie der nichteitrigen Sinusthrombosen. *Klinische Wochenschrift*. 1929;8:496–500.

331 Vitorović M. Psihične motnje v zvezi z generativnimi procesi: puerperij, laktacija. In: *Učbenik Psihiatrija*. Ljubljana: DUU Universum; 1978. p. 243–248.

332 Gueye M. *Les psychoses puerpérales en milieu Sénégalais: à propos de 92 observations*. Thèse, Dakar; 1976.

333 Weber of Sonnenstein. Schwangerschafts- und Puerperalpsychosen. Jahresbericht der Gesellschaft für Natur und Heilkunde zu Dresden. 1876: 131–143.

334 Brockington IF, Cox JL, Garret-Gloanec N, Apter G. Perinatal mental disorders. In: Salloum IM, Mezzich JE, editors, *Psychiatric Diagnosis: Patterns and Prospects*. Chichester: Wiley, Blackwell; 2009.

335 Hansen T. *Om forholdet mellem puerperal Sindssygdom og puerperal Infection.* Thesis, Kopenhaagen; 1888.

336 Behr of Hildenheim. Aetiologie der Puerperalpsychosen. *Allgemeine Zeitschrift für Psychiatrie.* 1876;56:802–814.

337 Hoppe H. Symptomatologie und Prognose der im Wochenbett entstehenden Geistesstörungen (zugleich ein Beitrag zur Lehre von der acuten hallucinatorischen Verwirrtheit). *Archiv für Psychiatrie und Nervenkrankheiten.* 1893;25:137–210.

338 Keyserlingk H. Zum Krankheitsbild der Wochenbettpsychosen. *Archiv für Psychiatrie und Nervenkrankheiten.* 1962;203:632–647.

339 Runge W. Die Generationspsychosen des Weibes. *Archiv für Psychiatrie und Nervenkrankheiten.* 1911;48:545–690.

340 Werner C. *Die Paranoia.* Stuttgart: Enke; 1911.

341 Meynert T. Amentia, die Verwirrtheit. *Jahrbücher für Psychiatrie.* 1890;9:1–111.

342 Vogel WFE. *Beitrag zur Klinik der Puerperalpsychosen und zur Prognose der Katatonie.* Inaugural-Dissertation, Breslau; 1908.

343 Steinmann I. Die Verursachung der Wochenbettpsychosen. *Archiv für Psychiatrie und Nervenkrankheiten.* 1935;103:552–579.

344 Shdarow. Die puerperalen Psychosen, vom ätiologischen, klinischen und forensichen Standpunkt, Moskau. (1896) Summarised in *Neurologisches Zentralblatt.* 1898. p. 278.

345 Mitkus W. Psicozy poporodowe. *Polska Gazeta Lekarska.* 1927;6:553–555, 578–580, and 598–600.

346 Inguirami L. Sulla prognosi delle psicosi puerperali. *Neopsichiatria.* 1957;23:287–308.

347 Haasz I, Haasz-Lux A. Postpartalne psihoze. *Lijecn Vjesn.* 1964;86:35–43.

348 Libusová E, Šmid J. Podíl iatropatogenie na vzniku poporodní psychózy. *Československa Gynaekologie.* 1967;33:109–112.

349 Pogády J, Hudáková G, Rybauská A Niektoré klinické ukazovatele pri popôrodnych psychózach. *Casopis Lékaru Ceských.* 1968;107:1010–1012.

350 Kraepelin E. *Psychiatrie: ein Lehrbuch für Studierende und Ärzte.* Volume 1. Leipzig: Barth; 1909. p. 520.

351 Pichot P. The birth of the bipolar disorder. *European Psychiatry.* 1995;10:1–10.

352 Angst J, Perris C. The nosology of endogenous depression. *International Journal of Mental Health.* 1972;1:145–158.

353 Brockington IF, Roper A, Buckley M, Copas C, Wigg P, Farmer A, et al. Bipolar disorder, cycloid psychosis and schizophrenia: a study using 'lifetime' psychopathology ratings, factor analysis and canonical variate analysis. *European Psychiatry.* 1991;6:223–236.

354 Reardon DC, Cougle JR, Rue VM, Shuping MW, Coleman PK, Ney PG. Psychiatric admissions of low-income women following abortion and childbirth. *Canadian Medical Association Journal.* 2003;168:1253–1256.

355 Munk-Olsen T, Laursen TM, Pedersen CB, Mors O, Mortensen PB. New parents and mental disorders: a population-based study. *Journal of the American Medical Association.* 2006;296:2582–2589.

356 Wernicke C. *Grundriss der Psychiatrie.* 2nd ed. republished under Lanczik M, Arts N, editors, Nijmegen: Arts & Boeve; 1906.

357 Kleist K. Autochthone Degenerationspsychosen. *Zeitschrift für die gesamte Neurologie und Psychiatrie.* 1921;69:1–11.

358 Leonhard K. *Aufteilung der endogenen Psychosen und ihre differenzierte Ätiologie.* Berlin: Akademie; 1968.

359 Perris C. A study of cycloid psychosis. *Acta Psychiatrica Scandinavica, supplement.* 1974;253.

360 Brockington IF, Perris C, Kendell RE, Hillier VE, Wainwright S. The course and outcome of cycloid psychosis. *Psychological Medicine.* 1982;12:97–105.

361 Grosse U. Diagnostische Beurteilung der im Puerperium ausbrechenden Psychosen. *Psychiatrie, Neurologie und Medizinische Psychologie.* 1968;20:222–225.

362 Winter F. *Die Wochenbettpsychosen.* Inaugural-Dissertation, Marburg; 1908.

363 Chevalier-Lavoure, Voivenel. Quelques observations nouvelles de psychoses puerpérales. *Comptes Rendus de la Société d'Obstétrique et de Gynécologie et de Pédiatrie.* 1910;12:238–245.

364 Hoch A, Kirby GH. A clinical study of psychoses characterised by distressed perplexity. *Archives of Neurology and Psychiatry.* 1919;1:415–458.

365 Schwingenheuer J. Über Generationspsychosen. *Archiv für Psychiatrie und Neurologie.* 1953; 190:150–165.

366 Raty-Vahsen D. À propos de psychoses du 'post-partum'. *Acta Psychiatrica Belgica.* 1982;82:596–616.

367 Davidson J, Robertson E. A follow-up study of postpartum illness, 1946–1978. *Acta Psychiatrica Scandinavica.* 1985;71:451–457.

368 Sayers S. Nursing care study: puerperal psychosis. *Nursing Times.* 1976;72: 774–776.

369 Fallgatter AJ, Schnizlein M, Pfuhlmann B, Heidrich A. Klinische Aspekte der Wochenbettpsychosen: Übersicht mit drei Fallbeispielen. *Nervenarzt.* 2002;73:680–685.

370 Mendhekar DN, Srivastava PK, Jiloha RC. Recurrence of puerperal psychosis in both pre- and post-partum periods: a case report. *Indian Journal of Psychiatry.* 2002;44:76–78.

371 Bågedahl-Strindlund M. Parapartum mental illness: an interview follow-up study. *Acta Psychiatrica Scandinavica.* 1997;95:389–395.

372 Heron J, Craddock N, Jones I. Postnatal euphoria: are 'the highs' an indicator of bipolarity? *Bipolar Disorders.* 2005;7: 103–110.

373 Sharma V, Burt VK, Ritchie HL. Assessment and treatment of bipolar II postpartum depression: a review. *Journal of Affective Disorders.* 2010;125:18–26.

374 Rabinowitsch M. *Über die Beziehung des Generationsgeschäftes des Weibes zur*

Schizophrenie. Inaugural-Dissertation, Jena; 1928.

375 Appleby L, Warner R. Spousal allegations of incest during transient psychotic episodes. *British Journal of Psychiatry.* 1991;159:886–887.

376 Saunders EB. Association of psychoses with the puerperium. *American Journal of Psychiatry.* 1929;85:669–680.

377 Meschede of Königsberg. Cyklischer Verlauf einer Psychose in funftägigen Perioden. *Neurologische Centralblatt.* 1903;22:1019–1020.

378 Bennewitz of Berlin. Geschichte eines periodischen, intermittirenden Wahnsinns im Wochenbette. *Hufelands Journal der Practischen Heilkunde.* 1837;84:83–97.

379 Dickson JT. A contribution to the study of the so-called puerperal insanity. *Journal of Mental Science.* 1870;16: 379–390.

380 Hattingen *Mania puerperalis intermittens. General Bericht der Königlich Rheinischen Medicinal-Collegii,* Koblenz. 1838: 96.

381 Parkes D. Bromocriptine. *New England Journal of Medicine.* 1979;301:873–878.

382 Brook NM, Cookson IB. Bromocriptine-induced mania? *British Medical Journal.* 1978;1:790.

383 Vlissides DN, Gill D, Castelow J. Bromocriptine-induced mania? *British Medical Journal.* 1978;1:510.

384 Charbonnier JF, Planche R. Bromocriptine et manie du post-partum. *Actualités Psychiatriques.* 1981;7:59–61.

385 Canterbury RJ, Haskins B, Kahn N, Saathoff G, Yazel JJ. Postpartum psychosis induced by bromocriptine. *Southern Medical Journal.* 1987;80: 1463–1464.

386 Kemperman CJF, Zwanikken GJ. Psychiatric side effects of bromocriptine therapy for postpartum galactorrhoea. *Journal of the Royal Society of Medicine.* 1987;80:387–388.

387 Daw JL. Postpartum depression. *Southern Medical Journal.* 1988;81:207–209.

388 Iffy L, Lindenthal J, Szodi Z, Griffin W. Puerperal psychosis following ablaction with bromocriptine. *Medicine & Law.* 1989;8:171–174.

389 Durst R, Dorevitch A, Ghinea C, Ginath Y. [Bromocriptine-associated postpartum psychotic exacerbation]. *Harefuah.* 1990;118:203–204.

390 Fisher G, Pelonero AL, Ferguson C. Mania precipitated by prednisone and bromocriptine. *General Hospital Psychiatry.* 1991;13:345–346.

391 Reeves RR, Pinkofsky HB. Postpartum psychosis induced by bromocriptine and pseudoephedrine. *Journal of Family Practice.* 1997;45:164–166.

392 Pinardo Zabala A, Alberca Munoz ML, Gimenez Garcia JM. Psicosis posparto asociada a bromocriptina. *Anales Medica Interna.* 2003;20:50–51.

393 Misdrahi D, Chalard R, Verdoux H. Épisode maniaque induit par la bromocriptine en post-partum: à propos d'un cas. *Journal de Gynécologie, Obstétrique et Biologie Réproductive.* 2006;35:79–81.

394 Lake CR, Reid A, Martin C, Chernow B. Cyclothymic disorder and bromocriptine: predisposing factors for postpartum mania. *Canadian Journal of Psychiatry.* 1987;32:693–694.

395 Chateau A. *Psychose puerpérale et bromocriptine.* Thèse, Paris; 1982.

396 Lipper S. Psychosis in patient on bromocriptine and levodopa with carbidopa. *Lancet.* 1976;ii:571–572.

397 Le Feuvre CM, Isaacs AJ, Frank OS. Bromocriptine-induced psychosis in acromegaly. *British Medical Journal.* 1982;285:1315.

398 Valdes J, Otazo R, Bulnes J. [A case of toxic psychosis caused by bromocriptine] *Actas Luso-españolas de Neurologia, Psiquiatria y Ciences Afines.* 1989;17:386–390.

399 Turner TH, Cookson JC, Wass JAH. Psychotic reactions during treatment of pituitary tumours with dopamine agonists. *British Medical Journal.* 1984;289: 1101–1103.

400 Serby M, Angrist B, Lieberman A. Mental disturbances during bromocriptine and lergotrile treatment of Parkinson's. *American Journal of Psychiatry.* 1978; 135:1227–1229.

401 Hippocrates (5th Century BC). *Epidemics.* Volume 1. Book III, cases 10 and 11. Translated by WHS Jones (1931), p. 235–236.

402 Chappert M. *Contribution à l'étude des psychoses puerpérales: 80 cas de psychoses du post partum chez les musulmanes algériennes.* Thèse, Paris; 1962.

403 Whalley LJ, Roberts DF, Wentzel J, Wright AF. Genetic factors in puerperal affective psychoses. *Acta Psychiatrica Scandinavica.* 1982;65:180–193.

404 Chkili T, El Khamlichi A. Les psychoses puerpérales en milieu Marocain: à propos de cent observations. *Tunisie Médicale.* 1975;6:375–391.

405 Durand-Comiot ML. La psychose puerpérale? Étude en milieu sénégelais. *Psychopathologie Africaine.* 1977;13: 269–334.

406 Ouedraogo A. *Approche étiopathogénique des psychoses puerpérales au Sénégal.* Dakar: Mémoire pour le Certificat d'Études; 1987.

407 Pires N, Filho HP. Psicoses Puerperais. *Arquivios de Neuro-psiquiatria.* 1950; 8:47–64.

408 David HM, Rasmussen NK, Host E. Postpartum and post-abortion psychotic reactions. *Family Planning Perspectives.* 1981;13:88–89 and 91–92.

409 David HP. Post-abortion and post-partum psychiatric hospitalization. In: *Abortion: Medical Progress and Social Implications.* Ciba Foundation, symposium 115. London: Pitman; 1985, p. 150–164.

410 Munk-Olsen T, Laursen TM, Pederson CB, Lidegaard Ø, Mortensen PB. First-time first-trimester induced abortion and risk of readmission to a psychiatric hospital in women with a history of treated mental disorder. *Archives of General Psychiatry.* 2012;69:159–165.

411 Di Florio A, Jones I, Forty L, Gordon-Smith K, Craddock N, Jones I. Bipolar

disorder, miscarriage, and termination. *Bipolar Disorders*. 2015;17:102–104.

412 Roldan F. *Bipolar disorder of early onset: effect of pregnancy and abortion on the illness*. Masters thesis, Birmingham; 1994.

413 Girot de Dinan. Aliénation mentale occasionée par la présence d'une mole dans la matrice. *Archives Général de Médecine*. 1828;18:562–563.

414 Ferguson J. The insanity following exhaustion, acute diseases, injuries etc. *Alienist & Neurologist*. 1892;13:407–438.

415 Lienau A. Über künstliche Unterbrechung der Schwangerschaft bei Psychosen in psychiatrische, rechtliche und sittliche Beleuchtung. *Archiv für Psychiatrie und Nervenkrankheiten*. 1914;53:915–942.

416 Sharma V, Sommerdyk C, Sharma S. Post-abortion mania. *Archives of Women's Mental Health*. 2013;16:167–169.

417 Ellery RS. Psychosis of the puerperium. *Medical Journal of Australia*. 1927;i: 287–292.

418 Pérez ML, Guiroy AJ. Psicosis puerperal a repetición. *Semana Medica*. 1932;39: 689–692.

419 Kogerer H, Pawlicki L. Schwangerschaft und Schizophrenie. *Psychiatrisch-neurologische Wochenschrift*. 1934;36: 253–256.

420 Hemphill RE. Incidence and nature of puerperal psychiatric illness. *British Medical Journal*. 1952;ii:1232–1235.

421 Da Silva L, Johnstone EC. A follow-up study of severe puerperal psychiatric illness. *British Journal of Psychiatry*. 1981;139: 346–354.

422 Mahe V, Montagnon F, Nartowski J, Dumane A. Post-abortion mania. *British Journal of Psychiatry*. 1999;175:389–390.

423 Chrobak. Abortus und psychose. *Zentralblatt für Gynäkologie*. 1907; 31:248–249.

424 de Berger J. *Puerperarum mania et melancholia*. Thesis, Göttingen; 1745.

425 Bartens of Bonn. Über den Einfluss der Schwangerschaft auf den Verlauf der Geistesstörung. *Allgemeine Zeitschrift für Psychiatrie*. 1884;40:573–583.

426 de Gorsky Z. *Considérations sur la folie puerpérale*. Thèse, Paris; 1888.

427 Hopker SW, Brockington IF. Psychosis following hydatidiform mole in a patient with recurrent puerperal psychosis. *British Journal of Psychiatry*. 1991;158: 122–123.

428 Euthius JA (1694) *De muliere alias mente sana, gravida demente. Miscellanea Curiosa sive Ephemeridum Medico-Physicarum Germanicarum Academiae Naturae Curiosorum*. Decuriae III:II, observation 4 on p. 10–11.

429 Holm RA. Om Puerperalafsindighed. *Hospitals-Tidende*. 2nd series. 1874;15: 229–242, 245–250, 262–267, and 273–282.

430 Reinhardt R. *Beitrag zur Lehre von den Puerperalpsychosen*. Inaugural-Dissertation, Leipzig; 1907.

431 Jolly P. Beitrag zur Statistik und Klinik der Puerperalpsychosen. *Archiv für Psychiatrie und Nervenkrankheiten*. 1911;48:792–823.

432 Tuke JB. On the statistics of puerperal insanity as observed in the Royal Edinburgh Asylum, Morningside. *Edinburgh Medical Journal*. 1864;10: 1013–1028.

433 Lübben KH. *Zur Statistik der Puerperal Psychosen*. Inaugural-Dissertation, Halle; 1872.

434 Clouston TS. Puerperal insanity, lactational insanity, the insanity of pregnancy. Lecture XV. *Clinical Lectures in Mental Diseases*. 4th ed. London: Churchill; 1896. p. 544–574.

435 Pedler GH. Puerperal mania. *West Riding Lunatic Asylum Medical Reports*. 1872;2: 137–156.

436 Quensel F. Psychosen und Generationsvorgänge beim Weibe. *Medizinische Klinik*. 1907;50:1509–1515.

437 Schou M. Lithium treatment during pregnancy, delivery and lactation: an update. *Journal of Clinical Psychiatry*. 1990;51:410–413.

438 Brockington IF, Oates M, Rose G. Prepartum psychosis. *Journal of Affective Disorders*. 1990;19:31–35.

439 Combs JD. Psychoses associated with childbearing. *Diseases of the Nervous System.* 1956;17:166–169.

440 Menzies WF. Puerperal insanity. *American Journal of Insanity.* 1893;50:147–185.

441 Boudrie G. *Étude sur les causes de la folie puerpérale.* Thèse, Paris; 1878.

442 Kleinsman AC, Knoppert-van de Klein EAM. Bipolaire stoornis en zwangerschap: ervaringen uit de praktijk. *Tijdschrift voor Psychiatrie.* 2006;48:147–152.

443 Cortyl G. *Étude sur la folie puerpérale.* Thèse, Paris; 1877.

444 Elfes K. *Katatonie mit besonderer Berücksichtigung des Verlaufs in der Gravidität.* Inaugural Dissertation, Kiel; 1912.

445 Trixler M, Gati A. The role of genetic factors in the outcome of postpartum affective psychoses. Satellite symposium at 8th Congress of the World Psychiatric Association in Budapest; 1988.

446 Goldenberg RL. Epidemiology and causes of preterm births. *Lancet.* 2008;371:75–84.

447 England S, Richardson B, Brockington IF. Postpartum psychosis after short gestation. *Archives of Women's Mental Health.* 1998;1:143–146.

448 Sack F. *Beitrag zur Lehre von den Generationspsychosen des Weibes.* Inaugural-Dissertation, Kiel; 1919.

449 Tulchinski D, Ryan KJ. *Maternal-fetal Endocrinology.* Philadelphia: Saunders; 1980.

450 Hübner K. *Art und Verlauf von Psychosen nach dem Wochenbett.* Inaugural-Dissertation, Tübingen; 1938.

451 De Leo D, Galligioni S, Magni G. A case of Capgras delusion presenting as a postpartum psychosis. *Journal of Clinical Psychiatry.* 1985;46:242–243.

452 Jilbert AR, Williams AE. Postnatal psychosis: a patient's experience with comments by the consulting psychiatrist. *Journal of Australian College of Midwives.* 1994;7:26–30.

453 Bell TS. Puerperal mania. *Transylvanian Journal of Medicine and the Associate Sciences.* 1833;6:182–186.

454 Hadley HG. A case of puerperal psychosis recovering from four attacks. *Journal of Nervous & Mental Disease.* 1841;94: 540–541.

455 Gödtel R. *Über Psychosen im Wochenbett und ihre Rezidivhäufigkeit.* Inaugural-Dissertation, Mainz; 1965.

456 Boutet A. Récidive de manie après 36 ans, chez une malade antérieurement atteinte de manie d'origine puerpérale. *Encéphale.* 1913;8:181–184.

457 Burns J. *The Principles of Midwifery including the Diseases of Women and Children.* London: Longman, Hurst, Rees, Orme & Brown; 1809. p. 275–279 and 319–321.

458 Gregory MS. Mental diseases associated with childbearing. *American Journal of Obstetrics & Gynecology.* 1924;8: 420–430.

459 Paquet DH. *Les psychoses puerpérales dans l'Ile de la Réunion: à propos de 106 observations.* Thèse, Paris; 1970.

460 Makanjuola ROA. Psychotic disorders after childbirth in Nigerian women. *Tropical and Geographical Medicine.* 1982;34: 67–72.

461 Munk-Olsen T, Jones I, Laursen TM. Birth order and postpartum psychiatric disorders. *Bipolar Disorders.* 2014;16: 300–307.

462 Gilmore A. Insanity in the puerperium. *Journal of Nervous & Mental Disease.* 1892;19:408–418.

463 Ideler KW. Über die Vesania puerperalis. *Annalen des Charité Krankenhaus zu Berlin.* 1851;2:121–182.

464 Hurt VL. *Contribution à l'étude des psychoses puerpérales.* Thèse, Bordeaux; 1911.

465 Masieri N. Contributo allo studio della patogenesi delle psicosi puerperali. *Rivista Italiana di Ginecologia.* 1925;4:163–183.

466 Ménaché M. Contribution à l'étude des psychoses de la lactation. *Nourrisson.* 1929;17:43–44.

467 Fumarola A. Disturbi mentali e periodi sessuali della donna. *Annali de Ostetricia e Ginecologia.* 1935;57:269–296.

468 Blinov A, Goian L, Ornstein I. Les psychoses puerpérales. *Bullétin de la Société Roumaine de Neurologie, Psychiatrie, Psychologie et Endocrinologie*. 1936;17: 112–138.

469 Martin MGL. *Étude sur la folie puerpérale*. Thèse, Lille; 1880.

470 Williardts JCF. *Dissertatio de metastasi lactea*. Inaugural-Dissertation, Tübingen; 1770.

471 Loiseau C. *De la folie sympathique*. Thèse, Paris; 1856.

472 LeGrande du Saulle H. De l'influence de la grossesse, de l'allaitement et du sevrage sur le développement de la folie. *Annales Médico-psychologiques. Third series*. 1857;3:297–303.

473 Révolat, père. Mania puerpérale intermittente. *Annales Médico-psychologiques*. 1847;9:310–311.

474 Joyce PR, Rogers JRM, Anderson ED. Mania associated with weaning. *British Journal of Psychiatry*. 1981;139:355–356.

475 Di Florio A, Jones L, Forty L, Gordon-Smith K, Robertson-Blackmore E, Heron J, et al. Mood disorders and parity – a clue to the aetiology of the postpartum trigger. *Journal of Affective Disorders*. 2014; 152–154:334–339.

476 Bergink V, Bouvy PF, Vervoort JSP, Koorengevel KM, Steegers EAP, Kushner SA. Prevention of postpartum psychosis and mania in women at high risk. *American Journal of Psychiatry*. 2012;169:609–615.

477 Van Swieten GLB. The Commentaries upon the Aphorisms of Dr. Herman Boerhaave. Volume 11. 1754: 50–51 and 150–164.

478 Westphal C. Endocarditis ulcerosa im Puerperium, unter dem Schein von Puerperalmanie auftretend. *Archiv für Pathologische Anatomie und Physiologie und für Klinische Medicin*. 1861;20: 542–551.

479 Casiano ME, Hawkins DR. Major mental illness and childbearing: a role for the consultation-liaison psychiatrist in obstetrics. *Psychiatric Clinics of North America*. 1987;10:35–51.

480 Hess M. *Über die sogenannten Puerperalpsychosen*. Inaugural-Dissertation, München; 1938.

481 Heidema ST. Puerperaalpsychosen. *Psychiatrische en Neurologische Bladen*. 1932;36:627–635.

482 Seurs L, Mierzejewska A, Claes SJ. Paranoïde psychose geïnduceerd door corticosteroïden: gevalbeschrijving en literatuuroverzicht. *Tijdschrift voor Psychiatrie*. 2011;53:37–46.

483 Karanikas E, Antoniadis D, Garyfallos GD. The role of cortisol in first episode of psychosis: a systematic review. *Current Psychiatry Reports*. 2014;16:503.

484 Svoboda L. Laktační psychosa při lupus erythematodes léčeném ACTH. *Československa Psychiatrie*. 1957;53: 106–110.

485 Johnson I. Steroid-induced prepartum psychosis. *British Journal of Psychiatry*. 1996;169:522–526.

486 Stedman TJ, Price J. Two cases of papillary carcinoma of the thyroid associated with psychosis and violence. *Australian & New Zealand Journal of Psychiatry*. 1988;22: 202–206.

487 Rochaix P. *Contribution à l'étude des troubles mentaux d'origine puerpérale*. Thèse, Lyon; 1913.

488 Butts NF. Psychodynamic and endocrine factors in postpartum psychoses. *Journal of the National Medical Association*. 1968;60:224–227.

489 Jurczyńska J, Zieleniewski W. [Clinical implications of occurrences of antithyroid antibodies in pregnant women and in the postpartum period]. *Przeglad Lekaarski*. 2004;61:864–867.

490 Amino N, Tada H, Hidaka Y. The spectrum of postpartum thyroid dysfunction: diagnosis, management and long-term prognosis. *Endocrine Practice*. 1996;2: 406–410.

491 Amino N, Mori H, Iwatani Y, Tanizawa O, Kawashima M, Tsuge I, et al. High prevalence of transient post-partum thyrotoxicosis and hypothyroidism. *New England Journal of Medicine*. 1982;306:849–852.

492 Jansson R. Autoimmune thyroiditis. *Acta Universitatis Upsaliensis*; 1984: number 492.

493 Kupka RW, Nolen WA, Post RM, McElroy SL, Altshuler LL, Denicoff KD, et al. High rate of autoimmune thyroiditis in bipolar disorder: lack of association with lithium exposure. *Biological Psychiatry*. 2002; 51:305–311.

494 Carney CP, Jones LE. Medical comorbidity in women and men with bipolar disorders: a population-based controlled study. *Psychosomatic Medicine*. 2006;68: 684–691.

495 Eaton WW, Pedersen MG, Nielsen PR, Mortensen PB. Autoimmune diseases, bipolar disorder, and non-affective psychosis. *Bipolar Disorders*. 2010;12: 638–646.

496 Bokhari R, Bhatara VS, Bandettini F, McMillin JM. Postpartum psychosis and postpartum thyroiditis. *Psychoneuroendocrinology*. 1998;23: 643–650.

497 Stowell CP, Barnhill JW. Acute mania in the setting of severe hypothyroidism. *Psychosomatics*. 2005;46:259–261.

498 Brownlie BEW, Rae AM, Walshe JWB, Wells JE. Psychoses associated with thyrotoxicosis – 'thyrotoxic psychosis': a report of 18 cases, with statistical analysis of incidence. *European Journal of Endocrinology*. 2000;142:438–444.

499 Bursten B. Psychoses associated with thyrotoxicosis. *Archives of General Psychiatry*. 1961;4:267–273.

500 Lazarus A, Jaffe R. Resolution of thyroid-induced schizophreniform disorder following subtotal thyroidectomy: case report. *General Hospital Psychiatry*. 1986;8:29–31.

501 Abbasi B, Sharif Z, Sprabery LR. Hypokalaemic thyrotoxic periodic paralysis and hypercapnic respiratory failure. *American Journal of the Medical Sciences*. 2010;340:147–153.

502 Øestergaard Jensen O. Thyreotoxisk krise simulerende acut psykose: to tilfaelde. *Ugeskrift for Laeger*. 1950;112: 1721–1722.

503 Lee S, Chow CC, Wing JK, Leung CM, Chiu H, Chen CN. Mania secondary to thyrotoxicosis. *British Journal of Psychiatry*. 1991;159:712–713.

504 Tagami T, Hagiwara H, Kimura T, Usui T, Shimatsu A, Naruse M. The incidence of gestational hyperthyroidism and postpartum thyroiditis in treated patients with Graves' disease. *Thyroid*. 2007;17: 767–772.

505 Andersen SL, Olsen J, Carlé A, Lauerberg P. Hyperthyroidism incidence fluctuates widely in and around pregnancy and is at variance with some other autoimmune diseases: a Danish population-based study. *Journal of Clinical Endocrinology & Metabolism*. 2015. 100: 1164–1171.

506 Vanderpump MPJ. The epidemiology of thyroid disease. *British Medical Bulletin*. 2011;99:39–51.

507 Peachell GE. A case of insanity associated with pregnancy and previous exophthalmic goitre. *Journal of Mental Science*. 1923;69:83–86.

508 Chisholm ID. *Psychiatric in-patients with hyperthyroidism*. Academic DPM thesis, London; 1966.

509 Dahale AB, Chandra PS, Shenne L, Thippeswamy H, Desai G, Reddy D. Postpartum psychosis in a woman with Graves' disease: a case report. *General Hospital Psychiatry*. 2014;36:761.e7-8.

510 Johnstone JC. Case of exophthalmic goitre with mania. *Journal of Mental Science*. 1884;29:521–529.

511 Abély P, Sizaret P, Laine B. Considérations sur un état maniaque post-puerpéral récidivant. *Annales Médico-psychologiques*. 1947;105:379–382.

512 Retzeanu A, Tomorug E, Elias S. Psihoza periodică la o hipertiroidină în timpul sarcinii. *Neurologia Psichiatria Neurochirurgia*. 1960;5:305–308.

513 Winokur G. Postpartum mania. *British Journal of Psychiatry*. 1988;153:843–854.

514 Doucet S, Jones I, Letourneau N, Dennis CL, Blackmore ER. Interventions for the prevention and treatment of

postpartum psychosis: a systematic review. *Archives of Womens Mental Heath.* 2011;14:89–98.

515 Essali A, Alebed S, Guul A, Essali N. Preventive interventions in postnatal psychosis. *Schizophrenia Bulletin.* 2013;39:748–750.

516 Sharma V, Smith A, Mazmanian D. Olanzapine in the prevention of postpartum psychosis and mood episodes in bipolar disorder. *Bipolar Disorders.* 2006;8:400–404.

517 Wisner KL, Hanusa BH, Peindl KS, Perel JM. Prevention of postpartum episodes in women with bipolar disorder. *Biological Psychiatry.* 2004;56:592–596.

518 Newport DJ, Stowe ZN, Viguera AC, Calamaras MR, Juric S, Knight B, et al. Lamotrigine in bipolar disorder: efficacy during pregnancy. *Bipolar Disorders.* 2008;10:432–436.

519 Linden S, Rich CL. The use of lithium during pregnancy and lactation. *Journal of Clinical Psychiatry.* 1983;44: 358–361.

520 Czeizel A, Rácz J. Evaluation of drug intake during pregnancy in the Hungarian case-control surveillance of congenital anomalies. *Teratology.* 1990;42: 505–512.

521 Bodén R, Lundgren M, Brandt T, Reutfors J, Andersen M, Kieler H. Risks of adverse pregnancy and birth outcomes in women treated or not treated with mood stabilisers for bipolar disorder: population-based cohort study. *British Medical Journal.* 2012;345: e7085.

522 van Foreest P. *Puerperas nonnunquam phreniticas fierit and sineglectim habeantur, sibi ipsis vim inferre.* In: *Observationum et curationum Medicinalium.* Lugduni Batavorum: Plantini; 1609.

523 Godding WW. Puerperal insanity. *Boston Medical & Surgical Journal.* 1874;10: 317–319.

524 Conolly J. Clinical lectures on the principal forms of insanity. Lecture 13. Description and treatment of puerperal insanity. *Lancet.* 1846;i:349–354.

525 Waters ATH. On the use of chloroform in the treatment of puerperal insanity. *Journal of Psychological Medicine.* 1857; 10:123–135.

526 White EW. On puerperal insanity. *Kings College Hospital Reports.* 1895;3:21–26.

527 Main TF. Mothers with children in a psychiatric hospital. *Lancet* ii: 1958;845–847.

528 Douglas G. Psychotic mothers. *Lancet* i: 1956;124–125.

529 Joy CB, Saylan M. Mother and baby units for schizophrenia. *Cochrane Database Systematic Reviews.* January 24, 2004: CD006333; 2007.

530 Bardon D. A mother and baby unit in a psychiatric hospital. *Nursing Mirror.* December 8, 1977: 30–33.

531 Lindsay JSB, Pollard DE. Mothers and children in hospital. *Australian & New Zealand Journal of Psychiatry.* 1978;9: 73–76.

532 Margison FR. *Assessing the use of a psychiatric unit for mothers and their babies: risks to the babies.* MSc thesis, Manchester; 1981.

533 Worthington TB. A case of puerperal mania, ending in, and apparently cured by an epileptic fit. *Journal of Mental Science.* 1881;27:396–398.

534 Cerletti U. L'Elettroschock. *Rivista Sperimentale di Freniatria.* 1940;1:209–310.

535 Gentis G. *Les psychoses puerpérales et leur traitement par la cardiazolthérapie.* Thèse, Paris; 1939.

536 Haas RM. *Les psychoses puerpérales.* Thèse, Paris; 1939.

537 Jacobs B. Aetiological factors and reaction types in psychoses following childbirth. *Journal of Mental Science.* 1943;89:242–250.

538 Mori L, Mingozzi M. L'elettroshock in gravidanza. *Annali dell'Ospedale Psichiatrico di Perugia.* 1944;1:1–20.

539 Von Hagen KO. Mental illness following pregnancy. *California and Western Medicine.* 1943;58:324–327.

540 Ross MT. Electric shock therapy in manic depressive psychosis. *New York State*

Journal of Medicine. November 1, 1943: 2055–2057.

541 Feldman F, Susselman S, Lipetz B, Barrera SE. Shock treatment of psychoses associated with pregnancy. *Journal of Nervous & Mental Disease.* 1946;103: 494–502.

542 Lafon R, Billet J, Billet B. N'abusons-nous pas des thérapeutiques psychiatriques et endocriniennes modernes dans le traitement des psychoses puerpérales? *Sud Médical & Chirurgical.* 1953;86: 2592–2596.

543 Impastato DJ, Gabriel AR. Electroshock therapy during the puerperium. *Journal of the American Medical Association.* 1959;163:1017–1022.

544 Baker AA, Morison M, Game JA, Thorpe JG. Admitting schizophrenic mothers with their babies. *Lancet.* 1961;ii:237–239.

545 Sneddon J, Kerry RJ. Puerperal psychosis: a suggested treatment model. *American Journal of Social Psychiatry.* 1984;4:30–34.

546 Reed P, Sermin N, Appleby L, Faragher B. A comparison of clinical response to electroconvulsive therapy in puerperal and non-puerperal psychoses. *Journal of Affective Disorders.* 1999;54:255–260.

547 Forray A, Ostroff RB. The use of electroconvulsive therapy in postpartum affective disorders. *Journal of Electroconvulsive Therapy.* 2007;23: 188–193.

548 Babu GN, Thippeswamy H, Chandra P. Use of electroconvulsive therapy (ECT) in postpartum psychosis – a naturalistic prospective study. *Archives of Women's Mental Health.* 2013;16:247–251.

549 Miller LJ. Use of electroconvulsive therapy during pregnancy. *Hospital & Community Psychiatry.* 1994;45:444–450.

550 Anderson EL, Reti IM. ECT in pregnancy: a review of the literature from 1941 to 2007. *Psychosomatic Medicine.* 2009;71:235–242.

551 Sherer DM, D'Amico ML, Warshal DP, Stern RA, Grunert HF, Abramowicz JS. Recurrent mild *abruptio placentae* occurring immediately after repeated electroconvulsive therapy in pregnancy. *American Journal of Obstetrics & Gynecology.* 1994;165:652–653.

552 Barnes TR, Katona CL. Susceptibility to drug-induced hypotension in puerperal psychosis. *International Journal of Clinical Psychopharmacology.* 1986;1: 74–76.

553 Price DK, Turnbull GJ, Gregory RP, Stevens DG. Neuroleptic malignant syndrome in a case of post-partum psychosis. *British Journal of Psychiatry.* 1989;155:849–852.

554 Verwiel JMM, Verwey B, Heinis C, Thies JE, Bosch FH. Succesvolle elektroconvulsietherapie bij een zwangere vrouw met het maligne nurolepticasyndroom. *Nederlands Tijdschrift voor Geneeskunde.* 1994;138:196–199 and correspondence.

555 Scott Russell C, Lang C, McCambridge M, Calhoun B. Neurolelptic malignant syndrome in pregnancy. *Obstetrics & Gynecology.* 2001;98:906–908.

556 Martínez-Fernández G, Plaza Moral A, Miró Descarga P, Arguís Gimmeno MJ, Gomar Sancho C. Distonía aguida durante trabajo de parto secondaria a haloperidol. *Revista Española de Anesesiologia y Reunimación.* 2004;51:229–230.

557 Silbermann RM, Beenen F, de Jong H. Clinical treatment of postpartum delirium with perfenazine and lithium carbonate. *Psychiatria Clinica.* 1975;8:314–326.

558 Cookson JC. Post-partum mania, dopamine, and oestrogens. *Lancet.* 1982; ii:672.

559 Iruela LM, Ibañez-RojoV, Gilaberte I, Oliveros SC. New possible indications for pimozide. *Journal of Clinical Psychiatry.* 1992;53:172–173.

560 Kornhuber J, Weller M. Postpartum psychosis and mastitis: a new indication for clozapine? *American Journal of Psychiatry.* 1991;148:1751–1752.

561 Weller M, Kornhuber J. Differentielle Neurolepsie bei schizophrenen Psychosen im Wochenbett: vorteile des atypischen Neuroleptikums Clozapin. *Nervenarzt.* 1992;63:440–441.

562 Gödecke-Koch T, Holze I, Wilhelm-Gössling C, Dietrich DE, Emrich MH. Clomethiazol als Adjuvans bei der Behandlung erregt-gehemmter Verwirrtheitspsychosen. *Fortschrift für Neurologie und Psychiatrie.* 2001;69:278–283.

563 Mendhekar DN, Sunder KR, Andrade C. Aripiprazole use in a pregnant schizoaffective woman. *Bipolar Disorders.* 2006;8:299–300.

564 Slone D, Siskind V, Heinonen OP, Monson RR, Kaufman DW, Shapiro S. Antenatal exposure to the phenothiazines in relation to congenital malformations, perinatal mortality rate, birth weight and intelligence quotient score. *American Journal of Obstetrics & Gynecology.* 1977;128: 486–488.

565 Diav-Citrin O, Shechtman S, Ornoy S, Arnon J, Schäfer C, Garbis H, et al. Safety of haloperidol and penfluridol in pregnancy: a multicentre prospective, controlled study. *Journal of Clinical Psychiatry.* 2005;66:317–322.

566 Goldstein DJ, Corbin LA, Fung MC. Olanzepine-exposed pregnancies and lactation: early experience. *Journal of Clinical Psychopharmacology.* 2000;20: 399–403.

567 Gentile S. Clinical utilization of atypical antipsychotics in pregnancy and lactation. *Annals of Pharmacotherapy.* 2004;38: 1265–1271.

568 McKenna K, Koren G, Tetelbaum M, Wilton L, Shakir S, Diav-Citrin O, et al. Pregnancy outcome of women using antipsychotic drugs: a prospective comparative study. *Journal of Clinical Psychiatry.* 2005;66:444–449.

569 Reis M, Kallén B. Maternal use of antipsychotics in early pregnancy and delivery outcome. *Journal of Clinical Psychopharmacology.* 2008;28:279–288.

570 Ennis ZM, Damkier P. Pregnancy exposure to olanzapine, quetiapine, risperidone, aripiprazole and risk of congenital malformations: a systematic review. *Basic & Clinical Pharmacology & Toxicology.* 2015;116:315–320.

571 Coppola D, Russo LJ, Kwarta RF Jr, Varughese R, Schmiider J. Evaluating the postmarketing experience of risperidone use during pregnancy. *Drug Safety.* 2007;30:247–263.

572 Habermann F, Fritzsche J, Fuhlbrück F, Wacker E, Allignol A, Weber-Schöndorfer C, et al. Atypical antipsychotic drugs and pregnancy outcome. *Journal of Clinical Psychopharmacology.* 2013;33:453–462.

573 Newport DJ, Calamaras MR, DeVane CL, Donovan J, Beach AJ, Winn S, et al. Atypical antipsychotic administration during late pregnancy: placental passage and obstetrical outcomes. *American Journal of Psychiatry.* 2007;164:1214–1220.

574 Newham JJ, Thomas SH, MacRitchie K, McElhatton PR, McAllister-Williams RH. Birth weight of infants after maternal exposure to typical and atypical antipsychotics: prospective comparison study. *British Journal of Psychiatry.* 2008;192:333–337.

575 Hammond JE, Toseland PA. Placental transfer of chlorpromazine. *Archives of Disease in Childhood.* 1970;45:139–140.

576 Nielsen HC, Wiriyathian S, Rosenfeld R, Leveno K, Garriott JC. Chlorpromazine excretion by the neonate following chronic in utero exposure. *Pediatric Pharmacology.* 1983;3:1–5.

577 L'Hirondel J, Venezia R, Rousselot P, Daridon F, Fellouse JC. Ictère neonatal à la chlorpromazine. *Archives Françaises de Pédiatrie.* 1968;25:1171–1177.

578 Srokol PW, Jones WN. Infant jaundice after phenothiazine drugs for labor: an enigma. *Obstetrics & Gynecology.* 1962;20:124–127.

579 Hill RM, Desmond MM, Kay JL. Extrapyramidal dysfunction in an infant of a schizophrenic mother. *Journal of Pediatrics.* 1966;69:589–595.

580 Tamer A, McKey R, Arias D, Worley L, Fogel BJ. Phenothiazine-induced extrapyramidal dysfunction in the neonate. *Journal of Pediatrics.* 1969;75:479–480.

581 Levy W, Wisniewski K. Chlorpromazine causing extrapyramidal dysfunction in the newborn infant of a psychotic mother.

New York State Journal of Medicine. 1974; 74:684–685.

582 O'Connor M, Johnson GH, James DI. Intrauterine effect of phenothiazines. *Medical Journal of Australia* 1981;i: 416–417.

583 Handal M, Matheson I, Bechensteen AG, Lindemann R. [Antipsychotic agents and pregnant women: a case report] *Tidsskrift for den Norske Laegeforen*. 1995;115: 2539–2540.

584 Sexson WR, Barak Y. Withdrawal emergent syndrome in an infant associated with maternal haloperidol therapy. *Journal of Perinatalogy*. 1989;9:170–172.

585 Collins KO, Comer JB. Maternal haloperidol therapy associated with dyskinesia in a newborn. *American Journal of Health – System Pharmacy*. 2003;60: 2253–2254.

586 Mohan MS, Pataole SK, Whitehall JS. Severe hypothermia in a neonate following antenatal exposure to haloperidol. *Journal of Paediatrics and Child Health*. 2000;36:412.

587 Akar M, Kasapkara CS, Özbek MN, Tüzün H, Aldudak B, Kanar B. Transient nephrogenic diabetes insipidus caused by fetal exposure to haloperidol. *Renal Failure*. 2014;36:951–952.

588 Gardiner SJ, Kristensen JH, Begg EJ, Hackett LP, Wilson DA, Ilett KF, et al. Transfer of olanzapine into breast milk, calculation of infant drug dose, and effect on breast-fed infants. *American Journal of Psychiatry*. 2003;160:1428–1431.

589 Abou-Saleh MT, Coppen A. Puerperal affective disorders and response to lithium. *British Journal of Psychiatry*. 1983;142:539.

590 McKenzie M, Deakin JFW. Puerperal affective psychosis: is there a case for lithium prophylaxis? *British Journal of Psychiatry*. 1993;162:564–565.

591 Stewart DE. Prophylactic lithium in postpartum affective psychosis. *Journal of Nervous and Mental Disease*. 1988; 176:485–489.

592 Stewart DE, Klompenhouwer JL, Kendell RE, Van Hulst AM. Prophylactic lithium in puerperal psychosis: the experience of 3 centres. *British Journal of Psychiatry*. 1991;158:393–397.

593 Austin MPV. Puerperal affective psychosis: is there a case for lithium prophylaxis? *British Journal of Psychiatry*. 1992;161: 692–694.

594 van Gent EM, Verhoeven WMA. Bipolar illness, lithium prophylaxis and pregnancy. *Pharmacopsychiatry*. 1992;25:187–191.

595 van Gent EM. Puerperal affective psychosis: is there a case for lithium prophylaxis? *British Journal of Psychiatry*. 1993; 162:564.

596 Cohen LS, Sichel DA, Robertson LM, Heckscher E, Rosenbaum JF. Postpartum prophylaxis for women with bipolar disorder. *American Journal of Psychiatry*. 1995;152:1641–1645.

597 Nora JJ, Nora AH, Toews WH. Lithium, Ebstein's anomaly, and other congenital heart defects. *Lancet*. 1974;ii:594–595.

598 Weinstein MR, Goldfield MD. Cardiovascular malformations with lithium use during pregnancy. *American Journal of Psychiatry*. 1975;132:529–531.

599 Weinstein MR. Lithium treatment of women during pregnancy and in the post-delivery period. In: Johnson FN, editor, *Handbook of Lithium Therapy*. New York: Springer; 1980. p. 421–429.

600 Park JM, Sridaromont S, Ledbetter EO, Terry WM. Ebstein's anomaly of the tricuspid valve associated wth prenatal exposure to lithium carbonate. *American Journal of Diseases of Childhood*. 1980;134:703–704.

601 Allan LD, Desai G, Tynan MJ. Prenatal echocardiographic screening for Ebstein's anomaly for mothers on lithium therapy. *Lancet*. 1982;ii:875–876.

602 Long WA, Willis PW. Maternal lithium and neonatal Ebstein's anomaly: evaluation with cross-sectional echocardiography. *American Journal of Perinatology*. 1984;1:182–184.

603 Steffelaar JW, van Wesemael JWJ. Anomalie van Ebstein van de tricuspidalisklep na expositie aan lithium

voor de geboorte. *Nederlands Tijdschrift voor Geneeskunde.* 1991;135:996–997.

604 Jacobson SJ, Jone K, Johnson K, Ceolin L, Kaur P, Sahn D, et al. Prospective multicentre study of pregnancy outcome after lithium exposure during first trimester. *Lancet.* 1992;339:530–533.

605 Gültekin F, Baskin E, Gökalp A, Dogan K. A pregnant woman with Ebstein's anomaly: case report. *Materia Medica Polona.* 1994;26:149–151.

606 Robert E, Guibaud P. Maternal valproic acid and congenital neural tube defects. *Lancet.* 1982;ii:937.

607 Diav-Citrin O, Shechtman S, Tahover E, Finkel-Pekarsky V, Arnon J, Kennedy D, et al. Pregnancy outcome following *in utero* exposure to lithium: a prospective, comparative, observational study. *American Journal of Psychiatry.* 2014; 171:785–794.

608 Ortigado Matamala A, García García A, Jiménez Bustos JM. Anomalia de Ebstein y exposición en el embarazo. *Anales de Pediatría.* 2006;65:626–627.

609 Arnon RG, Marin-Garcia J, Peeden JN. Tricuspid valve regurgitation and lithium carbonate toxicity in a newborn infant. *American Journal of Diseases of Childhood.* 1981;135:941–943.

610 Edmonds LD, Oakley GP. Ebstein's anomaly and maternal lithium exposure during pregnancy. *Teratology.* 1990;41:551–552.

611 Cohen LS, Friedman JM, Jefferson JW, Johnson EM. A reevaluation of risk of *in utero* exposure to lithium. *Journal of the American Medical Association.* 1994;271:146–150.

612 McKnight RF, Adida M, Budge K, Stockton S, Goodwin GM, Gesses JR. Lithium toxicity profile: a systematic review and meta-analysis. *Lancet.* 2012;379:721–728.

613 Eika B, Skajaa K. Acute renal failure due to bilateral obstruction by the pregnant uterus. *Urologia Internationalis.* 1988;43:315–317.

614 Vacaflor L, Lehmann HE, Ban TA. Side effects and teratogenicity of lithium carbonate treatment. *Journal of Clinical Pharmacology.* 1970;10:387–389.

615 Wilbanks GD, Bressler B, Peete CH, Cherny WB, London WL. Toxic effects of lithium carbonate in a mother and newborn infant. *Journal of the American Medical Association.* 1970;213:865–867.

616 Aoki FY, Ruedy J. Severe lithium intoxication. *Canadian Medical Association Journal.* 1971;105:847–848.

617 Woody JN, London WL, Wilbanks GD. Lithium toxicity in the newborn. *Pediatrics.* 1971;47:94–96.

618 Piton M, Barthe ML, Laloum D, Davy J, Poilpre E, Venezia R. Intoxication aiguë par le lithium. *Thérapie.* 1973;28: 1123–1133.

619 Schou M, Amdisen A, Steenstrup OR. Lithium and pregnancy. II. Hazards to women given lithium during pregnancy and delivery. *British Medical Journal.* 1973; ii:137–138.

620 Casparie AF, Miedema K, Peters PJ, Troostwijk AL, van Woerden LL. Lithiumintoxicatie tijdens de zwangerschap. *Nederlands Tijdschrift voor Geneeskunde.* 1974;118:1406–1409.

621 Karlsson K, Lindstedt G, Lundberg PA, Selstam U. Transplacental lithium poisoning: reversible inhibition of fetal thyroid. *Lancet.* 1975;i:1295.

622 Morrell P, Sutherland GR, Buamah PK, Oo M, Bain HH. Lithium toxicity in a neonate. *Archives of Disease in Childhood.* 1983;58:539–541.

623 Jenniskens-Bruins JJ, Gerards LJ. Lithiumintoxicatie bij een pasgeborene. *Tidschrift voor Kindergeneeskunde.* 1992;60:76–78.

624 Nishiwaki T, Tanaka K, Sekiya S. Acute lithium intoxication in pregnancy. *International Journal of Gynecology & Obstetrics.* 1996;52:191–192.

625 Flaherty B, Krenzelok EP. Neonatal lithium toxicity as a result of maternal toxicity. *Veterinary & Human Toxicology.* 1997;39:92–93.

626 Pinelli JM, Symington AJ, Cunningham KA, Paes BA. Case report and review of the

perinatal complications of maternal lithium use. *American Journal of Obstetrics & Gynecology.* 2002;187:245–249.

627 Malzacher A, Engler H, Drack G, Kind C. Lethargy in a newborn: lithium toxicity or lab error? *Journal of Perinatal Medicine.* 2003;31:340–342.

628 Blake LD, Lucas DN, Castello-Cortes A, Robinson PN. Lithium toxicity and the parturient: case report and literature review. *International Journal of Obstetric Anesthesia.* 2008;17:164–169.

629 Newport DJ, Viguera AC, Beach AJ, Ritchie JC, Cohen LS, Stowe ZN. Lithium placental passage and obstetrical outcome: implications for clinical management during late pregnancy. *American Journal of Psychiatry.* 2005;162:2162–2170.

630 Tunnessen WW, Hertz CG. Toxic effects of lithium in newborn infants: a commentary. *Journal of Pediatrics.* 1972;81:804–807.

631 Stothers JK, Wilson DW, Royston N. Lithium toxicity in the newborn. *British Medical Journal.* 1973;iii:233–234.

632 Olmedillas Alvaro MJ, Labay Matias MV, De Miguel Pardo C, Valero Adan MT, Martin-Calama J, Valle Sanchez F. Intoxicación por litio en un recién nacido. *Anales Españoles de Pediatria.* 1988;29:330–332.

633 Kozma C. Neonatal toxicity and transient neurodevelopmental deficits following prenatal exposure to lithium. *American Journal of Medical Genetics.* 2005;132A: 441–444.

634 Kallén B, Tandberg A. Lithium and pregnancy. *Acta Psychiatrica Scandinavica.* 1983;68:134–139.

635 Troyer WA, Pereira GR, Lannon RA, Belik J, Yoder MC. Association of maternal lithium exposure and premature delivery. *Journal of Perinatology.* 1993;13:123–127.

636 Schou M. What happened to the lithium babies? *Acta Psychiatrica Scandinavica.* 1976;54:193–197.

637 Viguera AC, Newport DJ, Ritchie J, Stowe Z, Whitfield T, Mogielnicki J, et al. Lithium in breast milk and nursing infants: clinical implications. *American Journal of Psychiatry.* 2007;164:342–345.

638 Stevens D, Burman D, Midwinter A. Transplacental lithium poisoning. *Lancet.* 1974;ii:595.

639 Wilson N, Forfar JC, Godman MJ. Atrial flutter in the newborn resulting from maternal lithium ingestion. *Archives of Disease in Childhood.* 1983;58:538–549.

640 Zegers B, Andriessen P. Maternal lithium therapy and neonatal morbidity. *European Journal of Pediatrics.* 2003;162:348–349.

641 Filtenborg JA. Persistent pulmonary hypertension after lithium intoxication in the newborn. *European Journal of Pediatrics.* 1982;138:321–323.

642 Amdisen A. In the discussion of a paper by Sedvall G. *Acta Psychiatrica Scandinavica, supplement.* 1969;207, p. 67.

643 v. Brenndorff AI, Ertelt W. [Lithium-intoxication in a newborn] *Monatsschrift für Kinderheilkunde.* 1978;126:451–453.

644 Mizrahi EM, Hobbs JF, Goldsmith DI. Nephrogenic diabetes insipidus in transplacental lithium intoxication. *Journal of Pediatrics.* 1979;94:493–495.

645 Nars PW, Girard J. Lithium carbonate intake during pregnancy leading to a large goitre in a premature infant. *American Journal of Diseases of Childhood.* 1977;131:924–925.

646 Frassetto F, Tourneur Martel F, Barjhoux CE, Villier C, Bot BL, Vincent F. Goitre in a newborn exposed to lithium in utero. *Annals of Pharmacotherapy.* 2002;36: 1745–1748.

647 Ang MS, Thorp JA, Parisi VM. Maternal lithium therapy and polyhydramnios. *Obstetrics & Gynecology.* 1990;76:517–519.

648 Krause S, Ebbesen F, Lange AP. Polyhydramnios with maternal lithium treatment. *Obstetrics & Gynecology.* 1990;75:504–506.

649 Skausig OB, Schou M. Diegivning under lithiumbehandlung. *Ugeskrift for Laeger.* 1977;139:401–404.

650 Cunnington MC, Weil JG, Messenheimer JA, Ferber S, Yerby M, Tennis P. Final results from 18 years of the International Lamotrigine Pregnancy Register. *Neurology.* 2011;76:1817–1823.

651 Tomson T, Bonizzoni E, Craig J, Lindhout D, Sabers A, Perucca E, et al. Dose-dependent risk of malformations with antiepileptic drugs: an analysis of data from the EURAP epilepsy and pregnancy registry. *Lancet Neurology*. 2011;10: 609–617.

652 Diav-Citrin O, Shechtman S, Arnon J, Ornoy A. Is carbamazepine teratogenic? A prospective controlled study of 210 pregnancies. *Neurology*. 2001;57:321–324.

653 Matolon S, Schechtman S, Goldzweig G, Ornoy A. The teratogenic effect of carbamazepine: a meta-analysis of 1255 exposures. *Reproductive Toxicology*. 2002;16:9–17.

654 Jentink J, Dolk H, Loane MA, Morris JK, Wellesley D, Garne E, et al. Intrauterine exposure to carbamazepine and specific congenital malformations: systematic review and case-control study. *British Medical Journal*. 2010;341: c6581, p. 1–7.

655 Vajda FJE, O'Brien TJ, Graham J, Lander CM, Easie MJ. Associations between particular types of fetal malformation and antiepileptic drug exposure in utero. *Acta Neurologica Scandinavica*. 2013;128: 228–234.

656 Veiby G, Daltveit AK, Schjølberg S, Stoltenberg C, Øyen AS. Vollset SE, et al. Exposure to antiepileptic drugs in utero and child development: a prospective population-based study. *Epilepsia*. 2013;54:1462–1472.

657 Robert E, Rosa F. Valproate and birth defects. *Lancet*. 1983;ii:1142.

658 Leading article. Valproate, spina bifida, and birth defects. *Lancet*. ii:1404–1405.

659 Samrén EB, van Duijn CM, Koch S, Hiilesmaa VK, Klepel H, Bardy AH, et al. Maternal use of antiepileptic drugs and the risk of major congenital malformation: a joint Euroean prospective study of human teratogenesis associated with maternal epilepsy. *Epilepsia*. 1997;38:981–990.

660 Artama M, Auvinen A, Raudaskoski T, Isojärvi I, Isojärvi J. Antiepileptic drug use of women with epilepsy and congenital malformations in offspring. *Neurology*. 2006;64:1874–1878.

661 Vajda FJE, Hitchcock A, Graham J, O'Brien T, Lander C, Eadie M. The Australian register of antiepileptic drugs in pregnancy: the first 1002 pregnancies. *Australian & New Zealand Journal of Obstetrics & Gynaecology*. 2007;47:468–474.

662 Vajda FJ, Graham J, Roten A, Lander CM, O'Brien TJ, Eadie M. Teratogenicity of the newer antiepileptic drugs – the Australian experience. *Journal of Clinical Neuroscience*. 2012;19:57–59.

663 Lisi A, Botto LD, Robert-Gnansia E, Castilla EE, Bakker MK, Bianca S, et al. Surveillance of adverse fetal effects of medications (SAFE-Med): findings from the International Clearinghouse of Birth Defects Surveillance and Research. *Reproductive Toxicology*. 2010;29: 433–442.

664 Kini U, Adab N, Vinten J, Fryer A, Clayton Smith J. Dysmorphic features: an important clue to the diagnosis and severity of fetal anticonvulsant syndromes. *Archives of Disease in Childhood, Fetal & Neonatal Edition*. 2006;91: F90–F95.

665 Campbell E, Kennedy F, Russell A, Smithson WH, Parsons L, Morrison PJ, et al. Malformation risks of antiepileptic drug monotherapies in pregnancy: updated results from the UK and Ireland Epilepsy and Pregnancy Registers. *Journal of Neurology, Neurosurgery and Psychiatry*. 2014;85:1029–1024.

666 Tanoshima M, Kobayashi T, Tanoshima R, Beyene J, Koren G, Ito S. Risks of congenital malformations in offspring exposed to valproic acid *in utero*: a systematic review and cumulative meta-analysis. *Clinical Pharmacology & Therapeutics*. 2015;98:417–441.

667 Wilson RD, Davies G, Désilets V, Reid GJ, Summers A, Wyatt P, et al. The use of folic acid for the prevention of neural tube defects and other congenital abnormalities. *Journal of Obstetrics & Gynaecology of Canada*. 2003;25:959–973.

668 Kjaer D, Horvath-Puhó E, Christensen J, Vestergaard M, Czeizel AE, Sørensen HT, et al. Antiepileptic drug use, folic acid supplementation, and congenital abnormalities: a population-based

case-control study. *British Journal of Obstetrics & Gynaecology*. 2007;115:98–103.

669 Rodriguez-Pinilla E, Arroyo I, Fondevilla J, García MJ, Martínez-Frias ML. Prenatal exposure to valproic acid during pregnancy and limb deficiencies. *American Journal of Medical Genetics*. 2000;90:376–381.

670 Clayton-Smith J, Donnai D. Fetal valproate syndrome. *Journal of Medical Genetics*. 1995;32:724–727.

671 Eriksson K, Viinikainen K, Mönkkönen A, Äikiä M, Nieminen P, Heinonen S, et al. Children exposed to Valproate in utero – population based evaluation of risks and confounding factors for long-term neurocognitive development. *Epilepsy Research*. 2005;65:189–200.

672 Moore SJ, Turnpenny P, Quinn A, Glover S, Lloyd DJ, Montgomery T, et al. A clinical study of 57 children with fetal anticonvulsant syndromes. *Journal of Medical Genetics*. 2000;37:489–497.

673 Williams G, King J, Cunningham M, Stephan M, Kerr B, Hersh JH. Fetal valproate syndrome and autism: additional evidence of an association. *Developmental Medicine and Child Neurology*. 2001;43:202–206.

674 Rasalam AD, Hailey H, Williams JHG, Moore SJ, Turnpenny PD, Lloyd DJ, et al. Characteristics of fetal anticonvulsant syndrome associated autistic disorder. *Developmental Medicine and Child Neurology*. 2005;47:551–555.

675 Thisted E, Ebbesen F. Malformations, withdrawal manifestations, and hypoglycaemia after exposure to valproate in utero. *Archives of Disease in Childhood*. 1993;69:288–291.

676 Ebbesen F, Jörgensen A, Hoseth E, Kaad PH, Möller M, Holsteen V, et al. Neonatal hypoglycaemia and withdrawal symptoms after exposure in utero to valproate. *Archives of Disease in Childhood, Neonatal Edition*. 2000;83: F124-$129.

677 Tomson T, Battino D, Bonizzoni E, Craig J, Lindhout D, Perucca E, et al. Dose-dependent teratogenicity of valproate in mono- and polytherapy. *Neurology*. 2015;85:866–872.

678 Tucker WI. Progesterone treatment in postpartum schizo-affective reactions. *Journal of Neuropsychiatry*. 1962;3: 150–153.

679 Kane FJ Jr, Daly RJ, Ewing JA, Keeler MH, Flowers CE. Oral contraceptives as psychopharmacologic agents. *Current Psychiatric Therapies*. 1966;6:219–221.

680 Atkinson S, Atkinson T. Puerperal psychosis – a personal experience. *Health Visitor*. 1983;56:17–19.

681 Meakin CJ, Brockington IF. Failure of progesterone treatment in puerperal mania. *British Journal of Psychiatry*. 1990;156:910.

682 Wilson AE, Christie T. Puerperal insanity; notes of cases treated by injections of ovarian extract (whole gland) from the Dundee Mental Hospital, Westgreen. *British Medical Journal*. 1925;ii:797–798.

683 Sichel DA, Cohen SL, Robertson ML, Ruttenberg A, Rosenbaum JF. Prophylactic oestrogen in recurrent postpartum affective disorder. *Biological Psychiatry*. 1995;38:814–818.

684 Ahokas A, Aito M. Role of estradiol in puerperal psychosis. *Psychopharmacology*. 1999;147:108–110.

685 Robert E, Francannet C. Comments on 'teratogen update on lithium' by J Warkany. *Teratology*. 1990;42:405.

686 Anon. Merkwürdiger Fall von Kindbettwahnsinn mit Verwundung des Herzbeutels, des Magens, der Leber und mit Durchschneidung der äufseren Brust – so wie der linken Speichel-Pulsader. *Hufelands Journal der Practischen Heilkunde*. 1829;5:3–44.

687 Ferguson J. The insanity following exhaustion, acute diseases, injuries etc. *Alienist & Neurologist*. 1892;13:407–438.

688 Pollák J. Psychosisok a terhesség, szülés és gyermekágy alatt. *Orvosi Hetilap*. 1929;44:1100–1104.

689 Frumkes G. Mental disorders related to childbirth. *Journal of Mental Science*. 1934;79:540–552.

690 Trixler M, Jadi F, Wagner M. Postpartum psychosisok: katamnesztikus vizsgálatok

1930–1980. *Ideggyógyászati Szemle.* 1981;34:555–562.

691 Rhode A, Marneros A. Zur Prognose der Wochenbettpsychosen: Verlauf und Ausgang nach durchschnittlich 26 Jahren. *Nervenarzt.* 1993;64:175–180.

692 Allwood CW. *An investigation into puerperal psychosis occurring in African women admitted to Baragwanath hospital.* MD thesis, Pretoria; 1992.

693 Spinelli MG. Postpartum psychosis: detection of risk and management. *American Journal of Psychiatry.* 2009;166:405–408.

694 Hatters-Friedman S, Sorrentino R. Commentary: postpartum psychosis, infanticide, and insanity – implications for forensic psychiatry. *Journal of the American Academy of Psychiatry and Law.* 2012;40:326–332.

695 Brockington IF. *What is Worth Knowing about 'Puerperal Psychosis'.* Bredenbury: Eyry; 2014.

696 v. Krafft-Ebing R. *Lehrbuch der gerichtlichen Psychopathologie mit Berücksichtigung der Gesetzgebung von Oesterreich, Deutschland und Frankreich.* Stuttgart: Enke; 1875. p. 275–276.

697 Editorial. Lord Denman on a case of infanticide. Lancet. 1848;i:318–319.

698 Matheson JCM. Infanticide. *Medico-legal Review.* 1941;9:135–152.

699 Dolenc M. Vierfache Kindesabschlachtung durch die Mutter infolge eines Raptus melancholicus. *Archiv für Kriminal-anthropologie und Kriminalistik.* 1913;51:48–52.

700 Hume D. *Commentaries on the law of Scotland, respecting the description and punishment of crimes.* Bell, Edinburgh; 1797, reproduced in Hunter R, McAlpine I, editors, *Three Hundred Years of Psychiatry.* Oxford: Oxford University Press; 1963. p. 557.

701 Trigueros G. Sobre un caso de psícosis puerperal. *Revista Frenopatica Española,* September 1906: 281–284.

702 Gosselin JY, Bury JA. Approche psychopathologique d'un cas d'infanticide. *Canadian Psychiatric Association Journal.* 1969;14:473–480.

703 Dayan J. Considérations sur la 'folie maternelle'. *Journal de la Psychanalyse de l'Enfant.* 1977;21:234–267.

704 Philippi. Mord und Mordversuch im Zustande des Wahnsinns. *Hitzig's Annalen.* 1830;8:362.

705 Ketai RM, Brandwin MA. Childbirth-related psychosis and familial symbiotic conflict. *American Journal of Psychiatry.* 1979;136:190–193.

706 Colasson F, Haller C, Orget J, Salzard C, de Tourris H, Giraud JR. Aspects actuels des psychoses aiguës du post-partum. *Revue Française de Gynécologie et Obstétrique.* 1981;76:69–474.

Menstrual Psychosis

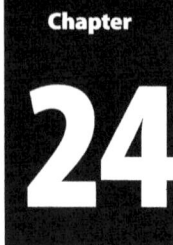

The Catamenial Process

As context it is necessary briefly to rehearse the neuro-endocrinology of the menstrual cycle, and its normal and abnormal variants. This is a summary of chapter 1 of *Menstrual Psychosis and the Catamenial Process*[1], which reviews the evidence, with more than 200 references; this bibliography mainly lists new studies.

The menstrual cycle depends on events at four levels – hypothalamus, pituitary, ovaries and uterus.

The Hypothalamus

The hypothalamus occupies the floor of the third ventricle in intimate relationship with the pituitary gland. It controls autonomic, endocrine and behavioural functions including the body temperature, the osmolarity of body fluids, thirst, appetite and weight, circadian rhythms and sexual activity.

Its most anterior part contains the gonadorelin neuronal network. These cells originate in the olfactory placode, whence they migrate to their hypothalamic locus; failure to migrate leads to Kallman syndrome (congenital eunuchoidism and anosmia). They are distributed diffusely in the preoptic area and mediobasal hypothalamus with extensive projection to the median eminence[2]. The number of neurons is only 1,500–2,000, a small fraction of those in the anterior hypothalamus. They receive signals from at least 10,000 neurons in 26 brain areas, integrating information about the internal homeostatic milieu and environment, thus ensuring that reproduction and behaviour are coordinated[3]. They are stimulated or inhibited by at least 25 neurochemical agents[3], and are influenced by neuronal–glia interactions[4,5]. It is now thought that the generation of their pulsatile output involves the arcuate nucleus in the mediobasal hypothalamus, the site of expression of three peptides – neurokinin B (which stimulates) and dynorphin (which inhibits) GnRH release, both of which act through the third peptide, kisspeptin[2].

The gonadorelin neuronal network is the hypothalamic gonadostat, the pathway through which the brain regulates the secretion of gonadotropins; lesions that prevent the production of GnRH arrest reproductive maturation and function. These cells secrete gonatotropic hormone releasing hormone (GnRH, gonadorelin), discovered in 1971 by the Nobel laureates Schally[6] and Guillemin[7]. GnRH is a decapeptide with the following amino acid sequence:

> (pyro)glutamic acid[1] – histidine[2] – tryptophan[3] – serine[4] – tyrosine[5] – glycine[6] – leucine[7] – arginine[8] – proline[9] – glycine[10] – NH_2

It reaches the pituitary *via* a portal venous system[8], a private conduit enabling minute quantities of hormones to reach their target cells, without dilution by the systemic circulation. The effect of GnRH on the anterior pituitary is to stimulate the secretion of the gonadotropic hormones. In order to have this effect, its secretion must be pulsatile. A 'pulse' is a discharge of about 10 µg/minute for six minutes, resulting in a 100-fold rise in portal blood concentration. GnRH has a half-life of only five minutes. Throughout adult life, day and night, GnRH pulses are secreted every one to several hours. A low frequency of pulses leads to hypothalamic amenorrhoea, which has many causes, including mutations in several genes, nutritional deprivation, chronic disease, depression, anorexia nervosa, exercise and stress.

Synthetic gonadorelin agonists have been developed, substituting glycine in position 6 or 10, or leucine in position 7, by other amino acids. Administered by injection or nasal insufflation, they lack pulsation, and act by stimulating then blocking the pituitary receptors. They are used to inhibit menstruation in a wide variety of diseases. They have no direct side effects, and no dangers from overdose, but the lack of oestrogens results in bone loss and other symptoms, which can be countered by oestrogen add-back therapy or the synthetic steroid tibolone; calcium supplements also help. Recently a non-peptide gonadorelin antagonist (Elagolix), which can be administered orally, has been developed[9].

The Pituitary

This is the body's 'master gland'. It lies immediately below the hypothalamus, protected by a depression in the skull (the *sella turcica*). It is composed of two embryologically distinct parts: the posterior lobe is neural, a continuation of the hypothalamic infundibulum: it produces vasopressin (anti-diuretic hormone) and oxytocin. The anterior part (adenohypophysis) is glandular, derived from an outgrowth (Rathke's pouch) of the oral ectoderm; it contains the intermediate lobe, which secretes melanocyte-stimulating hormone, and the anterior lobe, which secretes growth hormone, adrenocorticotropic hormone, thyrotropic hormone and – hormones concerned with female reproduction – the gonadotropic hormones, follicle-stimulating hormone (FSH) and luteinising hormone (LH), and prolactin (PRL).

FSH, discovered in 1927, is a glycoprotein, with a sugar component and a protein component with two polypeptide subunits – an α unit with 92 amino acids, and a β unit with 118 amino acids. The α unit is shared with three other hormones – LH, human chorionic gonadotropin (hCG) and thyroid stimulating hormone (TSH), the difference in biological activity depending on their β units. FSH has a half-life of three to four hours, and its pulsation is less prominent than that of LH. Released into the blood, it binds to receptors on the ovary's granulosa cells.

LH is structurally similar to FSH, but its β unit has 121 amino acids (identical to part of the hCG β unit). Its half-life is only 20 minutes. Secretion is pulsatile, and the amplitude, duration and frequency of these pulses regulate events during the menstrual cycle. Released into the blood, it acts on receptors on the ovary's thecal cells, and then the corpus luteum, which it drives during the two-week luteal phase. The modified androgen danazol inhibits both gonadotropic hormones.

After conception, hCG takes over control. It is secreted by the trophoblast, and then the placenta; large amounts may be produced by hydatidiform moles. It is similar in structure to LH, with an additional 28 amino acids to its β unit. It maintains the corpus luteum during early pregnancy.

PRL is a single chain polypeptide with 199 amino acids, similar to growth hormone. It is produced by the anterior pituitary, under the influence of TSH and oestrogen. It is inhibited by dopamine neurons of the arcuate nucleus. Secretion is pulsatile, and has a diurnal rhythm with a sleep-related peak. Although it is necessary for normal luteal function, its chief effect is to stimulate maturation of the mammary glands and (after delivery) to produce milk. Suckling activates receptors around the nipple, signalling the hypothalamus to increase prolactin secretion and release oxytocin. Hyperprolactinaemia, which has various causes, suppresses the menstrual cycle through a direct effect on GnRH neurons, thus reducing the frequency and amplitude of LH pulses. The therapeutic agents bromocriptine and cabergoline suppress PRL secretion.

Oxytocin is produced by neurosecretary cells in the supra-optic and paraventricular nuclei of the hypothalamus, and released from the posterior pituitary. It is a nona-peptide with the following sequence of amino acids:

cysteine^1 – tyrosine^2 – isoleucine^3 – glutamine^4 –
asparagine^5 – cysteine^6 – proline^7 – leucine^8 – glycine^9

It is structurally similar to vasopressin, which has phenylalanine^3 instead of isoleucine, and arginine^8 instead of leucine; oxytocin also has a mild anti-diuretic action (see page 62). Its half life is about three minutes. Its receptors are found mainly in the mammary gland and uterus, but also in many parts of the CNS. Its main actions are on lactation and uterine contraction, but it is also released at orgasm, and may be important in maternal and other relationships. In the menstrual cycle, its blood level is increased during the follicular phase, reaches a peak one day after the LH surge, and declines during the luteal phase. It has a role in the release of prostaglandin PGF_{2a} for luteolysis.

The Ovaries

These almond-sized organs are located on each side of the uterus. There is an outer cortex containing follicles at various stages of development and a medulla containing blood and lymphatic vessels and nerve fibres. Each follicle (700,000 at birth) contains primary oocytes; these are germ cells that have started their first meiotic division, but stopped in prophase. At puberty, under the influence of FSH, several oocytes start to develop each month, but only one completes meiosis, forming a haploid gamete (the Graafian follicle). This escapes into the fallopian tubes, where its further development is arrested unless it is fertilized. After the escape of the ovum, the follicle is converted to the corpus luteum, which after seven to nine days begins to degenerate, unless sustained by hCG from the trophoblast. The corpus luteum maintains pregnancy until, after a few weeks, the placenta takes over.

Between the follicles is a stroma of supportive tissues that includes interstitial cells, which secrete sex steroid hormones in response to LH and hCG. The steroid hormones are progesterone and three forms of oestrogen.

The oestrogens are made from androstenedione by aromatase. The main follicular secretion is 17β oestradiol. During pregnancy, more oestriol is produced, and after the menopause (and in women with polycystic ovary syndrome) more oestrone. Oestrogens are produced by the ovary, then the corpus luteum and (in pregnancy) by the placenta. They have many actions, including:

• Proliferation of the endometrial glands, cornification of the vagina and increased fluidity of the cervical mucus

- Secondary sexual development
- Feedback control of the pituitary, which is negative and positive at different stages of the menstrual cycle
- Reduction of bone resorption – hence the advance of osteoporosis after the menopause
- In the brain, blocking dopaminergic receptors, and interacting with catecholamine, serotonin and possibly cholinergic receptors

Oestrogens have a mild antidepressant action. Clomiphene, tamoxifen and aromatase inhibitors act as anti-oestrogens. Clomiphene has been used in the treatment of several menstrual disorders, and has been associated with psychosis, usually with a 'functional' psychosis[10–17], sometimes with memory disorder and confusion[18].

Progesterone is derived from cholesterol, *via* pregnenolone; it is in turn converted into androgens, and androgens into oestrogens. It is produced by the gonads, especially the corpus luteum and placenta (from the eighth week of pregnancy). It requires continuous LH secretion. Its actions include:

- Development of the endometrium to its secretory stage, preparing for implantation
- Through an action on the hypothalamic thermo-regulatory centre, elevation of basal body temperature during the luteal phase
- During pregnancy, maintaining the endometrium and decreasing the contractility of the myometrium (thus preventing premature labour)
- It is also active at the mid-cycle in triggering the mid-cycle surge. In the luteal phase it causes a slowing of the GnRH pulse rate and decrease in its amplitude

It is moderately sedative. A closely related steroid (alphaxalone) is an anaesthetic, possibly through action on γ-aminobutyric acid (GABA) receptors.

The ovary produces three other hormones: inhibins A and B and activin, discovered in the 1980s. They are glycoproteins, consisting of two di-sulfide linked subunits, sharing an α unit, and differing in their β units; activin has two β units. Inhibin A is secreted, under the control of LH, by the granulosa cells and later by the corpus luteum, endometrium and trophoblast. Inhibin B is also produced by the follicle, endometrium and trophoblast. Inhibin levels are high in the follicular phase and luteal phases, inhibiting pituitary production of FSH. Activin is produced by the gonads, pituitary, placenta and other organs; it has the opposite action, enhancing FSH synthesis.

The Uterus

The womb is lined by the endometrium, which, under the influence of oestrogen and progesterone, undergoes the monthly cyclical changes that prepare for the fertilized ovum. It has a surface layer of columnar epithelial cells, and an underlying stroma permeated by blood vessels. During the follicular phase, the mucosa thickens and the tubular glands lengthen, but remain straight. During the luteal phase, the glands become coiled and the stroma more vascular. When the ovarian steroid levels fall, the mucosa and its blood vessels necrose, and menstrual bleeding occurs.

The vaginal mucosa consists of stratified squamous epithelium, surrounded by a muscular layer and loose connective tissue. There are no glands, and lubrication is provided by glands in the uterine cervix. The epithelial cells contain glycogen, which breaks down into lactic acid, lowering vaginal pH to 3 to protect against bacterial invasion. The vaginal wall is cornified under the influence of oestrogen.

Prostaglandins are the only hormone produced by the endometrium. They are unsaturated carboxylic acids, derived from the fatty acid arachidonic acid, with 20 carbon atoms ('eicosanoids'), including a 5-carbon ring. They are ubiquitous. Because of their short half-life, they have local effects, but no blood-borne distant effects. They have a variety of actions, including participation in the inflammatory response and blood clotting. Their endometrial concentration is increased in the luteal phase, and during the first 48 hours of the menses they are released into the systemic circulation. Their effect is to stimulate the contraction of the myometrium, and induce vasospasm and necrosis of the mucosa. Their synthesis is blocked by aspirin and other non-steroidal anti-inflammatory agents.

The Normal Adult Menstrual Cycle

The typical cycle lasts four weeks (range 21–35 days). It is divided into follicular phase, mid-cycle gonadotropin surge, luteal phase, ischaemic phase and menstrual bleeding. Variation in cycle length is due to variation in the follicular phase, with a relatively constant luteal phase. The main hormonal events are as follows:

The Follicular Phase

The follicles develop, ending with maturation of the most advanced oocyte:

- GnRH pulsation initially has a low frequency (one every 1½–2 hours) favouring FSH secretion. It then increases to 1/hour, favouring LH.
- FSH has a mean level of 100–200 ng/ml. Towards the end of the phase, oestradiol and inhibin B cause a decline.
- LH has a mean level of <100 ng/ml, with increasing pulse frequency and amplitude.
- Oestrogen levels rise to their first peak of about 30 pg/ml, just before the mid-cycle surge.
- Serum progesterone is low (<1.8 μg/ml) until just before the mid-cycle.

The Mid-Cycle Gonadotropin Surge

This results in the release of the oocyte from the mature Graafian follicle:

- When oestradiol has reached a critical level for 1½–2 days, the responsiveness of the pituitary gonadotropes reaches a peak, and the oestrogen feedback loop becomes temporarily positive.
- This is followed by a small rise of progesterone, secreted by the pre-ovulatory follicle, augmenting the effect of oestrogen.
- There is a surge of GnRH, with increasing pulse frequency and amplitude.
- There is a synchronous pulsatile burst of LH and FSH, lasting about 30 hours.

Luteal Phase

This lasts 12–16 days. The follicle turns into the corpus luteum, and its production switches from oestradiol to progesterone:

- The GnRH pulse interval increases to one every three to five hours, with a steady decrease in amplitude
- Oestrogen and inhibin A check FSH secretion, whose levels fall to about 100 ng/ml
- LH also falls

- In the mid-luteal phase, oestrogen rises to a plateau
- Progesterone rises to 10–19 µg/ml in three to five days (more than 10 times its follicular level) and remains high for four to six days

Ischaemic Phase

(this is the last two days of the luteal phase):

- Oestrogen falls to its nadir, and progesterone falls precipitously to <1 ng/ml.
- Through the action of oxytocin and prostaglandins, the corpus luteum starts to degenerate (luteolysis).
- GnRH pulse frequency is minimal.
- FSH begins to increase 24 hours before bleeding.

Menstrual Bleeding

The endometrium is shed. In normal cycles, this is progesterone withdrawal bleeding, and, in anovulatory cycles, oestrogen withdrawal bleeding. The usual duration of menstrual flow is four to six days. The average loss is 30 ml, of which most occurs in the first three days. FSH peaks 24 hours after its onset.

Menstruation in the Life Cycle

Childhood

The gonadorelin pulse generator is active in the foetus and newborn infant, but afterwards there is a long period of gonadal dormancy, with a nadir at six years. During this time the pulse generator is inhibited by a 'neurobiological brake'[2], probably involving γ-aminobutyric acid and gonadal steroids. The mean oestrogen level is 2.2 pmol/l. Prepubertal girls have much higher FSH levels than LH levels.

Puberty

This is a transitional state, in which the young female grows rapidly and develops body hair and breasts. Breast development is stimulated by oestrogen, but the growth of body hair depends on adrenal hormones (adrenarche). Many factors influence puberty onset, including light, temperature and stress. Adequate nutrition, with sufficient fat, is signalled by increased serum leptin (discovered in 1994). At about the age of seven, the hypothalamic gonadostat is awakened. The GnRH neurones become less sensitive to inhibition, and come under the stimulus of glutamate and kisspeptin among other complex factors. At first, a pulsatile pattern appears at night, then a circadian rhythm develops. As a result:

- FSH is produced in increasing quantities. Initially its level is 10–20 times that of LH. It reaches a plateau.
- As GnRH pulses increase, so do the number of LH receptors in the gonadotrope. The mean waking LH increases 60-fold, as a result of increased pulse amplitude (9-fold) and pulse frequency (4-fold). The FSH/LH ratio falls to unity.

Menarche

This is the first menstrual bleed. Its age varies from population to population, and from time to time. It has fallen steadily from the late teens to the age of 13 or even earlier. It is affected by a large number of genes[2], is earlier in obese girls, and delayed in chronic malnutrition, illness, and vigorous physical training. The reasons for the onset of menstrual bleeding are not known. This dramatic event is often only a stage in achieving mature cycles.

Three studies have measured hormonal events at this time.

In the first, 112 American girls were followed from the age of 12 years, through puberty at 13, and up to 16[19]: every six months FSH, LH and oestradiol were measured in 24-hour urine specimens. FSH peaked at 12 µg/24 hours at the menarche, and then fell progressively to 5 µg/24 hours. LH reached the high level of 75 µg/24 hours, and remained high during the next three years. Oestrogen rose rapidly in the six months before the menarche, and continued to climb afterwards.

In the second study, six healthy pubertal girls, who had not menstruated, were followed for two years from the age of 11 to 13[20]. During this time, daily urine samples were collected, and five girls reached the menarche. Almost all had LH surges before the menarche, with amplitudes that did not differ significantly from that of adult controls. There was a small increase in progesterone, but only two girls had oestrogen and progesterone increases, matching the LH surges.

In the third study, nine pubertal girls aged 8–15 were compared with six adult women in respect of their response to transdermal oestrogen. Although the LH surge was smaller in magnitude, there was no difference in percentage change from nadir to peak, demonstrating that pre-menarchal girls have an LH surge in response to oestrogens[21].[a]

Adolescent Cycles

The early menstrual cycle is often long and irregular. In the first 2–3 years, with large individual differences, a high, but decreasing, proportion of cycles are anovulatory. Even when ovulation takes place, the follicle is relatively small with short luteal phases and low progesterone level. The maximum proportion of normal cycles is not reached until 26–30 years. The landmark of ovulation may involve a positive oestrogen feedback loop.

Pregnancy

During pregnancy the pituitary-ovarian axis is suppressed, and pituitary gonadotropins are undetectable. The placenta takes over, producing hCG, whose peak blood levels (35–120 IU/ml) are reached at 10 weeks gestation, after which it declines slowly to a nadir (5–20 IU/ml) at about 20 weeks. Oestrogen rises from about 2 ng/ml to 15 ng/ml. Progesterone rises by the 5th week, falls until the 9th week and rises again to a plateau of 125 ng/ml at the 32nd week.

The Postpartum Period

After delivery of the placenta, hCG, oestrogen and progesterone are rapidly cleared. During the first two puerperal weeks, gonadotropin secretion remains low. For 16–25 days the

---

[a] I am grateful to Professor Santoro for information about these studies.

pituitary fails to produce FSH in response to GnRH, and for 35 days fails to produce LH, after which it resumes its gonadotropic function. In bottle-feeding women the first menses occurs at 55–60 days, with a range of 20–120 days. But it is often anovulatory – the first ovulation is unlikely before the 10th postpartum week[22]; in almost all mothers, however, the second cycle is ovulatory[23].

Lactation

Breastfeeding maintains prolactin levels, which inhibit the ovarian response to FSH stimulation[24]. But most lactating mothers start menstruating again, depending on the frequency and amount of breastfeeding: Shaaban[25] reported that 73 per cent, and Vestermark[26] 57 per cent, started menstruating before weaning, with amenorrhoea averaging 34 weeks in those who persisted in breastfeeding; Chao's[22] review concluded that amenorrhoea persisted for about nine months. Measurements of prolactin, FSH, LH, oestradiol and progesterone have shown that this menstruation is often abnormal – in Shaaban's study, 7/19 had anovulatory cycles and another 5 luteal phase deficits. The first menstrual period is often anovulatory, and the early cycle length is prolonged with short luteal phases; Perez[27] found that only 24/200 women ovulated while on full breastfeeding.

The Menopause

In the late reproductive phase, follicular phases are shorter, and there are higher serum oestrogen levels (especially oestrone), FSH and LH, and lower luteal progesterone. Fertility declines, menstruation becomes irregular and anovulatory cycles are frequent.

Abnormal Menstruation

Anovulatory Bleeding Cycles

It was realized in the nineteenth century that menstruation could occur without ovulation. The first human case was published in 1927. Women with anovulatory cycles are infertile. Their menstrual periods are irregular, with prolonged and sometimes profuse bleeding. There is no corpus luteum and the endometrium is non-secretory. In the absence of progesterone, bleeding is due to oestrogen withdrawal; but the same mechanism – shut-off of the coiled arteries – is at work. Hormonal studies show low levels of FSH, premature and blunted LH surge, and low prolactin. Progesterone is absent, or less than 3 ng/ml. Body temperature is monophasic.

Luteal Phase Defects

Some women ovulate in the normal way, but have decreased progesterone secretion or effect. This is a subtle disorder, difficult to diagnose and probably underrecognized. These women are infertile, but have regular menses. Their follicles are small, the luteal phase short (eight days or less), with low levels of luteal progesterone (<10 ng/ml); the body temperature is monophasic. There is often a history of miscarriages and an early menopause is relatively frequent. As in amenorrhoea, its frequency is raised in female athletes and in women under stress or the influence of drugs, metabolic disease or chronic illness.

Polycystic Ovary (PCO) Syndrome

This is the most common cause of abnormal menstruation, affecting 5–10 per cent of women. The ovaries are enlarged with many cysts. The clinical features are infertility, absent, infrequent or irregular menses, hirsuitism and other signs of masculinization, obesity and non-insulin-dependent diabetes. There is an increased incidence of endometrial cancer, ischaemic heart disease and obstructive sleep apnoea. Its hormonal features are:

- Rapid GnRH pulse frequencies, favouring LH synthesis, with higher LH pulse amplitude and frequency, raised follicular phase LH and raised LH/FSH ratio
- Raised serum androgens
- Reduced oestrogen production, low levels of progesterone, and raised prolactin
- Hyperinsulinaemia and insulin resistance

There is some evidence of an association between PCO and bipolar disorder[28,29].

Congenital Adrenal Hyperplasia

Congenital adrenal hyperplasia is another cause of infertility and virilization, resulting from autosomal recessive disorders affecting the synthesis of cortisol from cholesterol, so that androgens are synthesized instead. These patients have ambiguous genitalia.

Hyperandrogenism

The normal level of androgen is 29 ng/ml. Women with twice this level have acne and hirsuitism, prolongation of the follicular phase (20 *versus* 17 days), short luteal phase (11 *versus* 13 days), disturbed menstruation and reduced fertility.

Medicine and Menstruation

There are claims that about 30 medical and surgical disorders are affected by the menstrual cycle, as discussed in chapter 2 of *Menstrual Psychosis and the Catamenial Process*[1], with more than 300 references. Apart from immune phenomena such as allergy to progesterone, there is substantial evidence for only 7 diseases – asthma, diabetes mellitus, endometriosis, epilepsy, hypersomnia, migraine and porphyria. These are reviewed with the following aims:

- To look for disorders that might be associated with menstrual psychosis
- To learn from the investigatory strategies and therapeutic experience of physicians
- Where the cause is known, to study the temporal pattern, in the menstrual cycle and life cycle, and response to treatment

Asthma

An association between asthma and the menstrual cycle has been recognized for 100 years. In some the onset, or a striking exacerbation, occurs at the menarche, but in others it starts late in reproductive life. Typically the attacks occur in the premenstrual phase, sometimes continuing after the onset of the menses and sometimes improving with the cessation of bleeding; but a few had their worst attacks during the menses, or at the mid-cycle. Clinical observations are supported by at least 10 questionnaire studies, showing that a large minority of female patients report a menstrual effect, usually premenstrual aggravation. In a recent study, self-identified premenstrual asthma was claimed by 92/756 (17 per cent) of asthmatic women[30]. The best evidence is from the measurement of forced expiratory peak flow: almost all studies showed a fall in peak flow at some stage in the cycle – the luteal phase, the 2–3 days immediately preceding the menses, the whole paramenstrual period or during menstrual flow. In some patients who had not noticed a deterioration, it could be demonstrated objectively.

There is conflicting evidence on hormonal associations, and the effect of pregnancy. As for response to treatment, oral contraceptives, progesterone and oestrogen have been effective in individual cases, but larger studies disagree whether oestrogen is detrimental, beneficial or neutral. Two patients responded to danazol and three to gonadorelins, of whom two relapsed when this treatment was interrupted, as in this example[31]:

> A 32-year old had recurrent premenstrual asthma. Treatment with Goserelin reduced her asthma and the need for prednisolone prophylaxis; there were no admissions to hospital in the next 14 months.

Thus some women with asthma show a menstrual effect, but menstrual asthma cannot contribute to the aims of this enquiry, because the timing is variable and cause unknown.

Diabetes Mellitus

If insulin-dependent diabetes develops in childhood, the menarche is often delayed. There-after, menstrual disorders, such as amenorrhoea, oligomenorrhea, polymenorrhoea and polycystic ovary syndrome, are common. Both hyper- and hypoglycaemic attacks can be related to menstruation.

Premenstrual Hyperglycaemia

An increase in insulin requirement in the premenstruum or during the menses was first noted in 1907; a number of cases of premenstrual ketoacidosis have been reported, as in this example[32]:

> A girl developed diabetes at 13. During her teenage years a clear-cut pattern emerged: on the first day of her menses, she became thirsty and giddy, required double the dose of insulin and even so developed glycosuria and ketosis. On the day after the cessation of bleeding she suffered from hypoglycaemia.

A meta-analysis of six studies showed that 55 per cent had a perimenstrual increase in blood sugar, or attacks of ketosis unexplained by infection or a lapse in treatment.

Premenstrual Hypoglycaemia

This is less common. One study found that 23/200 women complained of more frequent hypoglycaemic attacks at the menses, as in this example[33]:

> A 48-year old had suffered from diabetes for 40 years; she had diabetic nephropathy and was blind. At 45 her diabetic control became erratic at the menses, with recurrent hypoglycaemia and loss of consciousness just before and during menstrual flow. Reduction of insulin during the premenstruum failed to alleviate these episodes. She was treated with depot leuprorelin: two weeks afterwards she had two attacks, but then no more.

Onset before the Menarche

At a paediatric diabetic clinic, 7/52 girls had cyclical changes in control, lasting two to five days, before the first menstrual bleed[34]. One had cyclical hypoglycaemia and six hypergly-caemia, as in this example:

> A girl developed diabetes at 7½, well controlled by insulin injections. Two months before her 13th birthday, she suddenly developed keto-acidosis with intense thirst and vomiting. These symptoms returned four weeks later. A pattern emerged of sudden increases in blood glucose (requiring 15–30% more insulin) lasting two days, at 26-day intervals. Nine episodes were successfully treated by a temporary increase in medication. Ten months after the onset, she menstruated for the first time, after which the cyclical disturbance stopped.

In one girl this disturbance began at the age of nine, and, in another, 40 episodes were observed. It stopped at the menarche in three girls, and continued in three others, with the same cycle length; the seventh girl had not yet reached her menarche. One case was diagnosed retrospectively, when it was realized that her natural cycle was 56 days.

Endometriosis

Endometriosis is the name given to deposits of endometrial tissue outside the uterus. Most are in sites that can be reached by menstrual fluid – the uterine ligaments, rectovaginal septum, sigmoid colon, appendix, small intestine, bladder, umbilicus, cervix, vagina, vulva, ovaries, hernia sacs, laparotomy scars or lymph nodes. Distant deposits require dissemination through the lymphatics or blood stream. Pulmonary lesions can cause menstrual haemoptysis or pneumothorax. Other deposits can cause cyclical renal failure due to ureteric deposits, and sciatica or recurrent subarachnoid haemorrhage due to deposits in the spinal cord. There are three reports of cerebral manifestations[35-37]:

> A 20-year old, with a 3-year history of right-sided occipital headaches, occurring once or twice/month *unrelated* to the menstrual cycle and without a history of endometriosis, presented with a seizure. MRI-scan showed a right parietal lesion that proved to be an endometrial deposit.

> A 31-year old presented with Jacksonian seizures occurring every 30 minutes for 12 hours on the first day of her menses. CT scan showed three lesions and a cystic mass was removed, which proved to be endometrium.

> A 41-year old, who suffered from dysmenorrhoea, presented with paroxysmal headache, pain in the right side of the face and sensory abnormalities of the right arm associated with the menses; she was cured by Goserelin.

Ectopic endometriosis has been treated with oestrogens, Danazol or gonadorelin agonists. Pregnancy, hysterectomy and oöphorectomy may be beneficial.

Epilepsy

The relationship between epilepsy and menstruation was noted long ago. Marrotte[38], reviewing literature, traced it to Forestus (sixteenth century), who described a premenstrual seizure in a nun. In the English literature premenstrual convulsions were first described by Perfect[40].

Clinical Observations

Epilepsy can be precisely timed and counted. This is also true of epileptic discharges on the EEG (which are more frequent than fits), but only one patient has been shown to have EEG dysrhythmia exaggerated during the menses[41]; the bulk of the evidence is taken from calendar studies. Three patterns have been reported[42]:

- The most common is a paramenstrual increase, involving the last two to four days of the luteal phase and the menses themselves. With wide variations in frequency, this is present in about half of epileptic women.
- A few patients suffer from mid-cycle or ovulatory epilepsy.
- A different pattern has been observed in anovulatory or luteal-deficient cycles, with a reduction of seizures during the menses.

There may be a special relationship between menstruation and complex partial (temporal lobe) epilepsy; *petit mal* can also be exacerbated by the menses.

Mechanism

The interaction between epilepsy and the menstrual process is complex:

- Seizures, as a cerebral disturbance, may affect the hypothalamic pituitary axis.
- Epilepsy, especially temporal lobe epilepsy, is associated with menstrual disorders, such as polycystic ovary syndrome or hypogonadotropic hypogonadism.
- There may be a reciprocal interaction between antiepileptic drugs and the menstrual process.

- There is much evidence for the effect of progesterone:
  - Progesterone and its metabolites (such as pregnanolone and allopregnanolone[43]) are potent ligands of γ-aminobutyric acid receptors and have anticonvulsant effects similar to those of benzodiazepines and barbiturates.
  - Intravenous progesterone can reduce EEG dysrhythmia.
  - Some patients with catamenial epilepsy have lower luteal phase progesterone or its metabolites.

  Thus, in ovulatory cycles, paramenstrual epilepsy could be explained by withdrawal of progesterone and its metabolites. In luteal deficiency, high oestrogen/progesterone ratios could increase fit frequency
- In contrast, oestrogen lowers the seizure threshold. Within minutes of an intravenous injection, it can increase EEG dysrhythmia. Anovulatory cycles may be more common in epileptic women, with an increase in seizures.

Treatment

Progesterone is a rational treatment for patients with premenstrual exacerbation, anovulatory cycles or luteal defects[44]. Gonadorelins are appropriate for seizures related to ovulatory cycles, and have been effective in a number of patients, especially those with paramenstrual seizures. In some patients clomiphene has been effective.

Table 25.1 Cyclical epilepsy before the menarche

First author	Details
Brière de Boismont (1842)[47]	We have observed a young woman, who suffered a seizure every month for a year. They ceased at the menarche.
Muskens (1926)[48]	A 15-year old had an increase in seizures every four weeks for three months. When she menstruated for the first time her seizures ceased.
	A 13-year old started having seizures; in two years she had 13 fits, occurring every 4–6 weeks. At the age of 15 she menstruated for the first time, and seizures ceased for six months. They then returned during the menses.
	A 7-year old suffered seizures every 4–8 weeks; after her menarche all seizures ceased. The follow-up period was six years.
Livingstone (1954)[49]	In his experience of over 4,000 epileptic children, he saw eight epileptic girls in whom epilepsy started before the age of five, and in whom the seizures recurred regularly every four weeks. Following the onset of menstruation the seizures continued to occur only in association with the menstrual cycle.
Almqvist (1955)[50]	An 11-year old, suffering from learning disability, had a rhythmic pattern of seizures. Three years later she menstruated for the first time, and the pattern continued, linked to the menses.
	Another girl with learning disability had a rhythmic pattern of seizures before her menarche at 14. After that, the pattern continued, linked to the menses.

Occurrence in the Life Cycle

Cessation of seizures has been reported during amenorrhoea and in pregnancy[45]; but the opposite effect has been described. The menopause has no overall effect. There are reports of epilepsy starting at the menarche. In one series of 100 patients, six had their first seizure on that very day[46]. Of interest in the present context are reports that cyclical epilepsy can start before the menarche. The observations of four authors, published more than 60 years ago, are shown in Table 25.1 (on page 292).

In four of these patients, monthly seizures ceased at the menarche. It is interesting that these laconic reports, deeply buried in the literature, not only support the pre-menarchal occurrence of a disorder of the central nervous system, but also show that this can start in the first decade.

Hypersomnia

This is a rare sleep disorder, which was afforded only a sentence in the massive *Principles and Practice of Sleep Medicine*[51]. It was described 250 years ago[52]:

> An 18-year old, at the approach of her menses, developed lethargy and drowsiness. The same returned with greater force at the next two menses. It increased in severity, and was succeeded by *délire hystérique*, when she became furiously manic, and refused food and drink. Dr Pomme resorted to drastic measures: he plunged her into a cold bath, with the effect that she was induced to eat and drink after 12 hours. Spending eight hours in the bath each day, and wearing underwear soaked in cold water (frequently refreshed), she recovered in two months.

Eighteen cases have been described. Most had episodes starting in the premenstrual phase[52-59], but a few had catamenial[56,60-62] or paramenstrual[63] onsets. In one patient, somnolence appeared to substitute for the menses[64]. I have a personal observation, associated with depression:

> A 35-year old developed fatigue, lack of energy, somnolence and depressive symptoms on the 2nd day of the menses, lasting 2–3 days. There was some diurnal variation, because she felt well on getting up, and worst ½ hour later until 3 pm. "The back of my legs felt like I had climbed a mountain. I just wanted to curl up and sleep anywhere"; she would fall asleep in the middle of a sentence. She was weepy and irritable, felt morbid, had no joy in the children, no appetite and "no future", avoided company, was forgetful and could not put her mind to anything. Her husband had to take over the housework and cooking. In addition, she had backache, numbness in the hands and face, loss of taste sensation, an altered time sense and hyperacusis. She heard suicidal command hallucinations inside her head – "Come on, Pam, you can turn the car round and that will be the finish". "It was a voice, it was that real". Her face looked drained and drawn with staring eyes, like premature senility.

In the only quantitative study[65], reporting on mental disorders in 10,000 women including 1,500 with infrequent or scanty menses, there is a brief description of four patients with abnormal somnolence, one of whom suffered from fatigue and sleepiness during the menses.

Similar cases have been described in pubertal boys: Stadler[66,a] described five boys with episodic twilight states, marked by dreamy self-absorption, disorientation, sleep walking and automatic behaviour followed by patchy memory loss; they were associated with periods of deep sleep lasting up to 48 hours; in two boys, three to five day episodes returned every four weeks.

Of particular interest is a group of five with onset at or before the menarche (Table 25.2).

---

[a] This important paper was reported at the third annual meeting of the German Society for Neurology and Psychiatry in September 1937; a summary appeared, but the full paper, with its references to earlier cases, seems to be unobtainable.

Table 25.2 Menstrual hypersomnia with onset at or before the menarche

First author	Details	Comment	Additional features
Möller (1883)[67]	Twenty months before her menarche, a 12-year old suffered from attacks of day-time sleepiness. One month after the menarche, she developed a psychosis with grandiose delusions and was admitted to the local asylum. Sleep attacks were more frequent and prolonged during the menses.	There was no monthly pattern before the menarche, then it was menstrual	Psychosis
Kleine (1925)[68]	A 15-year old began to suffer from a 3–4 day 'sleep attacks'. The first three occurred at exactly one month intervals, and the fourth one month later, coincident with the menarche. Attacks continued with the menses, except for one occasion when they occurred 14 days later. At the age of 16 they ceased. At 20 they returned two to four times/year, again with the menses.	The monthly pattern started before the menarche, and continued with menstrual onsets	
Billiard (1975)[69]	A 13-year old fell asleep on a girl guide outing, and slept for six days. On the third day she menstruated (probably for the first time, but this is not quite clear). One month later she had another attack that lasted three days, ending 12 hours before menstrual bleeding. She had four further attacks. Of the six attacks, four were premenstrual, one started before and continued during the menses, and one started on the third day of bleeding. A final episode consisted of behavioural changes (hostility and withdrawal) without hypersomnia. She had abnormally high levels of 5-hydroxy-indole-acetic-acid in the CSF after probenecid, suggesting an increased turnover of serotonin during hypersomnia. She improved with oestrogens.	The first episode was probably at the menarche, after which attacks were paramenstrual	Abnormal serotonin metabolism
Papy (1982)[70]	A 21-year old suffered from bulimia and hypersomnia from the age of 13. Attacks lasted four to five days. The first occurred before her menarche. From 13–15 she had 1–2 attacks/year lasting four days, but they became more frequent, with 12 attacks between 1968 and 1974, all starting four to six days after the onset of the menses. With oral contraceptive medication, attacks became less frequent, with only 4 in four years. Three occurred during the first half of the cycle, 1 when she discontinued oral contraceptives and 6 in 1979–80, when she stopped them completely. These all occurred in the mid-cycle, about the time of ovulation.	There was no monthly pattern before the menarche, after which they were menstrual and later at ovulation	Bulimia
Sugimoto (1991)[71,a]	A 12-year old suffered the first of seven episodes, which started with mutism and progressed to hypersomnia, lasting about seven days. In one attack she had a prodromal fever of 40°. The first four occurred at intervals of 29–35 days, then, after a month free of symptoms, she had her menarche. After five regular menses, she had three consecutive hypersomnias starting shortly before, and lasting throughout the menses.	The monthly pattern started before the menarche, and continued with late premenstrual onsets	Mutism

[a] Translated by Yumi Okomura.

Two developed hypersomnia before the menarche without a monthly pattern[67,68] – only after the first menstrual bleed did a menstrual pattern develop; one of these also developed a psychosis[67]. A third had onset at the menarche[69]. Two had monthly sleep attacks before the menarche, which continued with the same rhythm afterwards[70,71].

It has been suggested that cyclic increases in serum progesterone are responsible for these cases[72], but disorders related to progesterone cannot explain episodes starting before the menarche. There are several reasons for favouring a hypothalamic basis:

- One had a tumour of the *sella turcica*[54].
- Several had bulimia or hyperphagia[56,57,61,68], which can be a hypothalamic disorder.
- Persistent or periodic hypersomnia is found in lesions affecting the hypothalamus and neighbouring brain areas. They include *encephalitis lethargica*, African trypanosomiasis, tumours in the third ventricle, multiple sclerosis with periventricular plaques, thalamic stroke and trauma, surgery or irradiation affecting these areas.
- It is now known that peptide neurotransmitters (orexins, also known as hypocretins[73,74]), whose neurons are in the lateral and posterior hypothalamus, have a major role in sleep and wakefulness. Their deficiency is involved in narcolepsy with cataplexy and other hypersomnias[75].

Migraine

Migraine is a paroxysmal disorder in which throbbing headache (often unilateral) is associated with visual disturbances and vomiting. It is based on vasomotor instability of the craniocerebral or meningeal arteries. It can occur with or without an aura. The link with menstruation was first noticed in 1758[76]. Menstrual attacks occur in about 10 per cent of female sufferers, usually without an aura and often particularly severe. A survey of 5,000 women aged 30–34 discovered 237 cases (about 7 per cent)[77].

Mechanism

The role of oestrogens was suggested by a classic series of experiments in Sydney[78,79].

> Somerville studied the effect of injections of progesterone and oestrogen in five women with recurrent attacks related to six or more successive menses. When progesterone was injected at the end of the luteal phase, it delayed menstruation without affecting migraine. Similar injections of oestradiol delayed the onset of migraine by 3–9 days.

These observations have been supported by other research showing that attacks occur during the oestrogen-free week in women taking oral contraceptives or oestrogen-replacement therapy. Falling oestrogen levels may not be the only menstrual trigger. A role for prostaglandins has been argued: prostaglandin E_1 can trigger migraine-like headache in normal subjects and enters the systemic circulation in greater quantities during the first 48 hours after the onset of bleeding.

Occurrence in the Menstrual and Life Cycles

In the menstrual cycle, attacks of migraine occur close to the onset of the menses – shortly before or shortly afterwards. Rarely, they occur in the mid-cycle, when oestrogens are also falling sharply. As for the life cycle, the onset coincides with the menarche in 10–20 per cent. It may be worsened by oral contraceptives, especially if there is an aura. Pregnancy has a beneficial effect in about two-thirds, with return in the early puerperium; but it can worsen or begin during pregnancy, in which case it is more commonly preceded by an aura. The menopause has variable effects – improvement, or worsening, especially after a surgical menopause.

Treatment and Prophylaxis

Menstrual migraine does not always respond to conventional therapy with triptans (serotonin receptor agonists) or prostaglandin inhibitors. In resistant cases, oestrogens have been beneficial, as shown by double blind placebo-controlled crossover trials. Occasionally it has been necessary to resort to gonadorelin agonists.

Migraine Psychosis

Migraine has many central nervous complications, including strokes and coma. In addition it can present with transient psychoses. It is necessary to glance at this literature, because some cases of menstrual psychosis could conceivably be migraine psychoses. *Migränedämmerzustände* [migrainous twilight states] were described in the early twentieth century. Ranzow[80] collected 10 cases, lasting a few hours or at the most three days, followed by amnesia. Since then, more than 25 others have been described, mostly in children or adolescents. The incidence is about 3 per cent of migraine sufferers. It may be higher in certain families. The following cases had a possible link to the menses[81,82]:

> A 40-year old officer's widow, previously stable, suddenly complained of loss of memory. She seemed to be expecting her dead brother, and believed her furniture had been stolen. She recovered six hours later. Her menses started on the same day, and 24 hours later she had a severe attack of migraine.

> A 16-year old, from her menarche, habitually suffered from menstrual migraine, accompanied by twilight states lasting some hours. In one attack she shouted out some odd ideas – she would not die, was a decent young woman. She came to herself after some hours in the clinic.

In her monumental study of 500 migraine sufferers in Berlin, Ulrich[83] laconically described this case:

> A 12-year old with a migrainous sister suffered attacks lasting 3–4 days every four weeks for two years. There was a disturbance of consciousness with amnesia and behaviour verging on the criminal. She would run away and return at night with no memory of what she did, or with confabulation. Bilateral headache with vomiting always preceded and sometimes followed these episodes.

She commented:

> The natural history of this disturbance is of particular interest. The regular return at 4-weekly intervals suggests a relationship with sexual functioning – a kind of equivalent of her menses *that had not yet started*.

She supported this with another case in a 12-year old, who suffered headache and other symptoms at the beginning of each month; these attacks stopped some months later at her menarche.

Porphyria

In the synthesis of haemoglobin, myoglobin, cytochromes, catalase and peroxidase, seven enzymes are involved in transforming glycine into protoporphyrin IX (the molecule that binds iron); deficiency of each results in a specific form of anaemia or porphyria. Menstrual exacerbations have been reported in three of these enzyme deficiencies, but in two of them – variegated porphyria and hereditary coproporphyria – they are rare. Acute intermittent porphyria is the form commonly associated with cyclical effects. It is due to deficiency of the third enzyme in the chain – porphobilinogen deaminase, which catalyses the formation of hydroxymethylbilane from porphobilinogen. There are many genetic variants. It is more common in women, and can develop after puberty, but usually in the second to fifth decades. Porphoryns are excreted in the urine, which has a dark brown or port wine colour; the Watson–Schwartz test for urinary porphobilinogen is diagnostic. Patients suffer from attacks of colic, pain and weakness due to neuropathy, and about half develop seizures, hallucinations or delirium. Attacks are triggered by various drugs – barbiturates, alcohol, sulfonamides, phenytoin, sedatives, oral contraceptives and some antibiotics – as well as fasting and infection.

Since Waldenström's description[84], there have been many reports of paramenstrual exacerbations, with at least 40 individual cases. This is an example[85]:

> A 19-year old war bride embarked at Southampton to join her husband in the USA. At sea she developed nausea and vomiting, and was treated for sea sickness with barbiturates. She became confused and behaved in a childish fashion. In New York she was admitted to hospital with a diagnosis of acute dissociative reaction. She was crying and giggling, incoherent and disorientated. In a lucid interval she gave a history of previous attacks of abdominal pain, one so severe that she had an unnecessary laparotomy. Her urine was a deep wine-red in colour. She ran a remitting course with premenstrual exacerbations, developed an ascending paralysis, lapsed into coma and died on the 72nd day.

In a Finnish national sample, 29/95 sufferers reported attacks linked to the menstrual cycle. The onset is usually premenstrual, but may be catamenial, or both. In most the link with menstruation has been asserted without evidence from precise dating of menses and episodes. The only patient with sufficient data for statistical tests is Hopmann's[86] third patient:

> This patient was followed for seven years, during which she had 50 menstrual cycles. A chart showed that she had ten attacks of abdominal pain, six immediately premenstrual, three during menstrual flow, and one each after the menses or in the mid-cycle.

There seem to be no demonstrations of a menstrual effect on porphyrin excretion, except in one amenorrhoeic patient who suffered from attacks of porphyria after the resumption of menstruation: she had an increase in porphobilinogen coinciding with ovulation[87].

Attacks during pregnancy have been reported. One patient had attacks in five successive pregnancies. Two patients recovered after termination. Raised urinary prophyrins have been demonstrated during pregnancy. But less than 10% of pregnancies are affected. Attacks have also been associated with hysterectomy, oöphorectomy and ovarian radiotherapy.

Porphyria is a life-threatening disorder, and it has often been necessary to use draconian anti-menstrual treatment, including castration. Danazol cannot be prescribed because it can precipitate attacks. Gonadorelin agonists were first used in 1984 and have been beneficial in more than 15 patients. A successful innovation was to restrict treatment to the first 21 days and then add a progestin, with the idea that intermittent treatment allows follicle matur-ation and oestrogen production to occur during the treatment-free interval, while the progestin establishes regular menstruation. But gonadorelins are not always effective: in one series of seven patients, two did not respond, and there was no marked effect on δ-aminolevulinic acid or total porphyrin excretion.

Progesterone Allergy

This causes a variety of skin lesions – urticaria, erythema multiforme, eczema – and also angioneurotic oedema or anaphylactic reactions. There have been numerous case reports, and reviews of up to 50 cases. Some patients have been sensitized by prior treatment with artificial progestins. The diagnosis is made by parenteral challenge or other tests demonstrating sensitivity to progesterone.

The timing of these disorders, within the menstrual cycle and the life cycle, could illustrate the direct effects of progesterone.

- Most cases developed during the years of reproductive maturity, when luteal cycles are fully developed; but four patients first developed symptoms at the menarche.
- The eruption usually appears during the second part of the cycle, and resolves with the onset of bleeding, or shortly afterwards. But some patients have eruptions throughout the cycle, with premenstrual worsening. Occasionally, the onset has been just before the menses, when progesterone levels would normally be falling. In others, symptoms have started at the mid-cycle; in one of these the worst were during menstrual bleeding, but pruritus began during the small pre-ovulatory progesterone peak.
- The resolution of symptoms has sometimes occurred with menstrual bleeding. But sometimes symptoms have peaked during the menses[88] or continued after the end of menstrual flow.
- One would expect symptoms to be more severe during pregnancy, when progesterone levels are much higher. This is true in some, and a number began during pregnancy. In two of these, the disorder was present only during two pregnancies, clearing up during the puerperium. But others have improved during pregnancy, to start again in the puerperium.
- Six had their first symptoms in the puerperium, one after two births. All had cyclical relapses, which were premenstrual in four and mid-cycle in the other two.
- One patient was symptom-free during a six-year period of amenorrhoea.

Thus there is no consistent pattern. These patients have responded to desensitization, antihistamines and corticosteroids, menstrual suppression by oestrogens, the anti-oestrogen tamoxifen, salpingo-oöphorectomy[89], Danazol and gonadorelin agonists.

Summary

About 30 periodic medical disorders may be affected by the menstrual cycle, but in most the evidence is sketchy.

For some diseases, physiological analogues of the clinical state are available – spirometry in asthma, glucose tolerance tests in diabetes, EEG dysrhythmia in epilepsy and urinary porphoryns in porphyria. In spite of this, much of the evidence is gained from case lore, calendar studies or treatment response. The dating of the onset of symptoms and the menses is rarely adequate for statistical tests.

Psychiatrists can learn from exemplary strategies for investigation, such as Somerville's migraine studies, and studies of epilepsy, distinguishing between normal and abnormal menstrual cycles. They can also benefit from therapeutic experience, using oestrogens or intermittent GnRH analogues to interrupt the cycle.

Explanations of the menstrual link are only available for three disorders (migraine, epilepsy and allergy to steroid hormones). They alone can illuminate the temporal pattern of symptoms associated with specific causes. The lack of any consistent pattern in progesterone sensitivity discourages the hope that such clinical features can yield aetiological clues.

The most interesting finding is that four diseases have occasionally presented with monthly symptoms before the menarche – diabetes mellitus, epilepsy, hypersomnia and migraine psychosis. The evidence is meagre and buried in ancient literature, but collectively it confirms that the primitive menstrual cycle is capable of triggering a range of clinical phenomena. In three of them these episodes stopped abruptly at the first menstrual bleed. This corroborates the more extensive evidence for pre-menarchal menstrual psychosis (see page 310–313).

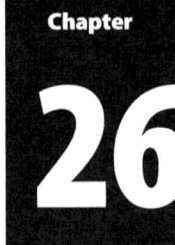

Chapter

Definitions and Classification

Menstrual Mood Disorder

It is necessary briefly to mention another, much more common, psychiatric disorder associated with menstruation: at the level of consultation, and strictly defined by prospective daily ratings, it affects 5 per cent of women. It has been given various names – premenstrual tension or syndrome, and late luteal or premenstrual dysphoric disorder. Its essence is the temporal association with the menstrual cycle of mood symptoms, sometimes accompanied by a somatic component (oedema or breast tenderness). The symptoms are common and found in many other disorders; there is some evidence, however, that anger and irritability are relatively specific. These are not the symptoms of a 'psychosis'. It is not a matter of severity: premenstrual depression may be suicidal, and premenstrual anger homicidal, while a menstrual psychosis can sometimes be relatively brief and mild in comparison.

The literature, amounting to thousands of publications, is a quagmire. The review in *Menstrual Psychosis and the Catamenial Process*[1] (10,000 words, with more than 400 references) was focused on areas with most relevance to menstrual psychosis, including severe disorders that might be a *forme fruste* of psychosis, genetic and biological investigations, and effective treatments. This reached the conclusion that menstrual mood disorder and the much more rare menstrual psychosis were probably distinct disorders, for the following reasons:

- Menstrual mood disorder occurs during normal, ovulatory cycles, while menstrual psychosis occurs in abnormal menstruation[90].
- The timing of menstrual psychosis is not only premenstrual, but can also be catamenial, or have onset in the mid-cycle.
- The association with bipolar disorder and postpartum psychosis is much stronger.
- There may also be a difference in treatment response, menstrual mood disorder responding to selective serotonin-reuptake inhibitors (SSRIs), Danazol and GnRH agonists, in contrast to the treatment response of menstrual psychosis (see page 342–344).

Nevertheless it is possible that occasional cases of menstrual mood disorder manifest psychotic symptoms such as delusions or brief hypomanic swings. It is surprising how seldom this occurs. This is a patient from my clinical practice, who developed brief hypomania after ECT:

A woman, as a child, was starved and beaten by her parents, sexually abused by several men including her brothers, and bullied at school. She made many suicide attempts and harmed herself by self-cutting, cigarette burns and head-banging. At the age of 12 she developed bulimia nervosa, and later abused ethanol, cannabis and glue. Diagnoses of hysterical or borderline personality disorder were made. During all her pregnancies, she was subjectively and objectively well. At 18 she gave birth to her first child. At 21 she contracted a stormy marriage. At 22 she gave birth to her 2nd child, and afterwards was hospitalized with postpartum depression and impaired bonding; she threatened to kill the baby, and attempted suicide by strangling, hanging and drowning, but recovered with ECT. At 27 she wounded a police officer, who was trying to prevent her from injuring herself; she was put on probation for three years. At 30 she was convicted of possession of an offensive weapon. She had a fruitless 6-month admission to a specialist unit for personality disorders. At 30 she wounded a security guard who was trying to stop her cutting herself; she was convicted and given a 3-year prison sentence. She was again pregnant, and felt "the best since my second child was born". Asked to see her, I predicted a recurrence of her puerperal illness. After the birth of her 3rd child, she developed severe postpartum depression with rejection of the baby, and was admitted to the Queen Elizabeth mother & baby unit. Treated with ECT, she had a 2-day episode of hypomania. She recovered and bonded to the baby. In August, in spite of lithium prophylaxis, she had a recurrence of self-harm, and menstruated shortly afterwards. Her husband confirmed that she had cyclical premenstrual deteriorations "like clockwork". For several months she had a pattern of relapses and prompt menstrual recovery. Treated with Goserelin injections, she became amenorrhoeic, and remained bright and cheerful. After two years in hospital, she was discharged at the end of her prison sentence. Her husband, and staff members, who had known her for years, said she was as well as she had ever been, comparable with her well state during pregnancy. She was transferred to her area consultant, who made a diagnosis of personality disorder, and withdrew the treatment. She relapsed and lost her children.

Definition of Menstrual Psychosis

The diagnosis requires:

- Acute onset, against a background of normality
- Duration measured in days or weeks, with full recovery
- Psychotic features – confusion, delusions, hallucinations, stupor and mutism, or a manic syndrome
- A circa-mensual periodicity, in rhythm with the menstrual cycle

Exacerbation of a chronic psychosis is excluded.

Evidence for the Menstrual Association

This chapter is a radical revision (not merely an abridgement) of the account given in *Menstrual Psychosis and the Catamenial Process*[1]. The 2008 monograph identified 80 cases with substantial evidence for the menstrual association, using statistical tests as a guide. In this revised analysis I employed simpler criteria based on the number of dated episodes:

- One or two episodes. Since women between the ages of 13 and 50 spend a third of their lives menstruating or in the premenstrual phase, two episodes could be coincidential. Although in 1982, a single relapse at the first postpartum menses awakened my interest in menstrual psychosis, all such cases have been rejected, with the exception of single episodes at the menarche (see page 313–315).
- Three or four episodes. At this frequency an association becomes plausible, especially if there is additional evidence, such as undated episodes observed in hospital. These are 'possible cases' – 188 in the literature and 18 in my series.

- Five or 6 episodes, or at least 10 undated episodes. This corresponds approximately to the 'established cases' in my 2008 monograph; there is an association between psychosis and menses 'on the balance of probability'. There are 85 'probable cases' in the literature and 11 in my series.
- Seven or more episodes, often with supportive evidence from undated episodes. In these 'confirmed cases', the diagnosis is beyond reasonable doubt. There are 19 in the literature and 4 in my series.

Classification

Two German authors have proposed a classification of menstrual psychoses– v. Krafft–Ebing[91] and Jolly[92]: v. Krafft–Ebing recognized *menstruale Entwicklungs-psychose* [menstrual development psychoses], *Ovulationspsychose* – under separate headings of single, relapsing and periodic cases – and *epochale Menstrualpsychose* – continuous bipolar disorders with switches timed to the menses. Jolly collapsed *Ovulationspsychose* into a single group of recurrent psychosis associated with the menses, preserved the 'epochal' cases, and employed three categories based on timing within the life cycle – circamensual psychosis starting before the menarche, onset with the menarche and onset at the menopause. In *Menstrual Psychosis and the Catamenial Process*, I developed these ideas, placing the patients under two broad divisions.

- Timing within the menstrual cycle
- Timing within the life cycle

Within the menstrual cycle, there were onsets in the mid-cycle, premenstrual phase, during menstrual bleeding ('catamenial') and over a broad span covering the premenstrual and catamenial phases ('paramenstrual'). Within the life cycle, there are five stages to consider:

- Before the menarche
- At the menarche
- Monthly psychosis during amenorrhoea
- Onset during pregnancy
- Onset after childbirth

There are also the special circumstances of monthly psychoses in the absence of a pituitary, after the menopause and in males.

In the present analysis, timing within the menstrual cycle has been re-grouped according to two hypothetical triggers –

- Ovulation and the mid-cycle gonadotropin surge, including episodes that end abruptly at the menses
- The collapse of luteal support leading to a cascade of steroid hormones and endometrial necrosis, associated with late luteal, catamenial and paramenstrual onsets

The term 'epochal menstrual psychosis' has been reserved for patients with continuous illness and menstrual switches.

The onset of psychotic symptoms will be determined partly by the trigger, and partly by episode latency, which depends on the pathogenetic process. Many cases demonstrate the variability of this latency. There are patients whose episodes shift from mid-luteal[93] or paramenstrual to mid-cycle onset, from mid-cycle to follicular[94] or from late luteal to catamenial onset[91]. Occasional cases give evidence of both triggers[95–98]. The 'epochal' group, with its switch from depression to mania and back, supports the idea of two critical moments in the genesis of episodes. It is not always possible to apply this schema for lack of information about dating within the 'premenstrual' phase.

Chapters 4 and 5 provide examples representative of each of these groups, and Chapter 6 of episodes linked to childbearing.

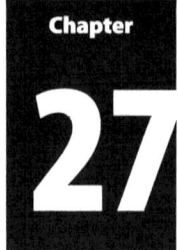

Timing within the Menstrual Cycle

The Mid-Cycle Trigger

There are 75 cases with a mid-cycle trigger in the literature including 11 'probable' and three 'confirmed'[93,99,100]; there was only one case in my series. Two will be summarized under postpartum cases, and the one from my series under the association with learning disability on page 337. Clinical Gem 27.1 (on page 305) shows Wollenberg's case[99], with 13 dated episodes and mean cycle lengths of 34 days for the menses and 33 days for mania; note that the illness started with several months of continuous mania.

The Late Luteal Trigger

There are more than 140 cases in the literature, including 39 'probable' and 6 'confirmed'[91,101–105]. In my series there are 27 cases, including 9 'probable' and 2 'confirmed', which are summarized under Runge psychoses (see pages 320–321) and the discussion of frequency on pages 323–333. Clinical Gem 27.3 on page 308 (of v. Krafft-Ebing[91,106]) describes 16 dated episodes.

Clinical Gem 27.2 (on pages 306–307) is the most remarkable in this literature, with 54 episodes[104,105]. She had a long and irregular cycle ranging from 32 to 50 days, with mean 40, later 35 days. In phase two (including the two menses that continued after the first irradiation), nine episodes were dated, supported by five earlier onsets simultaneous with the menses.

Epochal Menstrual Psychosis

There are 12 epochal menstrual psychoses in the literature - 6 'probable' (all in the Japanese literature, with charts rather than dates) and 2 'confirmed'[107,108]; Clinical Gem 27.4[107] (on page 309) is one of them.

Clinical Gem 27.1 Mid-Cycle Menstrual Psychosis

A young woman was calm and gentle, enjoyed her work, her schoolbook full of original and wise comments. Her menarche was at 15. In January 1889, aged 25, she became restless and sleepless, refused to get dressed, laughed a lot, and took it out of her cat, which she said was the Devil. Chastised by her mother, she said, "You have struck the loving Saviour". She wrote a letter to the Kaiser, and many poems. She felt confused and said she was going mad. Admitted to hospital she attacked the doctor and other patients, tried to abscond and had to be isolated; she was overactive, sleepless, laughing, dancing in the corridor and hoarse from singing. The episode continued through March and April, and it was not until May, the day after the onset of her menses, that she calmed down. A week later she became melancholic, switched to mania, and again settled in July when her menses appeared. She then embarked on a cyclical illness (as detailed below) related to 15 menstrual periods, with much variation in cycle length (range 19–45 days). There were 14 manic episodes, of which seven had a sudden onset that preceded the menses by 6–26 (mean 16) days. The course was variable: one episode cleared up after five days, but most transposed into depression of variable severity and duration, while two continued with a degree of liveliness until the next sudden onset, and one episode was followed by alternating mood states. She recovered in December.

Episode	Onset of mania	Onset of menses
1	July 17	July 29
2	August 23	August 29
3	September 23	October 13
4	October 31	November 25
5	December 7	December 19
6	January 12	January 21
7	February 1	February 9
8	February 27	March 14
9	March 28	April 19
10	April 25	May 15
11	May 26	June 20
12	July 2	July 22
13	August 5	August 25
14	September 20	

Clinical Gem 27.2 54 Episodes of Menstrual Psychosis

A 36-year old had eight children. She was a friendly person who kept herself to herself, but looked after the children well. In April 1911, she suddenly expressed the idea that her husband was King Ludwig of Bavaria, saved from the water. She prayed constantly, spoke in a stereotyped way, ran about aimlessly and misrecognized people; she lapsed into stupor, mute and immobile except for rhythmic hand movements. After 12 days she recovered, without the slightest trace of mental illness. These episodes continued for years, with a wide variety of clinical pictures. Onset and recovery were often sudden. The dating, summarised in the following, corresponds to three phases of observation. In phase 1 (the early stages) she had four episodes, then, in 1913, gave birth to her 9th child, whom she breast-fed. The 5th episode started in October, at the return of the menses, nine weeks after the birth. In these early attacks, the duration of attacks was recorded: it was long and variable; in general, stupors lasted 2–3 weeks and were followed by hypomania. Only at the end of this phase was a relationship with the menstrual cycle suspected. Phase 2 covers 12 episodes with fairly complete dating of onsets; this phase can be used for a study of the association. Phase 3 covers the period of amenorrhoea that followed irradiation of the ovaries: stupors continued without any change or reduction in severity, and with a periodicity similar to the menstrual cycle before the interventions; there were 28 further episodes at intervals varying between 30 and 67 days, with a mean 42 days. Surgical removal of the ovaries and uterus had no effect.

Phase 1. The early stages

Episode	Onset of psychosis	Duration	Comment
1	April 29, 1911	12 days	
2	May 20	33 days	
3	January 16, 1912	20 days	
4	February 26	64 days	
			On August 25 she gave birth
5	October 31, 1913	120 days	Onset at 1 postpartum menses
6	August 30, 1915	36 days	Sudden onset at the menses
7	November 16, 1916	68 days	Onset at the menses
8	January 9, 1918	107 days	
9	May 27		Simultaneous with the menses
10	June 29	27 days	Simultaneous with the menses
11	Late January 1919		Menstrual onset on January 22

Phase 2. Dating of onsets

Episode	Onset of psychosis	Onset of menses
12	April 19	April 18
13	A few days before May 23	May 23
14	July 11	July 12
15	August 19	August 25
16	Some days before October 7	September 30

Episode	Onset of psychosis	Onset of menses
17	Some days before November 9	November 16
18	December 18	December 18
19	January 22, 1920	January 22
20	March 2	(Onset during amenorrhoea)
21	April 8	April 10
22	May 25	May 28
23	Some days before June 30	June 29

Phase 3. After the interventions

Episode(s)	Onset of psychosis	Onset of menses
On August 19, 1920, her ovaries were irradiated		
24	August 21	August 21
25	Some days before September 30	September 29
26–31	November 5 December 14 January 26, 1921 March 7 April 16 May 17	Amenorrhoea from now on
On June 28, 1921, her ovaries were again irradiated		
32–39	June 29 August 24 October 15 December 5 February 10, 1922 March 19 April 20 May 25	
On June 28, 1922, her ovaries were removed		
40–49	July 2 August 3 September 23 October 26 November 29 January 15, 1923 February 24 April 4 May 9 July 7	
On August 7, 1923, her uterus was removed		
50–54	August 8 September 27 November 16 December 20 February 3, 1924	

Clinical Gem 27.3 Late Luteal Menstrual Psychosis

A woman had her menarche at the age of 16, and, in her late twenties, manic episodes lasting six and four months. At 29 she developed episodes of mania with insomnia, pressure of speech, in some episodes confusion, and a religious component that returned every month for two years. The onsets of menstrual flow and episodes were as follows:

Episode	Onset of menses	Onset and duration of episode
1	October 15, 1874	October 16–31
2	November 10	November 11–28
3	December 9	December 9–?
4	January 9, 1875	Uncertain onset–January 14
5	January 26	January 24–February 2
6	February 17	February 20–March 2
	March 12	Subclinical undated episode.
7	April 8	April 8–18
8	April 29	'With the menses'–May 12
9	May 19	May 21–30
10	June 11	June 14–24
11	July 7	July 8–18
12	July 30	July 31–August 10
13	August 21	August 22–September 3
14	September 20	September 21–26
15	October 17	October 19–29
16	November 11	November 17–27

This pattern continued for a further eight months (without dating), after which she recovered, although she remained amenorrhoeic until January 1877. This is case 12 in his 1878 paper[106] and *recidivierende Fall* 14 in his 1902 monograph[91].

Clinical Gem 27.4 Epochal Menstrual Psychosis

In his monograph *Die Manie*[107], Mendel described, as case 19, a young woman, whose menarche occurred at 16. In the summer of 1871 (aged 22), following a disappointment in love, she suffered from depression followed by a brief manic episode. She then embarked on a cyclical illness whose dates are shown in the following. The cycle length is short, with a range of 19–27 (mean 24) days. The eight manic episodes invariably started within 2 days of the cessation of menses, and lasted an average of 15 days. Depressions started on the same day that mania ended, or on the next day, 1–5 days before the onset of the menses; they lasted a mean of 8 days:

Menses	Mania	Depression
	November 12 –November 24	November 25 –December 3
November 28 –December 2	December 4 –December 17	December 18 –December 23
December 20 –December 23	December 24 –January 10	January 10 –January 18
January 13 –January 17	January 19 –February 8	February 8 –February 13
February 9 –February 13	February 14 –February 28	March 1 –March 8
March 4 –March 7	March 8 –March 24	March 25 –April 3
March 30 –April 4	April 4 –April 14	April 15 –April 21
April 18 –April 21	April 22 –May 10	
May 14 –May 17		

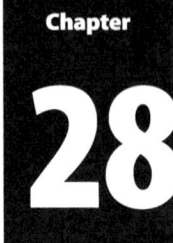

Timing within the Life Cycle

Onset before the Menarche

Starting in the last 30 years of the nineteenth century, German writers began to mention girls who developed periodic psychoses at monthly intervals before the menarche[109–111]. There are 26 in the literature (14 German, 8 Japanese, 2 Polish, 1 American and 1 Norwegian, but none in the French or British Commonwealth literature), plus 4 of my own; of these, 4 are 'confirmed'[101,112] and 8 'probable'[110,112–118]. In 6 the menarche had not been reached at the time of publication; in the rest the subsequent history was often informative with 4 mid-cycle and 8 late luteal onsets.

The first to be reported is unique because, in addition to at least four pre-menarchal episodes, she had a prolonged period of amenorrhoea after the menarche, during which the monthly episodes continued[110]:

> The 15-year old daughter of mentally ill parents began to suffer paroxysms of mania every four weeks with full recovery, including one episode two months before her menarche at 17. This was followed by amenorrhoea, but mania returned every month for six months, diminishing in severity. At 19, during another 9-month phase of amenorrhoea, she had a minor surgical operation on her arm, followed (the next day) by a brief episode of raving that ended with the return of the menses. She remained well during a 3-month follow-up period.

Because of the interest of this phenomenon, four cases will be summarized. Clinical Gem 28.1[101] had 10 episodes, at a mean interval of 25 days and duration of 6 days; some were mild, but the catatonic and manic features in episodes 4 and 10 establish this as a psychotic series. Her menarche concluded the series.

Schönthal[113] described Clinical Gem 28.2. There were eight events at approximately monthly intervals – psychosis, psychosis, menarche, psychosis, psychosis, depression, psychosis and her second menses, with a mean interval of 31 days; after the menarche, episodes had a late luteal trigger.

The next example is of interest because it is a 'confirmed' post-menarchal case; after two years of subclinical monthly episodes (as reported by her parents), she had a late menarche, but continued to suffer nine undated episodes (observed in hospital) clearing up at the beginning or ending of menstrual bleeding[112]:

> At the age of 14, a girl, whose sister suffered from mental illness, began to suffer 'peculiar attacks', when for 2–3 days she became mute, and did exactly what she wanted, impervious to persuasion; these attacks came on more or less every four weeks, or sometimes six weeks, with variable duration. After two years her family got used to them. The duration lengthened to 12 days, and the severity gradually increased to complete food refusal, gross restlessness and violence. At 19 she suffered attacks of *grand mal* epilepsy preceded by an aura, and had her menarche, after which her

Clinical Gem 28.1 Premenarchal Periodic Psychosis Ending at the Menarche

Under the name *primordiale menstruelle Psychose (die menstruale Entwicklungspsychose)*, Friedmann's[101] second case was a 15-year old, whose father suffered from mental illness. She was small and anaemic, and seemed young for her age. She was under strain while working in a sewing factory, and was tired and weepy for a fortnight, then suffered the series of 10 episodes summarized in Table 28.1:

Table 28.1 Friedmann's second case

Episode onset	Clinical details
1 (January 11)	She suddenly took to her bed, without any signs of fever or somatic disease. The next day she was anxious, weepy, staring and mute. On 23rd (after 12 days) she recovered, with partial loss of memory for the episode – she thought she had been ill for only four days, and remembered thinking she was going to die. She was left with a feeling of fatigue and pain in the limbs.
2 (January 28)	Her sleep was disturbed and she became inactive. On 31st, she was crouching fearfully in a wardrobe, sobbing, unresponsive and refusing food. She recovered on February 9th with a patchy memory of the episode, and a great need to sleep.
3 (February 19)	She spent a restless night staring at the ceiling, and said, "They are coming from up there". She spent the day muttering, and refused food. At night she was restless and wet her bed. On March 1st she recovered.
4 (March 14)	She relapsed with catatonic rigidity, lasting 10 days.
5 (April 6)	She relapsed, and recovered after 9–10 days.
6 (April 27)	She relapsed for eight days – the mildest episode yet.
7 (May 27)	She had an even milder episode lasting 5–6 days.
8 (June 27)	She had a very light episode, the only signs being disgruntlement and weariness. It lasted 3–4 days.
9 (At the end of July)	She had her 9th episode, which was like the last.
10 (August 23)	This time she was hypomanic – talkative, aggressive and running around. She rushed out and stole some worthless pencils and nails. She recovered after five days, and, questioned about her thefts, knew nothing about them.

On 24 September, 32 days after the last episode, she menstruated for the first time, and remained well.

Clinical Gem 28.2 Premenarchal Periodic Psychosis Continuing after the Menarche

In a long paper on early onset psychoses[113], the 7th illustrative case was a 15-year old, who suffered from 'chlorosis' (anaemia) during the previous six months. She was a cheerful, good-humoured girl. On June 24th she complained of headache and insomnia, refused to eat and started to shout, sing, pray and rush about the neighbourhood. Admitted to hospital she was anxious and bewildered, restless, incoherent and disorientated. She spoke little, wept, laughed and appeared to be listening to voices. She started hammering on the doors and windows, and had to be isolated. She began to improve on July 3rd and recovered by the 8th (15 days after the onset). On August 21st she relapsed and was admitted to hospital. This attack resembled the last, except that anxiety and confusion were greater; she was sleepless and restless, sighed, groaned and made defensive gestures, ate little and lost 6lb in weight. She recovered on September 2nd (after 13 days), and remembered seeing shapes and hearing voices. From September 20th - 25th she had her first menstrual period, and remained well. On October 21st she relapsed – weeping, anxious, eating nothing, restless, jumping and dancing, speaking rapidly and excessively, singing, praying, smearing and hitting out; she had to be isolated. She recovered on the 27th (after six days); it seemed like a dream. On November 25th, after a bad night in which she talked in her sleep, she became anxious and monosyllabic, and the next day was singing, dancing, crying, laughing and praying, and again had to be isolated; she recovered on the 29th (after four days); she said she had heard voices cursing and threatening her. On December 18th she suffered from headache and vomiting, and complained of depression and homesickness, but recovered on the 21st. On January 22nd in the next year she relapsed – unresponsive, sleepless, restless, singing and declaiming. She had rapid mood changes - cheerful and anxious, weeping and laughing. She recovered on February 2nd (after 10 days), with a patchy memory of the episode. From February 20th - 25th she had her 2nd menstrual period, and remained well, with regular menstruation, thereafter.

menses appeared regularly and lasted 3–7 days. The attacks then changed to premenstrual depression with mutism, stupor, explosions of anger, shouting, cursing and hitting out, and ideas of surveillance and poisoning. The onset was sudden and all symptoms cleared up at the end of menstrual bleeding, so that she was often admitted to hospital, only to be sent home again. At 20 she was hospitalized nine times (case 7).

The next example was reported to me by email in 2014 by an American obstetrician and gynaecologist, who described 25 monthly episodes of confusion and disorientation in her daughter, who suffers from learning disability. They began at the age of seven, with abrupt onset, 10–12 days course and full recovery. This is the earliest onset of a pre-menarchal menstrual psychosis, and recalls the early pre-menarchal onset of menstrual epilepsy[49] and menstrual hyperglycaemia[34]. The mid-cycle timing is based on the *mother's* menstrual cycle. Menstrual migraine psychosis is an alternative diagnosis.

> Her daughter was delayed in motor, speech and cognitive development, but is friendly, happy and enthusiastic. She suffers from food allergies and migraine. In September 2012 (aged seven) she began to have monthly 'spells', lasting 10–12 days. She became agitated, irritable and aggressive (throwing things, hitting out, spitting at her mother and smearing faeces). Her teacher noticed that these started every month on a Saturday, with exactly 12 days illness and 16 days normality; onset and recovery were sudden. In February 2013 the episode was worse, with mutism and refusal of food and drink. In July she had a second severe episode after eye surgery: she was screaming, thrashing around and banging into things, and required four men to control her. She was apparently disorientated and appeared not to recognize her mother. A full neurological investigation, including CSF, 48-hour EEG and MRI scan, was negative; the only laboratory finding was an antibody to immunoglobulin G. On day 10 she abruptly awoke and asked why she was in hospital. Further episodes occurred in August, October, November, December and January (2014), always on a Saturday. During one episode she had a stabbing pain on the left side of her head, and photophobia; with a possible diagnosis of cluster headache, she was treated with oxygen and other agents. In 2014, lamotrigine, verapamil and two forms of triptan were prescribed. From March there was a change: episodes came every 21 days, lasting 10–12 days with only 10–11 days normality. Her mother gave birth to a second child and, coincident with the first postpartum menses, a relapse occurred at the time of her mother's ovulation, with recovery 3–4 days after menstrual bleeding. The possibility of a menstrual neuropsychiatric disorder was considered and, in September, treatment started with Luprorelin depot injections. There was a dramatic improvement, although she still had mild episodes.

Premenarchal episodes might seem incredible, but are supported by the same phenomenon in four medical disorders - diabetes, epilepsy, hypersomnia and migraine psychosis, as described in Chapter 25. As for frequency, Takagi[116] collected five cases in teenage girls and one in a boy, one with good evidence.

Episodes at the Menarche

There are a number of nineteenth century works devoted to mental illness during 'puberty'. This is a life stage lasting years and the word should not be used to denote the first menstrual bleed. Most of this literature deals with disorders found in teenage girls – that is, adolescent psychiatry; for example, a thesis with the promising title *De la folie à l'époque de la puberté* presents four cases that have nothing to do with puberty or menstruation[119] and the same is true of Marro's[120] massive review.[a]

---

[a] I thank Chiara Bombardieri of the Biblioteca Scientifica C Livi for sending me this series of articles.

There are five reports of single brief episodes at the menarche[91,101,116,121,122], as in this example[122]:

> On July 3rd, a 16-year old complained of headache and buzzing in her head. She would eat nothing, and began to pray, sing and speak wonderful things. On the 9th, admitted to hospital, she was restless, perplexed and gave a dreamy impression. She followed the nurses and doctors around like a little dog. On the 12th her menses appeared for the first time. She remained anxious and weepy for three more days. On the 16th at the end of menstrual bleeding she recovered.

These cases hint at a causal link, but sporadic psychosis cannot be excluded. Two, however, were followed for many years[123,124]:

> In 1882 a 17-year old suddenly became disturbed; she was declaiming and frightfully worked up. On the following day she had her menarche and immediately returned to normal. She qualified as a schoolteacher and had no major episodes until 1910 when, aged 36, during a spell of amenorrhoea, she became manic for 3–4 weeks, followed by a paranoid phase. Three months later she threw herself out of a window (case 9).

> A 13-year old had her menarche and was hospitalized with a mild manic episode for 2 months. At 16 she had a second 2-month manic episode. She remained well for 23 years when, at 39, she developed an episode of agitation, logorrhoea and euphoria. She had a recent enlargement of the thyroid, with delayed and scanty menses.

The lack of recurrences in the course of 15–20 years strengthens the case for the menarche as a trigger. In addition, there are 11 cases in the literature, and one in my series, in which episodes at the menarche have started a periodic psychosis linked to the menses; two had numerous episodes. In the first example the evidence is from the statements of the patient, her relatives and a psychiatrist, without dates, but there were 13 episodes[125]:

> A 16-year old was admitted to Charenton Hospital with violent *délire*. She gave a history of similar brief episodes, of which the first had occurred two years earlier at the end of her first menses. This was followed by five monthly recurrences, starting 2–3 days before the menses and ending when bleeding stopped. In the following year she had four more premenstrual episodes. In the next year the attacks returned and, in hospital, three more episodes were observed, with onset 1–3 days before the menses and recovery at the end of bleeding (case 9).

This Ukrainian woman had 15 late luteal episodes[126]:

> A professor's daughter, aged 14, on the day of her menarche, suddenly became anxious for no reason, wept and sobbed and could not calm herself even by prayer. The most dreadful were her thoughts about the Blessed Virgin and her Saviour, that caused such despair that she hit her head against the wall, tried to throttle herself and jump out of the window [sufficient evidence of a religious delusion]. This lasted three days coincident with menstrual flux. She had another menses and an identical episode 28 days later, lasting four days. In the course of one and a half years she had 15 similar episodes. After a lapse of two years, the episodes returned, again at the menses, and she was still under treatment five years later.

Another account was presented in 25 pages with much detail on medical findings (blood pressure, proteinuria and red cell counts)[103]:

> Towards the end of her 14th year, a girl, whose brother developed *dementia praecox* at 16, became absent-minded, forgetful, contrary and irritable, and had to be removed from school. Three days before her menarche, she became disturbed, with flushing, headache and vomiting

that cleared up with the onset of bleeding. Three days before her second menses, she became manic, with insomnia, euphoria, practical jokes, laughing, shouting, dancing, disrobing, rushing about and confused speech. The same happened at the next menses. In 2½ years she had 19 episodes and only 19 menses, with a mean cycle length of 43 days, usually of mania, but also psychotic depression (slow, monosyllabic answers, mutism, stupor and ideas of poisoning), or atypical features (a dreamy state, with echolalia or stereotypies); she also had staccato, tic-like ('myoclonic') movements, a seizure, oedema of the face, hypertension and albuminuria, similar to pre-eclamptic toxaemia. Thirteen of these attacks were premenstrual, four during a 4-month amenorrhoea, at intervals of 23, 30, 41 and 50 days and two as part of a more continuous illness.

All cases starting with the menarche had late luteal timing, except for the following, which began at ovulation before the menarche[112]:

A 16-year old had not yet menstruated. On October 11th she suddenly became manic. From 25th–27th she had her menarche. On November 6th (10 days after the end of her 1st menses), she relapsed, and recovered with her 2nd menses (November 23rd–26th). On December 17th (21 days after the end of menstrual bleeding) she suddenly relapsed. After her next menses (27th–31st), she remained well (case 2).

Monthly Psychosis during Amenorrhoea

In 1848 these two cases were briefly mentioned[127,128]:

An article on the indications for bleeding mentioned a girl whose menses stopped two years after her menarche. Soon afterwards she had an attack of mania lasting 3–4 days, coinciding with her previous menses. Every month, at the same time, the *délire* returned. It disappeared after the application of leeches to her thighs. In the intervals her reason was almost perfect.

A 45-year old woman, who had never menstruated, suffered a circamensual psychosis lasting several days, and remained perfectly calm in the interim.

These are the first hint that monthly periodic psychoses can develop without menstrual bleeding. This Russian woman had eight episodes at a mean interval of 32 days (range 24–36 days)[129]:

An article from St Petersburg described a 17-year old, whose menarche was at the age of 13. Her menses stopped when she had a streptococcal sore throat with a fever of 40°. On April 27th she suddenly became restless, shouted and in a panic tried to run out of the house; within an hour she switched to stupor and mutism. This lasted until May 15th (18 days); in retrospect she described terrifying auditory hallucinations. Seven days later she suddenly screamed and was hyperactive for an hour, then switched to mutism and immobility. This lasted until June 16th (25 days). On the 24th she relapsed, but the end of this episode is unknown because her father discharged her from hospital on July 5th; she did, however, recover. On July 18th she suddenly relapsed, with shouts and attempts to flee; within an hour she was immobile, as if dead, and manifested waxy flexibility. She recovered on August 2nd (15 days). Identical attacks occurred from August 15th–28th (14 days), September 16th–October 4th (19 days), October 20th–November 6th (17 days) and November 26th–December 24th (28 days). She then remained well, but did not menstruate until April 6th in the next year.

In addition to these cases, in which the psychosis appeared only during amenorrhoea, 13 patients had at least three amenorrhoeic episodes during the course of a periodic psychosis with menstrual timing; 5 were 'probable' or 'confirmed cases'[91,98,130–134], as in this example[130]:

> An article entitled *Menstruation und Psyche* described, at a length of ten pages, a young woman whose menarche was at the age of 13. At 16 she began a series of 17 brief psychotic episodes, which were remarkable for the variety of clinical presentations (see page 334). Only five episodes were dated – all starting during a four day period around the onset of bleeding, plus a general statement that most episodes started 1–3 days before or after menstrual bleeding. There were 3-month and 6-month circamensual sequences – May–June–July 1920 and May–June–July–August–October 1921. Five attacks occurred during amenorrhoea, and these were the most severe.

The next patient[132] had eight episodes with intervals of 30, 30, 27, 35, 26, 28, 27 (mean 29) days. Two paramenstrual episodes were linked to the menses; the other six occurred during amenorrhoea:

> An article entitled *État maniaque périodique remplaçant les règles* described an 18-year old, who was always a little excited before her menses. On September 22nd, at the onset of bleeding that lasted only one day, she became excited and agitated, shouting and singing. She was sleepless and febrile (40°), her speech sordid and incoherent, and she required a strait-jacket. She recovered after 20 days. On October 22nd, on the day her menses were expected, she relapsed, and this episode lasted until November 4th (13 days). On November 21st, she suddenly relapsed, and recovered on the 30th (nine days). On December 19th she had a new period of agitation, lasting until the 31st (12 days). On January 23rd in the following year, she became manic until February 3rd (11 days). On 17th she began treatment with diencephalic radiotherapy. On February 18th agitation returned until March 1st (11 days). Progesterone treatment was started. On March 18th the next episode started but only lasted until the 24th (six days). On the 21st her menses reappeared, for only two days. On April 14th, she had a further attack without menstruation, lasting six days. She received another course of diencephalic radiotherapy. Normal menstruation reappeared in May and June, and she remained well.

In this example[133], there were 14 episodes, of which 8 occurred during amenorrhoea:

> The 20-year old daughter of a colleague, whose father and sister suffered from prolonged paranoia and depression, had her menarche at the age of 14, but, while working on an anti-aircraft battery in Vienna, became amenorrhoeic. After the war she started medical training in Graz, but developed melancholia and tried to hang herself. Thirty ECT had no effect. In June her menses ceased for ten months, and repeated hormonal interventions succeeded only once in provoking their return. During this period of amenorrhoea, her illness took on a regular, periodic quality, with a sudden change from confusion, restlessness and inaccessibility to complete and full recovery, allowing vacations at home. A chart showed the circa-mensual timing of episodes with onsets August 13th, September 6th, October 4th, October 27th, November 17th (premenstrual), December 9th, January 22nd 1948 (a doubled interval), February 12th, March 7th, March 30th (premenstrual from now on), April 22nd, May 17th, June 15th and July 14th. All six episodes that occurred during regular menstruation cleared up during menstrual flow. In July 1947, she dramatically improved (in spite of an acute allergic reaction) after an injection of a pint of blood from a woman in the 5th month of pregnancy.

Finally there are two patients whose pituitary was irradiated. One[135], who had 19 episodes after childbirth, is summarized on page 323. The other[136] (Clinical Gem 28.3 on the next page) is a unique case of a young woman, whose pituitary gland was destroyed first by a tumour and then by irradiation; she suffered six episodes of depression with persecutory delusions, at intervals of 39, 22, 31, 30 & 25 (mean 29) days.

Clinical Gem 28.3   Periodic Psychosis without a Pituitary

In his book entitled *Periodic Psychosis of Adolescence*[113], Yamashita's third case was a girl born in October 1966. At the age of seven she developed diabetes insipidus, and was found to have a large pinealoma, which was treated by irradiation. At nine she received growth hormone replacement. In 1983 (aged 16) her menses had not begun, so she was treated with oestrogen and progesterone, but stopped taking them in March 1986 (aged 19) because of headaches and insomnia during menstrual bleeding. She then became amenorrhoeic. On March 25th (one month after stopping the ovarian steroids) she became inactive and sleepless; she started talking ill of her family members (never before), and said there was a demon with a blood-red body and glittering eyes behind the door. When seen at the hospital on the 31st, she was expressionless and gave fragmentary answers. She slept well that night and had fully recovered by April 2nd (after eight days). On May 3rd she was again unable to sleep. She gave low monosyllabic answers after a long pause. When admitted on the 8th, she remained silent and showed no emotion. She thought orange juice was poisoned, and tried to drink out of the toilet; she was afraid of everyday sounds like the radio or windows being shut. She recovered by the 15th (12 days), and remembered feeling confused and thinking that staff were going to kill her. On the 25th she suddenly relapsed. She refused to see her family, eat or take medicine. She said her parents had been cremated, and a nurse had killed her mother, and poisoned the thermometer and her coffee; staff controlled the television programs, and a firework was a sign that the murder had been executed. She recovered on June 7th (13 days). On 25th she began to weep. Her face was flushed. She ceased eating or taking medicine. She recovered by July 12th (17 days). On 25th she became strangely rigid; her face was flushed. She could not sleep and said she had no parents. This episode was milder and she recovered on August 6th (12 days). On August 19th she ceased to smile, and was unable to speak to her parents. Her movements became slow, her face flushed. She asked, "Am I going to be cooked?" She had almost recovered by 30th (11 days). She was treated with carbamazepine, and remained well.[b]

---

[b] I thank Itaru Yamashita for sending me a copy of the English translation of his monograph.

The Menopause

With hardly any long-term observations, there is a dearth of information on the effect of the cessation of the menses. Only three 'probable or confirmed cases' had onset in the forties, none related to the menopause. Berthier[137] described recovery after the menopause:

> Gournay was admitted in 1847 with *délire* in the form of agitation followed by stupor, which occurred every month and lasted during the menses. The rest of the month she was calm and reasonable. In 1859 her menses became irregular, but each time they appeared she had an episode. In 1860 they appeared after 6 month's amenorrhoea and again she was psychotic throughout the bleeding. Then, at the age of 49, she passed the menopause and remained lucid, hard-working, sleeping and eating well and complaining only of mild headaches (case 210).

Another woman's periodic illness continued after the menopause[91]:

> Miss Labutta, who presented at the age of 32, had four dated menstrual episodes, plus a general statement about others which were not dated. With the menopause she continued to have mild 4–5 day episodes (*recidiverende Fälle* case 13).

There is no doubt that this disorder can survive an artificial menopause, because of the failure of oöphorectomy to arrest it[104,105,135,138]. One in my series experienced a worsening after the menopause:

> She suffered from a bipolar disorder with five episodes, of which one was a brief postpartum episode (onset day 4) and another was prepartum; this was followed by a late postpartum recurrence and then two years of regular bipolar mood changes with two weeks in each phase (diagnosed as 'rapid cycling'). At the age of 50, after her menopause, she started experiencing 'ups' (getting on top, more energetic, catching up on housework and correspondence, being more sociable, going to the theatre and sending toys to Byelorussia) and 'downs' (lack of energy, whiling away the day not doing much, watching the television, not sleeping well and overeating). This continued for years. During one relatively severe episode, she was admitted to hospital, where it was noted that every month she had a 2-week 'high' and a 2-week 'low'. After her menopause the 2-week switching worsened. She said, "Before the menopause my mood swings were not a problem".

Episodes can also start after the menopause[137,139]:

> A former patient, some years later, was brought back by her husband who could not contain her; she sowed disorder wherever she went, often with violence. At 50 she had her menopause, and her *délire* became periodic: every month for 4–5 days, at a time corresponding to her menses, she developed incoherent mania (case 211).

> Mrs F, aged 56, had her menopause three years earlier. She was talkative, incoherent and sometimes delirious or stuporose. It was noted that she had spells of confusion at regular intervals every three weeks, when she would be acutely confused for a week, then recover. She had previously had her menses every 21 days. She was cured by injections of ovarian extract.

Monthly Psychoses in Men

The first indication that men may also suffer from periodic monthly episodes of mental disorder was published in 1822: Gall[140] mentioned a man who, once a month for two to three days, was tormented by the impulse to commit a murder. There are 12 relevant cases (in the German, Dutch, American and Japanese literature), all but two of whom were teenagers. Two had a sequence of five episodes[141,142], including one whose monthly pattern depended on his mother's account; she described an almost exact regularity every 4 weeks, like a girl's monthly period. Three had seven episodes[143–145]:

> An 18-year old man developed delusions of persecution – he was neglected by his mother and laughed at by his work-mates; the police were after him, and his food was poisoned. He was confused, hallucinated and had flight of ideas. He improved, then, on July 26th, relapsed. He recovered but had a series of further relapses with onsets September 3rd & 23rd, October 23rd, November 29th and January 4th. The duration of episodes varied between 9 and 17 days. He improved with atropine.

> At the age of 28, a man, whose sister developed a chronic psychosis, had an episode of restlessness, insomnia, excitement, auditory and visual hallucinations, and mutism. After ten years attacks became more frequent, lasting 5–6 weeks. At 45 he suffered a series of seven 'abrupt psychic changes' (lasting 5–10 days) with onsets October 3rd, November 4th, December 7th, January 13th, February 11th, March 5th and April 3rd.

> An immature 16-year old boy, whose dysplastic, dull-minded father reached puberty only at 19, was himself held back at school, and preferred to play with girls. In August 1949 he became depressed and refused food, but recovered in a few days. From August to December this mood change returned every month for a week. He was admitted to hospital, where he had to be fed. He recovered on the 6th day, but relapsed into stupor three weeks later. The same happened a month later. He was treated with testosterone, and had only two two-day episodes in the next year. At 19 he was followed up and found to have matured as a man.

In this case[146] there is no dating, but many episodes were carefully studied.

> A feeble-minded obese 16-year old (more like an 11-year old) presented with sexual delusions and erotic behaviour. There was an alternation between stupor and agitation, with a few days of calm. The mean phase duration was four weeks, with 13–14 phases/year. For eight years, the author studied blood pressure, weight, temperature and blood sugar.

In this man it is difficult to deny the chart evidence of at least 40 monthly attacks[147].

> At the age of 16, a boy who suffered from migraine became strange and irritable. He was sleepless, overactive and destructive, and spoke in a confused way. Admitted to hospital he shouted, whistled and sang, was disorientated in time, had laughing fits, spoke incoherently or not at all. He recovered after several weeks. His future course was complex: a chart showed, in nearly 20 years, a multitude of similar episodes with durations ranging from two weeks to five months, and all sorts of intervals. The phase of interest is the triennium from 35–37, in which attacks came regularly every month and lasted 1–2 weeks. Treatment with thyroid brought them to an end.

As with amenorrhoea, recognition depends on a regular monthly sequence, without the anchor of the menarche or menstrual cycle. This does not appear to be an extremely rare phenomenon. Grahman[145] saw five cases in seven years.

Links between Menstrual Psychoses and the Psychoses of Childbearing

In the absence of other plausible aetiological clues, the link to menstrual psychosis deserves attention. The evidence is from several different sources – pregnancy onset, menstrual relapses after early postpartum episodes, 4–13 week onsets, menstrual cure, and the association of puerperal and menstrual psychoses at different phases of a woman's life.

Onset during Pregnancy (Runge Psychoses)

In 1911, the Kiel nosologist Runge[148], who wrote one of the most comprehensive accounts of *Generationpsychosen*, described this expectant mother who had five episodes of a monthly periodic disorder:

> A 20-year old single woman, whose mother and sister were mentally ill, became pregnant, with her last period at the beginning of March. Four weeks later, as soon as she missed her next period, she became disturbed with restlessness, pressure of speech and destructiveness; this lasted eight days. She relapsed a month later, tore her clothes and ran naked into the street, cycled off in garters and slip, hit out, bit, scratched and smashed windows, sang and spoke incoherently. Admitted to hospital on May 7th, she was disorientated, heard voices and said she had seen the Devil; by the 11th (after four days) she had recovered. On June 6th she relapsed, recovering on the 17th. On July 5th she relapsed, recovering by the 12th. On August 13th she relapsed, recovering on the 21st. She gave birth on November 30th (case 11 on pages 640–641 and 679–681).

Provided that this was a full-term pregnancy, her first episode was in the first month of gestation. Runge's diagnosis was 'hysterical psychosis', but Ewald[149] wrote,

> Runge gave an instructive example of an hysterical-delirious confusional state, which affected a single woman, starting in the first month and returning every four weeks, at a time her menses were expected.

He was the first to recognize this as a variant of menstrual psychoses. A second case was described by Dupouy[150], but with only two episodes:

> In January, a 19-year old single woman became pregnant for the first time. Towards the end of February she developed confusion and agitation, for which she was admitted to hospital: she showed continuous verbigeration and a state of dreamy confusion, lasting 15 days, after which she became lucid and calm. About four weeks later she had a new attack of excitement with agitation, euphoria, logorrhoea, incoherence, punning and joking, disrobing, shouting, singing, food refusal and insomnia. After eight days it cleared up again, and she returned to normal, remaining well for the rest of the pregnancy (case 4).

Twelve other authors have described manic or cycloid episodes, starting in the first month of pregnancy, which may have been single Runge episodes[151–162]. One had two possible

Runge episodes in different pregnancies, and one postpartum episode with relapses[160]. In my series there are six possible cases. One with a single episode was mentioned in the section on post-abortion psychosis (see pages 188–189). Another had a similar experience: she was "extremely high, on cloud 9 and talking loads" and was bleeding heavily when five to six weeks pregnant, so this was either a post-abortion psychosis or a Runge psychosis, depending on which occurred first – miscarriage or psychosis. Another was hospitalized with mania, and then had a two-month termination of pregnancy. Another became manic soon after conception and had three relapses during that pregnancy. Another had her first manic episode six weeks after conception, and continued to suffer brief episodes from then on, during two pregnancies and two postpartum periods. The sixth patient, with four or five episodes, follows (see Clinical Gem 29.1 on the next page).

The Runge psychosis is an example of a menstrual psychosis occurring during abnormal menstruation. Menstruation-like bleeding during pregnancy occurs when the gonadorelin neuronal complex resists heavy inhibition by chorionic gonadotropic hormones. There is no doubt that this can happen, because Lehsau[163], in his Münster *Inaugural-Dissertation*, collected 45 cases. Goecke[164] reviewed six German papers, with a total of 60,000 births and estimated the frequency as 1 per cent of pregnancies; 11/64 cases had six or more bleeds, nine of which were no less copious than normal menstruation. Outside the German literature it is seldom mentioned, but an American paper reported that 8/221 expectant mothers reported bleeding at the time the first post-conception menses was due; one bled for five consecutive days[165], and a Japanese author reported a mother who bled regularly every month during two pregnancies[166]. It is not known why menstruation-like bleeding occurs during pregnancy.

Confirmation that Runge psychoses are menstrual requires the simultaneous onset of psychosis and menstrual bleeding during pregnancy. This has not yet been observed.

Menstrual Relapses after an Early Puerperal Episode

It was noticed in the early nineteenth century that mothers who suffered puerperal psychosis, with onset during the first three weeks, worsened at the time of the menstrual periods[167]. This is Prichard's[168] observation:

> After the birth of the last child, a 40-year old mother, who had borne several children, developed an unusual degree of mental excitement. She talked in a loud voice, and in a more vehement manner than was natural to her. She was highly excited by every trifling circumstance, and even by imaginary causes. She was with difficulty restrained without absolute coercion. Her sleep was disturbed, and she had scarcely any intervals of tranquillity. These symptoms abated as she recovered strength, but recurred in a lesser or greater degree about the periods of the catamenia, at which times she displayed symptoms of mental alienation. She was gradually restored nearly to her usual degree of tranquillity, though still subject to returns of excitement at the periods of the catamenia.

Menstrual exacerbation lacks the sharpness and contrast of a relapse following recovery. In 1876 multiple menstrual relapses were described[169]:

> A 48-year old widow was admitted ten times to an asylum. The third admission followed 15 days after childbirth. She was in an excited state – loquacious with ideas of persecution and hypochondriasis; voices insulted her using dirty words. She shouted out prayers, had a mission to fulfil and would inaugurate an Israelite temple. She spent three months in the Salpêtrière; three

Clinical Gem 29.1 Puerperal, Menstrual and Runge Psychoses

This mother suffered a large number of brief manic or cycloid episodes, with acute onset and full recovery. In most, manic symptoms predominated: her mood was ecstatic, frightened or agitated. She was excited, hyperactive and distractible, requiring little sleep. Her speech was noisy and pressured; she was punning and jumping from topic to topic. At times she 'spoke in tongues' with neologisms and echolalia. She wrote confused poems, and kept a diary full of pseudoscientific jottings. Normally reserved, she became overfamiliar and disinhibited. She had religious delusions (that she was in Hell, was the Devil, must convert the world before the 2nd coming) and other themes (she had terminal leukaemia, had been carrying triplets and had an abortion forced on her).

The first two episodes, at the age of 16, had cycloid features. While at a Christian retreat, she believed a woman had put a curse on her. The world had come to an end, and Jesus had come to take away the believers, but left her behind. Her fear was so terrible that her father (an angel or a ghost) had to stay up with her all night; she was about to give birth to a dog. When her mother washed her hair, she was terrified that she was trying to drown her; and a family picnic was a pretext for sacrificing her. Colours were too bright, noises and voices distorted, and there were odd smells around. Seen by a psychiatrist, she was in a semi-stupor, preoccupied and perplexed. After a 9-day illness she recovered but relapsed a month later. She remembered these episodes as a time of fear and confusion. Both episodes began 2–3 days before her menses.

At the age of 24, during her 1st pregnancy, she menstruated once. She was delivered by emergency Caesarean section, and breast-fed for six weeks. On day 6 she suddenly became manic. She recovered quickly, but relapsed six times – 44 days, 82 days, 115 days, 137 days, 163 days and 198 days after the birth. There was statistical confirmation that these were premenstrual episodes.

The Runge psychosis developed during her 2nd pregnancy. She and her husband were in New Zealand when she conceived about December 21st. At the end of the year she flew home, a 36-hour flight. She was already high on arrival. Admitted to hospital on January 3rd, she was excited and confused, overactive, sleepless and elated. Her mind was being directed by a massive computer, and her actions affected everyone. She was preoccupied with the periodic table; all atoms had to have a fixed pattern otherwise the ceiling beams would collapse. The pregnancy was confirmed and treatment withheld, but within three days she improved. On the 28th she relapsed, higher than ever; her condition deteriorated so rapidly that she was sedated with haloperidol; by February 10th she had recovered. On the 22nd she relapsed again, recovering by March 8th. She had two minor relapses on March 24th and April 26th, after which she remained well during the rest of her pregnancy. In August she gave birth to her 2nd child. Two days later she developed puerperal mania, with two relapses.

During an observation period of 41 years after the first episode, she had other brief episodes. It is not certain that any of her episodes were unrelated to the reproductive process.

days after discharge she was readmitted for another nine months. She was always excited at her menses, and all her relapses coincided with their appearance (case 11).

A considerable number of such cases have been published, including 21 with at least three relapses. This has been called 'the menstrual relapse phenomenon'[170], but is better regarded as the onset of a menstrual psychosis after recovery from the puerperal episode. The extreme claim was made by Bailo[171] that 70 per cent had a tendency to premenstrual relapses for some months. It is one thing to make such a claim, another to prove it. There are the following considerations:

- To eliminate coincidential associations a sufficient number of episodes are required.
- Scepticism is so widespread and entrenched that hardly any psychiatrists are alert to the menstrual effect.
- Menstrual bleeding is a banal event, often missed by medical or nursing staff.
- Menstruation in the early puerperium or during the first postpartum year in lactating mothers is often abnormal (see page 287).
- The menstrual process can precipitate psychotic episodes without menstrual bleeding, for example, in girls before the menarche, or during amenorrhoea.

If there are many relapses, one can feel more confident about the connection with menstruation. There are 10 in the literature with more than 5 relapses. Two had 6[172,173], two had 7[174,175] and one had 8[176]. This mother had 12 relapses[93]:

A 24-year old gave birth, and 'just afterwards' became restless, sleepless and excited, with fits of rage. Admitted to hospital, she was overactive and believed she was being photographed and her conversation recorded. She recovered but, 14 days later, relapsed. During the next ten months she fluctuated between excited periods, lasting 10–14 days, and symptom-free intervals. When excited she was playful, heard voices, spoke different languages or dialects and had flight of ideas; sometimes she had catatonic features. At these times she was premenstrual, with swelling of the face and eosinophilia. The vaginal cytology showed hyperoestrogenic stimulation, confirmed by hormonal measurements. She failed to respond to ECT, but improved with androgens. Twelve episodes were timed. The relapses began premenstrually and shifted to the mid-cycle.

This mother had 13 relapses of a psychosis starting during labour[177]:

A 33-year old was mother of six infants. An attack of *manie* started during labour: she failed to recognize her husband or children, believed she was among strangers, broke out into *fureur* and threatened murder and arson; 15 days later she was still extremely agitated, sleepless, hitting out and insulting imaginary beings with incessant vociferation. After five weeks, when her menses reappeared, she deteriorated and had to be restrained in a strait jacket. She had two relapses, coinciding with the menses and lasting 8–10 days. During the next year the periodicity, alternating between calm and agitation, did not fail even once for eleven months; her regular menstrual bleeding was always accompanied by agitation (case 7).

This mother had at least 13 relapses[135]:

A 35-year old gave birth to her 2nd child. On day 3 she became excited and overactive. With ECT, she recovered. Her menses appeared at 23–26 day intervals. During the next 10 months she was tense, fearful and sleepless before and during each menstrual period. She was treated with oestradiol, corpus luteum and pituitary irradiation. Eleven months after the birth, she was readmitted mute and bewildered; she sank into stupor and required tube-feeding. After a brief illness she recovered with ECT. In spite of ovarian and pituitary irradiation, and hysterectomy, she continued to relapse every month for another year, and was admitted to hospital 13 times. She then recovered.

This mother had 33 episodes[100]:

> A 26-year old, whose mother suffered from postpartum depression, father from catatonia and brother from psychosis, developed a depressive psychosis after giving birth to her 1st child. After her 3rd birth she was admitted with depression and delusions with religious, persecutory and sexual themes; she believed God or the Devil would take her to heaven or hell, or arrange for her suicide, and that family members were promiscuous, or sexually abusing her children. She recovered in two weeks, but suffered 33 identical monthly depressions, all starting in the premenstrual phase, lasting 15 days and ending three days after the menses. During her 8th episode she set fire to herself, suffering 20% burns. Treatment that included lithium, oestrogens, progesterone and gonadorelin agonists was ineffective but she responded to bupropion.

There are some data relevant to the frequency of this phenomenon. Herzer[178], in a survey of 221 cases of puerperal psychosis collected at Basel during 25 years, had one mother who, following two separate deliveries, had 'relapses' coincident with the first appearance of the menses, and one who gave birth 10 times and suffered for three years from menstrual episodes. Rees[179], studying 31 patients with 'postpartum schizophrenia', found that 10 had relapses in the premenstrual phase; they occurred with both anovulatory and ovulatory bleeding. The Mie team[108] stated that 5 per cent of puerperal psychoses developed into periodically recurrent psychoses. Its frequency can also be estimated in my series of bipolar/cycloid mothers: only 15 had menstrual relapses, and only one as many as six.

4–13 week Postpartum Onsets

In Section 4 (pages 200–203) evidence was presented that postpartum psychosis can start, not only in the early puerperium, but later, in the 4–13 week, as observed in 399 cases in the literature and 41 mothers in my series. Marcé's intuition linked these late onsets to the resumption of menstruation[180]:

> The first postpartum menses exercises, on the development of puerperal insanity, an influence that Baillarger was the first to notice, and which my observations confirm *beyond doubt* [my italics]: of 44 mothers who developed puerperal psychosis, and who did not lactate, eleven became ill in the 6th week, precisely at the return of the menses. Sometimes the psychosis preceded the menses by 5–6 days, but it usually began at the onset of bleeding or during menstrual flow. I have also seen it break out when the menses were expected, but failed to appear. Mothers, who breast-feed for some months, become ill after weaning, very often at the moment the menses reappear after a long interval.

It is now known that ovulation does not occur before the 36th postpartum day (just over five weeks)[27], so that onset in the 6th week could not have a late luteal trigger; but it could be triggered by ovulation, if pathogenesis were short, or it was associated with anovulatory menstruation.

If Marcé's ideas are correct, these late onset cases should not be termed 'puerperal psychoses' – they are menstrual psychoses.

These 4–13 week onset postpartum episodes can follow a relapsing course, as in this example: with a history of bipolar menstrual mood swings, she had an episode starting at least 12 weeks post partum, with a relapse[181]:

> A farmer's wife, who had her menarche at 17, enjoyed good mental health up until her marriage. Since then, her mood became elevated in the premenstrual phase, rapidly changing to depression with the onset of bleeding. After the birth of her 4th child, these menstrual mood disturbances became psychotic. In spite of breast-feeding, her menses resumed after eight weeks. On the second

day of her second menses she became sleepless and had attacks of extreme fear believing that she was going to die, stamping her feet and praying, then talking for four hours; on the next day she expressed delusions of poisoning. Admitted to hospital she recovered in a few days. She was well for four weeks, but relapsed twelve hours before next menses; this episode lasted throughout menstrual flow and disappeared when it stopped (case 3).

In the literature, 9 per cent had at least one relapse, and 14 mothers more than 2 relapses. Huang[182] reported a patient with 4, Burger[183] with 6 and Delay[131] with 9 relapses. Ewald's patient[104,105], with 54 episodes, had one episode that started a few weeks after giving birth to her ninth child. This mother had 12 episodes[184]:

A 28-year old, whose mother suffered from a mental illness, was a strong-minded woman who helped in her husband's restaurant. After suffering a miscarriage and stillbirth, she gave birth to a second child on October 6th. A chart showed that she menstruated about November 10th, and developed a manic illness about December 1st, eight weeks after the birth. She became overactive and overtalkative, with flight of ideas, emotional lability, insomnia, auditory hallucinations and ideas of persecution. During this illness, about December 10th and January 4th, she had her second and third postpartum menses. She recovered in mid-January, but suffered from 12 relapses, as detailed below. After the first three, the illness changed to depression, but the last relapse switched to mania at the end of menstrual bleeding. Hormonal tests showed low FSH and progesterone levels, indicating anovulatory cycles. Treatment with clomiphene and hCG was started, and the disorder came to an end.

Episode onset	Onset of menses	Form of episode
1 February 5th	February 14th	Mania
2 March 18th	April 3rd	Mania
3 April 25th	May 1st	Mania
4 May 27th	June 4th	Depression
5 July 9th	July 9th	Depression
	August 9th	–
6 September 9th	September 13th	Depression
7 October 15th	October 14th	Depression
8 November 5th	November 9th	Depression
9 December 4th	December 9th	Depression
10 December 28th	January 4th	Depression
11 January 30th	January 30th	Depression
12 February 20th	March 3rd	Bipolar

Translated by Yumi Okumura

In my series, seven mothers, with onset 4–13 weeks after the birth, had a relapse, including one with two and one with three relapses.

Marcé's is a plausible hypothesis, which has survived not because of positive evidence, but because no one has volunteered any other explanation. Since the application of radio-immune assays to gonadotropic hormones (1967–1968), it has been possible to monitor the menstrual process, identify ovulation and detect abnormalities in the luteal phase. It should now be possible to confirm or refute the hypothesis that 4–13 week onsets are related to postpartum menstruation.

Note that the same cause has been suggested for relapses of early onset puerperal psychosis and 4–13 week onsets. The difference is that a 4–13 week onset is a menstrual psychosis after a normal puerperium, while relapses are menstrual episodes following an early puerperal episode. In the literature, 4–13 week onsets were more common (399 *versus* 289), but in my series relapses were more common – 74 cases (of which 61 were bipolar/cycloid) *versus* 41 (of which only 20 were bipolar/cycloid), suggesting that births complicated by postpartum psychosis are at higher risk of menstrual sequelae.

Menstrual Relapses after Late Postpartum Episodes

A relapsing pattern has been observed after psychoses that develop later than three months post partum. This mother had four postpartum episodes, with onsets one year, 10 months, 4 months and 29 days after the birth, two of which had four relapses[185]:

> The mother of five children, with the history of a brief psychosis when her youngest was one year old, gave birth to her 6th child. Ten months later, when breast-feeding, she had a recurrence. Admitted to hospital she was perplexed, misidentified people and had numerous hallucinations; after a month she recovered. Two years later she gave birth again. After four months breast-feeding, she had a recurrence and was readmitted, recovered, and relapsed four times. A fifth relapse was in the first month of her next pregnancy. She recovered in five weeks and remained well until the birth. After 29 days she became disturbed, violent and confused. Admitted to hospital, she misidentified the doctor as her brother. She again recovered after a month, but relapsed four times. She had four later episodes, unrelated to childbearing, but with some evidence of a menstrual influence.

This is another example: a mother, with a history of menstrual episodes, developed a psychosis four months after her first birth, while breastfeeding, three days before her first postpartum menses; she had several relapses[186]:

> A merchant's wife had her menarche at 18. Five years later, when menstruating, she became disturbed and confused. Her brother stated that she was regularly disturbed at her menses – restlessness at night, confused, singing, declaiming, breaking any glass she could lay her hands on, or disrobing. At 26 she had a menstrual episode of overactivity and confusion, and a month later her wedding had to be postponed because of an attack of confusion. On the evening of her marriage, she became confused again, and soon had two further episodes, when already pregnant. After the birth of her 1st child, she remained well for four months during the amenorrhoea that accompanied lactation. In the 5th month postpartum she became sleepless, and saw a skeleton, her dead father in heaven, and a wolf trying to bite her; in order to escape (not to attempt suicide), she jumped out of the window and fractured her calcaneum; she believed her son, mother and sister would die, and she was jumping into a grave. After her rescue, she believed she was in heaven; she failed to recognize her husband. She was admitted to the Charité hospital, with a diagnosis of *Tobsucht*. On January 5th (three days after the onset of this episode) her first postpartum menses began; by 12th (nine days later) she had recovered. On the 26th she relapsed, became depressed and mute, then began to rave, scratching and biting the attendants, and tearing her clothes. On February 1st her menses started, lasting a single day, and on 11th (16 days after the onset of the episode) she recovered. She had further relapses starting in late February, April, early and late May and June, and finally recovered in August.

A menstrual relapsing pattern has been noted after a weaning episode: Marcé[94], and independently LeGrand du Saulle[187], published this case, with seven episodes; note that the timing shifted from the mid-cycle to follicular phase:

> A 26-year old gave birth to a daughter. Her husband died of a spinal disease nine months later. She weaned the child at 13 months. After three weeks (August 1855) she had an attack of 'hysteria'. After five weeks her menses reappeared. From that time on, she suffered during the autumn and winter from 'a nervous state close to madness' with ill-temper, incessant lamentations, extreme emotionality and passionate tendencies towards the opposite sex. At the end of January she had another attack of manic excitation – agitation, loquacity, violence and disordered ideas – which cleared up with onset of the next menses (early February). She had a violent relapse on the 11th and her menses appeared on the 24th. On March 11th she had another relapse of extraordinary violence (requiring six people to control her) and her menses appeared on 23rd. On April 28th she had a milder relapse coincident with the menses. In May the menses appeared first (25th) and mania from 29th–31st. In June the menses appeared on 23rd, and she did not relapse until July 2nd. In July her menses appeared on 26th and she remained well.

Menstrual Cure

In the eighteenth century, Jani[188] described this case:

> A 40-year old, with nine children, went into labour with a transverse lie. The infant had to be turned, and died. On day 6 she reflected on her many household irritations, her husband's lack of tenderness and her bereavement. She doubted God's mercy, thought the Devil had come to get her, and shuddered and groaned with fear. Her insanity lasted six months, until her menses returned.

This is recovery from a postpartum psychosis on the return of the menses. There are eight instances of a more dramatic effect[168,189–193]. This Czech patient had menstrual recovery from three episodes[190]:

> At the age of 26, a schoolmaster's wife gave birth to her 1st child. On day 8 she suddenly developed unspeakable wistfulness, anxiety and insomnia, followed the next day by delusions and hallucinations. When her menses reappeared at six weeks, she suddenly recovered. Three years later she gave birth to her second child. On day 10 she developed fever, pain in the right groin, restlessness and anxiety, followed by persistent delusions and visions; she wanted to destroy everything around her. When her first menses appeared at six weeks, she improved and was discharged shortly afterwards. Nine years later she gave birth to her 3rd child. On day 12 she suddenly developed fever, pain in the right groin, thirst and insomnia. The following day she had a higher degree of fever, with abdominal pain and tenderness, together with terror, agitation, crying and wailing. Although the fever soon subsided, the mental disturbance continued: she was like a wild animal, ripping and destroying clothing and blankets. Admitted to hospital, she had delusions and visions, failed to recognize people, feared that she would be strangled and required restraint in a straitjacket. After the first postpartum menses she achieved peace of mind.

Delay[191] conducted a unique investigation. Before radio-immune assay (developed in 1956) made it easy to measure oestrogen and progesterone in the blood, he investigated menstrual function in mothers with postpartum psychosis by serial uterine biopsies. His 20 patients each had 2–4 biopsies/month, a total of 236 biopsies (about 11 per patient). He claimed that, with one exception (case 19), the appearance of authentic menses was contemporaneous with cure. In 6/19 menstrual bleeding was not associated with cure, but these (he claimed) were haemorrhages associated with ovulation.

The claim that the menses are both cause and cure is a paradox. The argument is that psychosis occurs during abnormal menstruation, and ends when normality is restored.

Women Who Suffer Menstrual and Childbearing Episodes in Different Epochs

In the literature there are 18, and in my series 7, mothers with onsets related to childbearing as well as unrelated menstrual episodes. It is convenient to arrange these under the headings of prepartum, early and late postpartum and post-abortion episodes.

Prepartum Psychoses

Six women, four from the literature and two from my series, suffered from episodes during pregnancy and later developed a series of menstrual episodes[106,194–196]. This mother from my series had two prepartum (and also early and late postpartum), and at least seven later menstrual episodes[197]:

> A woman whose father had recurrent depression treated by ECT suffered from premenstrual tension and premenstrual migraine. At the age of 23, in the 3rd trimester of her 1st pregnancy, she developed hypertension and antepartum bleeding. She became labile, irritable, euphoric, sleepless and overtalkative; hypomania was diagnosed, and chlorpromazine prescribed. After the birth she developed lethargy, insomnia and loss of weight, but recovered suddenly after six weeks. At 25, she gave birth to her 2nd child, followed by a similar mild illness that lasted three weeks. At 29, after the birth of her 3rd infant, she was "high" for two weeks, but not definitely abnormal. At 34, after the birth of her 4th infant, she became excited, agitated, confused, aggressive and overtalkative; she recovered in eight weeks. At 35 she became pregnant for the 5th time. She was admitted @ 36 weeks with hypertension. She became agitated, sleepless, overactive and overtalkative. A diagnosis of hypomania was made and she was treated with chlorpromazine. Two months after the birth she was again referred with insomnia and mutism, wandering about in a daze. She believed that she and her husband and children were dead, that she was being poisoned and had many other strange ideas. Treated at home with ECT, she recovered after four premenstrual relapses. In the next six years she developed a series of brief episodes, of which seven were dated and shown to be premenstrual.

Early Postpartum Psychoses

Four women, who suffered menstrual episodes in adolescence, later suffered early puerperal psychoses[198–201]; one from my series, who had two adolescent episodes one month apart, a Runge psychosis and six menstrual relapses has already been summarized (Clinical Gem 29.1 on page 322). None had unequivocal evidence of both menstrual and puerperal disorders. In addition, four mothers, including three from my series, suffered early post-partum psychoses and developed menstrual psychosis later in life[183,197]. This mother had two postpartum and six later menstrual episodes[183]:

> A 26-year old, whose mother suffered from religious paranoia, had a brief mental illness after her first child was born. After her second birth she suddenly became restless, began to shout and expressed suicidal ideas. Hospitalized three weeks postpartum, she was confused, springing out of bed, seizing hold of nurses and other patients, then mute and unreactive. She recovered, but two years later developed a regular 8–10 day illness with headache, confusion, insomnia and visual hallucinations, once with mutism and catalepsy; three episodes were documented and shown to have mid-cycle onset, and there were accounts by herself or her husband of at least three more (case 1).

4–13 Week Onset Postpartum Psychoses

In the literature two girls who suffered menstrual psychosis in adolescence developed late postpartum episodes[198,202]. This mother had two later 4–13 week onset episodes[202]:

> A 14-year old had an attack of mania, then, at the age of 16, melancholy, followed by several months of brief relapses at the time of her menses. She gave birth to two children. Four months after the first she developed mania, improved with ECT, then relapsed. Two months after the second she again developed mania with numerous relapses.

In addition, four mothers (including two of my own), who suffered late postpartum episodes, subsequently developed evidence of menstrual psychosis[203,204]. This is an example from the literature[203]:

> A 23-year old gave birth to her 1st and only child. Two months later she became agitated with delusions of persecution; she was not admitted to hospital, but her husband said she was *aliénée* for 3 months. She then developed a menstrual psychosis that lasted at least seven years: every month at her menses, always in the same way, she became irritable, bizarre, taciturn and, especially at night, clouded, with hallucinations of gun-shots and persecutory delusions – she would be set alight, her parents and husband killed – but only for 2–3 days; afterwards she was absolutely normal in conduct and appearance (case 5).

Post-Abortion Psychosis

Three women, who suffered post-abortion episodes, had menstrual episodes at another time[98,205,206]. One in my menstrual series suffered an episode after a mole pregnancy. The following patient had several post-abortion episodes as well as prepartum, late postpartum and menstrual episodes[206]:

> A 36-year old had her menarche at the age of 14. At 18 she suffered from typhus, complicated by a confusional state and a paranoid disorder that lasted three months. Ten months after the birth of her 1st child, when her menses reappeared, she had a series of transitory attacks of agitation. Nine months after the birth of her 2nd child, when four months pregnant, she had a miscarriage, followed by a maniaco-paranoid disorder. Not wishing to have any more children, she had nine terminations in seven years. Each time the menses reappeared after the curettage, she suffered from agitation, fantastic ideas, and disordered conduct; these episodes were brief, and did not lead to hospital admission. Seven years later, when five months pregnant, she was admitted in a state of intense agitation: she believed she had won enormous sums on the lottery and commanded the world. She rapidly recovered and the pregnancy was terminated. A week later the agitation reappeared, with urticaria, five days before the return of her menses. Two dated episodes occurred in the paramenstrual phase.

The weakness of much of this evidence justifies widespread scepticism, but its strength in some cases and the sheer number of examples indicate that this hypothesis is worth further examination.

The Recognition of Menstrual Effects in Women with Childbearing Psychoses

After I became aware of a possible menstrual link (1982), 38/233 (16 per cent) of my series of childbearing psychoses had menstrual effects. This high figure is underpinned by the higher rates reported by Marcé[207] (6/20) and Martin[177] (4/10). It is curious that this association is seldom mentioned. In an attempt to understand why, I studied the distribution of reports by generation and language group. Before 1900, menstrual effects were reported in 28/440 cases (nearly 7 per cent). After that date (and the death of v. Krafft-Ebing) this proportion fell to 48/1,566 cases (3 per cent). The phenomenon has received some recognition in France, Germany, Italy and the United States (about 4 per cent of cases), but not in the Netherlands (1 per cent). As for the British Commonwealth, it was reported by Scott[208] in Ireland, Tuke[209] and Easterbrook[198] in Scotland, and Dennerstein[173] in Australia, but the only time it has been reported in England was in 1983 *by the patient herself*[193].

A Menstrual Hypothesis

The links with menstruation are not only the most promising, but almost the only lead we have to the nature of the childbearing trigger of bipolar/cycloid disorders. Menstrual and puerperal psychoses have similar clinical features and are both complications of the female reproductive process. But there are few cases in which the association has been firmly established – 11 mothers with at least six premenstrual relapses, 2 with Runge psychoses and 8 with solid evidence of menstrual psychosis at different life stages. These are supplemented by a mass of poorly documented observations, plus hypotheses about 4–13 week onsets and the phasic course. In my series 40 per cent had one or other of these features – 48 had 4–13 week onset, 82 a relapsing course, 5 menstrual exacerbations, 19 menstrual relapses, 3 onset at the first menses, 6 Runge psychoses and 21 some evidence of menstrual psychosis unrelated to childbearing.

This raises the possibility that menstruation is involved in the triggering of *all* bipolar/cycloid disorders related to female reproduction. Childbearing psychoses have onset not only in the early puerperium, but also after abortion (including mole pregnancies), in the first trimester of pregnancy, after second trimester births, 4–13 weeks after the birth, and after weaning. All these events have a common theme – the resumption of the menstrual cycle after a period of inhibition. They all involve a cascade of hormones responsible for menstrual shutdown, but the hormones are different – for example, gonadotropic hormones early in pregnancy (when abortions occur), prolactin in breastfeeding mothers and oestrogens during anovulatory menstruation. Perhaps 'kick-starting' the menstrual process triggers the psychosis.

This unifying hypothesis has the merit of filling a vacuum. But only 2–3 per cent of patients have strong evidence of it and it cannot explain a prepartum trigger, active in mid- and late pregnancy. It seems unlikely that the resumption of menstruation could be the common factor in the whole 'family' of bipolar childbearing psychoses, and it has yet to be established that the connection between puerperal and menstrual psychoses is due to a shared trigger rather than a shared diathesis. Nevertheless, the hypothesis that the resumption of menstruation is *one* of the triggering factors deserves critical enquiry.

30

Investigations

Frequency of Menstrual Psychosis

There are two general statements and nine relevant surveys. Burger[183] stated that, in the last nine years in Bonn, he had five cases among 2,000 female hospital admissions. Krasowska[210] observed 20 Polish women with psychoses linked to the menstrual cycle, giving three examples. The surveys are difficult to compare, and give very different estimates. Four asylum surveys[186,211–213], all from the nineteenth century, give rates of 1–20/1,000 hospital admissions, which are much lower than the rate of puerperal psychosis, which, at that time, accounted for 8 per cent of female admissions. On the other hand, Mall[214] and the Mie team[95,108,215,216] found an astonishingly high proportion of cases.

> A study of 429 schizophrenic, 64 depressed and 46 epileptic women from Marburg (1938–1946), Tübingen (1946–1952) and Landeck (since 1952) demonstrated a relationship to the premenstrual period – 'in the overwhelming majority of cases': 26% of those which presented in the premenstrual period tended to recur with the next cycle[214].

> In a study of 219 women with episodic psychoses (stupor, confusion and oneiroid states), two had onset before the menarche, two at the menarche, five after abortion, one during pregnancy, two during labour, four postpartum, 14 during lactation and 164 related to menstrual cycle (mainly premenstrual)[95,108,215,216].

The Kitakyushu study[117,217] gives the only estimate of the number of adolescents affected:

> A prospective study of brief psychoses in adolescents attending a clinic in 1979–1992 (273 boys and 274 girls) found eleven with at least four episodes – two boys and nine girls; six were associated with the menstrual cycle.

Burckhart's study[218], focussing on bipolar and acute polymorphic psychoses, seems ideal but his criteria were too loose:

> He studied 48 manic depressive patients and 55 with atypical (cycloid or acute polymorphic) psychoses at Frankfurt university clinic in 1937–1939: menstrual onsets were found in 9/70 patients who were currently ill (five with manic depression and four with atypical psychoses), and 15/34 of those currently well, of whom eleven had atypical psychoses.

Enumerating the published cases, it is striking that a large proportion were published by a few clinicians. These authors have contributed 109/326 'possible cases' (one-third) and 46/119 'probable or confirmed cases' (a higher proportion):

Author	A[a]	B	C	Total
My series	18	12	4	34
v. Krafft–Ebing[91,106,219]	16	9	2	27
Takagi[116]	5	2		7
Leone[220]	2	5		7
Mie group[95,108,215,216]	4	3		7
Berthier[137]	4	1		5
Prengowski[221]	4	1		5
Yamashita[136,222]	2	3		5
Hegar[112]	1	2	1	4
Powers[195]	3	1		4
Krasowska[210]	3	1		4
All[11]	62	40	7	109

[a] A = 'possible cases', B = 'probable cases', C = 'confirmed cases'.

The number that have reached me from all sources is greater than 60, compared with 321 puerperal psychoses. An international panel (Action on Menstrual Psychosis), started in 2011, now includes 38 sufferers (or their parents) from six nations – the United Kingdom, United States, Australia, New Zealand, Switzerland and Sweden; this compares with several hundred in Action on Puerperal Psychosis, which was inaugurated in the early 1990s. It is obvious that the sufferers and parents who contact me are from the higher educational ranks – those that use the internet to seek solutions to medical problems.

Taking an overall view of the number of cases and publications, and the large series collected by a few individuals, it seems possible that hospital surveys understate the prevalence of this disorder. Its frequency may be only an order of magnitude less common than 'puerperal psychosis', whose incidence has been accurately measured at about 1/1,000 pregnancies[223,224]. My guess, therefore, is that menstrual psychosis (at the level of hospitalization) affects about 1/10,000 women. One should bear in mind several factors that depress this figure:

- The admission rate, or even the referral rate, may be reduced by the brevity of episodes.
- In so far as menstruation is only one trigger for periodic psychoses, the pattern of monthly attacks will be disturbed by the intrusion of episodes with other precipitants; 'confirmed' cases are relatively pure forms – even amenorrhoeic episodes obscure the pattern. The menstrual process may have a hidden influence on more chaotic illnesses.
- In so far as these disorders are bipolar, depressive episodes may outnumber manic or mixed episodes. The definition employed in this monograph excludes them.
- The prevalence of subclinical cases may be much higher. This is an example:

A 21-year old was referred with a history of several years of episodes that began a few days before the menses and continued for two days after the onset of bleeding. Twenty years later I interviewed her again. She gave a graphic description of a bipolar disorder beginning with depression, anxiety, irritability and somnolence that increased to spending the whole day in bed.

At menstrual onset she switched to a state of intense well-being, required only four hours' sleep, sought out company, and sometimes acted in an embarrassing way or made extravagant and useless purchases. These symptoms waxed and waned in severity, but continued month by month with a regular pattern that hardly ever spared a menstrual cycle. She sought advice, and took progesterone and other hormones, but never required hospitalization. She learned to adjust her life style to a predictable disorder. It did not prevent her from obtaining a consultant medical post.

National Contributions

There are astonishing differences in the numbers of cases ('probable or confirmed') reported by different nations. Top of the list, by a large margin, are cases from Germany and Austria (41, all but 5 of which were published before 1930), followed by Japan (21). The United States has contributed 12, France (where the disorder was first described) 9, the most recent in 1952, and Italy 6 cases. Canada, the Netherlands, Poland and Spain have contributed 2 each, and Australia, Puerto Rico (in Spanish), Russia, Taiwan and the Ukraine one each. Excluding my own, there is only one British case.

Clinical Features

The range of clinical pictures covers the whole spectrum of acute psychoses. Bipolar disorders, however, in all their conventional (and some unconventional) forms predominate. This is the more obvious if cycloid (acute polymorphic psychosis) is added to the bipolar rubric. These two presented with a polymorphic clinical picture[225,226]:

> A patient was anxious and perplexed, and her mood labile. At times she was retarded and mute, saying she "just wanted to die". At other times she was laughing and screaming, and so restless that eating was difficult and sleep erratic. She had auditory hallucinosis and passivity experiences, believed she was suspected of drug addiction, and repeated phrases with no clear reference.

> A patient was restless, irritable, and showed rambling excessive speech. Fear and confusion were mentioned several times. She had hallucinations, both auditory and visual, and referred to imaginary persons who criticized or threatened her.

These two presented with extreme anxiety[91,227]:

> A patient raved with anxiety – gasping, staring with horror, starting at every sound. She believed she, indeed everyone, would die, and described ghostly hallucinations and visions of fire.

> Against a background of melancholic mutism, a patient was agitated, hyperventilating and clinging on to people. She had delusions of damnation, and believed both food and drink were poisoned. She had terrifying hallucinations of devils and animals fighting. She failed to recognize her husband, and believed her visitor wore her husband's clothes but had a different face.

These two presented with catatonia as a salient symptom[228,229]:

> A patient became withdrawn and lapsed into stupor. She was confused and disorientated. Her thought content was bizarre and her speech unintelligible, and she responded to auditory and tactile hallucinations. She showed catalepsy and catatonic posturing, and echoed the examiner's questions.

> A patient believed her psychiatrist and co-workers were plotting against her and heard voices from her car radio. She manifested stereotypic movements including hand-clapping, staring, turning the shower on and off, blinking and lip-smacking.

The association with bipolar disorder raises questions about the frequency of menstrual episodes in bipolar women. There are three relevant studies:

Wehr[230] studied 47 women with 'rapid cycling affective disorder' (defined as four or more episodes per year), many of whom had postpartum episodes. There was no convincing relationship between manic-depressive cycles and the menses: nine began and 14 persisted after the menopause; only five had mood cycles similar in duration to menstrual cycles.

Leibenluft[231] followed 25 rapid-cycling women for three months with daily ratings: five women showed increased hypomania in the postmenstrual phase and six the reverse pattern; eight showed a statistically significant relationship between menstrual cycle and mood.

Shivakumar[232] studied 41 bipolar women for at least three months: eight had higher depression scores and five higher mania scores in the luteal phase.

These results agree that only a small proportion of bipolar women have a menstrual effect.

Nosology

In *Menstrual Psychosis and the Catamenial Process*[1], a diagnostic analysis of 78 'established cases' showed that 15 had mania and depression, either within an episode or in different episodes; 19 recurrent mania; 9 mania paired with other alternative syndromes and 9 hypomania with depression or stupor. Thus 58 (74 per cent) were easily identified as bipolar – a higher proportion than for puerperal psychosis (see pages 173–174). This association is so strong that menstrual psychoses may reveal the true span of the bipolar phenotype. Certain patients, with many episodes, illustrate the range of clinical pictures, as does this patient, who presented with six symptom groups[130]:

- She often had prodromal somatic symptoms – headache, chills, an unpleasant taste in the mouth, buzzing in the ears, aching in the finger tips or intense malaise. Her body felt smaller and her head crooked. She reported visual symptoms like migrainous *aurae* – seeing things with a coloured contour, coloured rings and spots, objects distorted or crooked, the walls and floor lop-sided, and furniture smaller. She came to recognize these prodromata, and sought medical help for the imminent episode.
- The 1st, 2nd, 3rd, 5th, 10th and 15th episodes had a manic picture – euphoria, distractibility, overactivity, dancing on tables, climbing on cupboards, running after doctors, mocking nurses, molesting patients, speaking continuously, singing and declaiming. She ran about in the nude and responded to the doctor with a flood of obscenities.
- The 4th episode was depressive, with guilt over sexual misdemeanours for which she feared her father would take legal action. The 15th episode switched from expansive mania to agitated depression with voices and hallucinations of black shapes.
- Aggression was prominent in the 9th episode – destroying crockery, violent to patients and staff, and cursing her mother, the nurses, all politicians and the English.
- She often expressed odd ideas (suspicions and presentiments rather than delusions) – that there were worms in her hand; that warming the cemetery would bring her grandfather back to life; that the French were invading – the walls crumbling because of explosions, and bullets hitting her; that her brother was locked in the cellar; that her food had been poisoned (so that she refused medicine and had to be force-fed). The 6th and 7th episodes were dominated by such ideas.
- In the 11th and 14th episodes the symptoms were catatonic, with monotonous excitation, stereotypies and mannerisms.

Organic Causes

Organic features such as disorientation and perseveration[92] have been reported. Visual hallucinations are rather common. Amnesia for the episode was mentioned by several patients[91,131,183,233]. Several patients, therefore, may have been suffering from an organic psychosis. Berkley's patient[234] had symptoms suggesting endometriosis, and a cerebral deposit is a possible explanation for her menstrual delirium. Kramer[228] described, under the name 'menstrual epileptoid psychosis', a patient with 'fainting spells' – falling, trances and myoclonic jerks – who was given a diagnosis of temporal lobe epilepsy; her menstrual psychosis responded to treatment with phenytoin. The following is another possible epileptic psychosis[212]:

> A patient with a history of epilepsy began to suffer, at the age of 43, from periodic mania with onset a few days after menstrual onset. She developed seizures at the menses, after which she was dazed and confused, misidentified people, had erotic tendencies and expressed grandiose ideas.

Hyperammonaemic psychosis is a rare and recently described cause of postpartum psychosis[235]. Two papers have reported similar episodes in relation to menstruation. This is one[236]:

> A cheerful lively girl suffered from von Recklinghausen's disease, along with several relatives on her father's side. Since her menarche (at the age of 13), around the time of each menses she had episodes of abdominal pain, anorexia and nausea, and became sleepless, excited and overtalkative. Investigated in hospital, she behaved like a baby, soiled the bed and complained of numbness of the hands and feet. At 18 she developed seizures and lapsed into coma. She was found to have hyperammonaemia, due to carbamoyl phosphate synthetase 1 deficiency, confirmed by liver biopsy. She was treated with haemodialysis and carnitine, which brought down her blood ammonia, but too late to prevent permanent brain damage.[a]

A second patient had liver arginase deficiency[237], and for 18 months lapsed into coma for three days at the onset of the menses, with raised ammonia levels.

Mucha[238] described an acute psychosis with many seizures and double incontinence, coinciding with the menarche – probably an incidental attack of encephalitis.

Stein[239] described a psychosis with marked organic features that recurred at the next menses:

> A 14-year old Yemenite-Egyptian woman developed disorientation, memory loss, abdominal swelling, muscle pain, spasticity, hyperreflexia, myoclonic jerks and loss of consciousness, switching to mania two days before the menses. It recurred two days before the next menses.

The association of organic features with learning disability will be discussed on page 337.

Natural History

Age of Onset

This was known in 113 'probable or confirmed cases'. It was in the first decade (at the age of seven) in one, the second decade in 69 (including 10 before the menarche and 3 at the menarche), in the third decade in 25, the fourth decade in 15 and fifth decade in only 3

---

[a] Translated by Yumi Okumura.

(which included a 44-year old man). Thus more than half presented as teenagers, and there was no evidence of an increase towards the menopause.

Lifetime Course

The evidence is fragmentary. No case description covers the whole reproductive period, starting with puberty, and proceeding through the menarche, pregnancies or abortions to the menopause. In most, the data on the present illness were limited to an observation lasting less than five years. In the literature, only a dozen patients had more than five years' continuous observation[98,104,105,108,136,138,197,206,216,240] or follow-up data 5–13 years after the index episodes[91,106,197,241]. Three from my series were followed beyond the menopause and one continued to suffer episodes. The evidence at present available gives the impression that, for most patients, menstrual psychosis is a brief, self-limiting phase, affecting only a small proportion of the 400 menses in a woman's life.

The Effect of Pregnancy

Pregnancy interrupts the menstrual process, and one would predict a cessation of episodes. Among the 'possible cases' of menstrual psychosis, there are 10 supportive observations, for example[200,201]:

> At the age of 21, a Vietnamese adoptee developed a brief polymorphic psychosis, accompanied by rapid blinking and stereotyped movements. She had five relapses, lasting 3–5 days, followed by brief depression and hypomania. She became pregnant and had the longest period of good health she had enjoyed for years. When the infant was born she suffered a puerperal psychosis.

There is little information from 'probable' or 'confirmed' cases. Of 23 who were parous before the onset of menstrual psychosis, only two had further pregnancies: One of these developed a Runge psychosis. Two mothers, who developed menstrual episodes later in life, had suffered prepartum psychoses. There is at present no instance of an established pattern of periodic episodes interrupted by pregnancy.

Associated Diseases

Occasional patients have suffered from medical disorders known to be affected by menstruation: four (including two from my series) had premenstrual migraine[91,210], and, in addition, one child might have suffered from migraine psychosis. Six (including one from my series) had hypersomnia[95,97,242–244], one of whom was male. Apart from the two patients, mentioned previously, thought to be suffering from epileptic psychosis, nine (including two from my series) had epilepsy or seizures of various kinds[96,112,113,229,245].

Gynaecological Illness

Various gynaecological disorders have been reported:

> Hyperprolactinaemia was noted in nine (including two from my series)[96,97,225,229,246–248]. This could have been secondary to treatment with neuroleptic drugs. One patient responded to treatment with bromocriptine[97].

> Luteal defects were noted in five[96,131,184,247,249].

> Anovulation was noted in 10[93,96,118,134,174,184,216,241,250,251].

In addition, one patient had low oestrogen levels throughout[95], and 4 (including one from my series) with no gynaecological measurements had amenorrhoeic episodes. The extensive Mie university studies[95,108,215,216] showed that anovulatory cycles were suspected in 44/60 cases studied; among their 219 patients with periodic psychoses, 137 had some form of menstrual abnormality, of which 61 had oligomenorrhoea and 25 amenorrhoea for at least three months. This is such a high proportion that it raises the possibility that these abnormalities are universal. Some patients were reported to have normal menstruation[95,197,252], but abnormalities can be intermittent, and sporadic measurements do not prove that menstruation was normal in a cycle affected by psychosis. An American study of two patients, however, suggests a more complex relationship to ovulation and the luteal phase[245]:

> A woman, whose mother suffered from a similar menstrual disorder, developed myoclonic seizures at the age of six, and was found to have carnitine deficiency (an inborn inability to metabolise long chain fatty acids). At her menarche she became aggressive (assaulting her parents), and experienced auditory hallucinations with incoherent speech, disorientation, loss of vocabulary and memory. In hospital she was sexually provocative. Her symptoms developed in the week before menstrual flow, and then remitted. She was found to have luteal peaks of LH and FSH, which were inappropriate in this phase of the cycle; these corresponded to her behavioural disorder. She responded to treatment with progesterone.

> At her menarche an 11-year old, who developed cerebellar ataxia and *grand mal* seizures in infancy, started to suffer a periodic psychosis, with aggression, withdrawal, self-mutilation and hallucinations, that continued for two years. Observation in hospital showed that symptoms occurred several days before her menses, with recovery at the end of menstrual bleeding. She also had raised LH, FSH and oestradiol five days before the menses. She recovered with leuprolide.

Learning Disability

In the literature, 12 patients had learning disability to some degree. It was mild (IQ of 80) in 3[115,226,241] and in one of my series. It was probably severe (though details were scanty) in 6 of v. Krafft–Ebing's cases[91,106] and 4 of others[92,173,204,253]. It was extreme in Grody's[237] case of urea cycle deficiency. One patient had microcephaly[226] and three hydrocephalus[91]. My series includes a surprising number, including these two:

> Her parents described insomnia, overactivity, incoherence and delusions. Her cognitive level was affected: she was unable to perform complex actions and had complete loss of memory for episodes.

> She became agitated, irritable and aggressive (throwing things, hitting out, spitting at her mother and smearing faeces). One episode was worse, with mutism and refusal of food and drink; she was screaming, thrashing around and banging into things, required four men to control her. She was apparently disorientated and appeared not to recognize her mother.

Four other parents and a doctor have contacted me by email; three daughters suffered from early childhood autism and one from Asperger's syndrome. This association seems to occur too frequently to be a chance phenomenon, and to differ from puerperal psychosis. It raises the question of a separate disease entity.

Family History

Twenty patients with 'probable or confirmed' menstrual psychosis had first degree relatives with a history of psychosis, affecting 9 fathers, 8 mothers and 12 siblings. Constant[245] described a patient whose mother suffered from 'perimenstrual schizophreniform psychosis'. Although none of the patients and their relatives had data of good quality, the frequency of family mental illness in these patients suggests that a genetic study would be productive.

Other Investigations

The extensive Japanese endocrinological studies have already been mentioned. The most recent paper from Mie included endocrine challenge tests using TRH, GnRH, the dexamethasone suppression test, insulin tolerance, and growth hormone response to insulin-induced hypoglycaemia, as well as the circadian rhythm of cortisol, studied in up to 23 patients[108].

Few cases have been published since the advent of neuro-imaging. One patient had neuro-imaging scans performed at the Mayo Clinic: the findings were normal.

There have been no necropsies.

Chapter

31

Causes

Menstrual psychosis is the consequence of events in the menstrual cycle, probably at the mid-cycle and onset of the necrotic phase, that interact with the bipolar and acute poly-morphic diatheses, and ignite a psychotic episode. These events could be at the pituitary–ovarian level or the hypothalamus.

At the Pituitary-Ovarian Level

This means that gonadotropins or ovarian steroid hormones themselves, without involving the hypothalmus, trigger episodes at long range through their blood-borne effects on the brain. Since episodes occur during amenorrhoeic cycles and before the menarche, progester-one can be ruled out, except as denominator in the oestrogen/progesterone ratio. Gonado-tropins have a plausible role in mid-cycle onsets; unusual levels of FSH have been noted before the menarche[19] and in the luteal phase of occasional patients[245], but there may be only one precedent for their involvement in the pathogenesis of any psychosis[254]. There are reasons, however, for implicating oestrogens, either through excess or through their rapid fall, since much research indicates their importance in schizophrenia[255], and they have occasionally appeared to precipitate a psychosis[256]. Abnormal oestrogen levels occur in anovulatory cycles. Their role is plausible in the late luteal phase, but less so in mid-cycle, premenarchal or amenorrhoeic onsets; before the menarche, oestrogen effects are seen in breast development, but the pituitary–ovarian axis is at the cadet stage and levels are relatively low. They will be much reduced in hypothalamic amenorrhoea. Unless monthly cycling originates in a 'clock' in the suprachiasmatic nucleus or in the intrinsic activity of GnRH neurons, it must depend on feed-back control, in which oestrogens have a major role. This, and the therapeutic efficacy of clomiphene (an anti-oestrogen, which acts on all oestrogen receptors including the hypothalamus) supports the involvement of oestrogens.

At the Hypothalamic Level

This means that neurochemical events linked to the GnRH neurons directly disturb a system involved in the bipolar/cycloid diathesis. This hypothesis is attractive for several reasons:

- It would explain the gynaecological disorders often found in these patients
- It is compatible with the occurrence of menstrual or monthly periodic psychosis:
  - Before the menarche (with arrest at the menarche)
  - At the menarche
  - During amenorrhoea
  - In early pregnancy

- After childbirth
- After ovarian irradiation or surgical castration[138,105]
- In patients whose pituitary has been destroyed[135,136]
- In men

Although the role of oestrogens is not ruled out, these are reasons for shifting the focus of aetiological enquiry from circulating oestrogens to the gonadorelin neuronal network, or the arcuate nucleus, in the hypothalamus.

Management

32

Clinical Investigation

From 150 years of observation, clear principles for the clinical study of these patients have emerged. First, one can dispose of two procedures widely used in clinical research:

- Semi-structured interviews exploring the gamut of psychotic symptoms. These require special training and take an hour or more to complete; although at some stage informal and unstructured evidence requires professional endorsement (to clarify words like 'delusion', 'hallucination' and 'confusion'), semi-structured interviews are neither necessary nor helpful in this disorder.
- Daily rating scales, such as the Moos Menstrual Distress Questionnaire[257]. These, conducted for two consecutive months, are mandatory for the diagnosis of premenstrual tension, but are inappropriate for menstrual psychosis. They do not cover psychotic symptoms, and two months is insufficient to establish the diagnosis; moreover, psychotic episodes do not usually appear every month.

The rating procedure must be simple enough to be completed by patient, relative or nurse over a long period, and for this a diary is appropriate. Nothing need be recorded during intervals of health, except the onset of menstrual bleeding; to this can be added the timing of ovulation, by measurement of the body temperature. During episodes there should be a brief daily description of the salient symptoms and behaviour changes. The use of narrative, describing behaviour and recording speech (as opposed to ratings and clinical jargon), gives the data a timeless value, which has enabled diagnoses to be made after the lapse of decades or centuries[258]. When matched to menstrual bleeding, this will (after some months) refute or confirm the diagnosis, and allow a measurement of duration and a rough grading of severity, which will be useful in assessing treatment response. It must be admitted that the dating of episode and menstrual onsets is often imprecise, but this error has to be accepted until we have better measures. Establishing the diagnosis in this way is an essential step for both scientific observation and clinical practice. The authors of many publications have not anticipated the scepticism with which their opinions and intuitions have been received, and the failure to provide dates is the reason why so few cases are now available for study, and excellent case studies are based on 'possible cases'[245]. As for clinical practice, it is not justifiable to deploy draconian treatments without a firm diagnostic basis, and it is good practice to delay intervention until a dated baseline has been obtained.

Since abnormal menstruation is frequent, and has a bearing on treatment, it is important to obtain a gynaecological opinion. This should include measurements of serum progesterone in the luteal phase, so that anovulation or luteal defects can be diagnosed.

Treatment and Prevention

There have been no treatment trials, but a recurrent disorder with a time base of a month allows the clinician to put various interventions to the test. Once a diagnosis has been made, and a baseline established, the clinician has a wide choice of therapies, including unconventional treatments that are not only palliative but curative. There are an opportunity and the obligation to find the best intervention for each patient (bespoke treatment). Cross-over trials can be undertaken, using the patient's own baseline as control, preferably with the double-blind discipline. In this way, each individual, and all such patients, will benefit from the increase of knowledge.

This review will focus especially on treatments used in 'probable' and 'confirmed' cases. In 'possible cases', with only three or four episodes, there is too much risk of spurious claims after recovery due to the natural history of the disease. Because of the tendency to spontaneous remission, one can be more confident of treatment failure than success.

The range of therapies include those that are conventional in psychiatric illness (ECT, neuroleptics and mood stabilizers), those acting on the menstrual cycle (sex steroid hormones, agents inhibiting the cycle, irradiation and castration) and unusual therapies used in one or two patients, such as atropine[143], intra-cerebral oxygen injections[174], adrenal steroids[98], verapamil (a calcium channel blocker)[100], bromocriptine[97], buproprion[100], phenytoin[228] and blood transfusion from a pregnant woman[133]. Treatment will be considered under the headings of sedation, ECT, mood stabilizers, sex steroids, suppression of the menstrual cycle and thyroid.

Sedation

In the late nineteenth century, excitement could be calmed by bromides, and v. Krafft–Ebing used them in an attempt to prevent recurrences. Since 1953 neuroleptic agents have been used routinely in manic or polymorphic psychoses as a first line of treatment. They have a tranquillizing role, but there are many examples of their failure to arrest the periodic illness; this includes second generation antipsychotic agents such as olanzapine[259] and quetiapine[260] and depot neuroleptics.

ECT

In the late 1930s, convulsive therapy was introduced. This often appeared to be effective in treating the acute episode, but the natural history of brief episodes is an alternative explanation. It is ineffective in preventing recurrences[93,131,133–135,170,173–176,197,210,220,240,241,250,252,261].

Mood Stabilizers

Lithium and anti-epileptic agents such as carbamazepine and valproate have a prophylactic role in bipolar disorders. But in menstrual psychosis most reports have been negative, although they were claimed to stop the illness in a male patient with three episodes[262]. In eight 'probable or confirmed' cases (including two from my series), lithium failed to prevent further episodes[100,182,225,240,245,263]. As for carbamazepine, there was temporary success in three cases[136,229,244]; others failed to respond[100,182,240]. Valproate has been used in one patient, in whom it was ineffective.

Sex Steroid Hormones

These include oestrogens, progesterone and their combination in oral contraceptives. In the form of crude ovarian extracts they have been available since 1899[233]. A temporary oestrogen effect has been claimed[174,210], but in other cases it had no effect[100,115,135,172,269,270]. Progesterone and related steroids have a rationale in the treatment of luteal defects, and can counterbalance oestrogens in anovulatory cycles. In a review of the treatment of periodic psychoses with premenstrual symptoms, 15/28 responded[215]. Successful treatment or prophylaxis with progesterone has been claimed in 10 patients in the literature and one in my series[172,193,225,245,246,264–268]; in one, there was a recurrence when injections of progesterone were withdrawn[261]. Four were 'probable cases'[225,246,261,266]. Some had a combination with other agents – progesterone and testosterone[210], progesterone and clomiphene[216,251] and progesterone and thyroid[108]. In other cases (including two from my series), it failed[95,96,100,131,135,174]. Oral contraceptive agents were effective in several 'probable cases'[182,220,237,271] but failed in others (including one from my series)[98,173,229,259,270]. Androgens appeared to be effective in 3 'probable cases': in one a testosterone implant coincided with the end of illness[174], and in another androgens plus ammonium chloride and salt restriction seemed to end the series[93]. They were effective in an immature male patient[145].

Arresting the Menstrual Cycle

From 1890 American surgeons began to use oöphorectomy to treat mental illness, and, from 1896, irradiation of the ovaries, pituitary or diencephalon became possible. Desperate clinicians resorted to these draconian treatments[104,105,272] but without effect, as confirmed in one woman in my series, whose womb and ovaries were removed. Pituitary gland injections have also been tried[130]. Clomiphene was introduced in the late 1950s, Danazol in 1971 and the gonadorelin analogues in 1977. Danazol has been used four times – once with success[173] and thrice without[100,240] including one from my series. Gonadorelin injections resulted in substantial improvement in a pre-menarchal patient, and probably also a Swedish girl, but failed in two others[100,240]; Human chorionic gonadotropin (hCG) failed to arrest the illness in one patient[115]. Cyproterone was effective in suppressing both menstrual cycle and a chaotic illness in one from my series. Aromatase inhibitors have not so far been tried.

The efficacy of clomiphene, which induces ovulation, has been claimed in 10 cases[96,98,184,251,216,249,272,273]; most were 'probable' and two were 'confirmed' cases[98,184]. This is an example[98]:

> Two patients received clomiphene 100 mg/day from the 3rd to the 7th day of the cycle. In the first, clomiphene delayed the attack by seven days and reduced its length to one quarter. In the second, irregular menstruation was replaced by a stable cycle of 33 days, and cyclical psychosis gave way to brief disturbances before ovulation and before the menses.

In three patients clomiphene was supplemented by other drugs. In one, ovulation was induced, but the luteal phase was defective; the patient improved, but was not cured until norethisterone (a progestin) was added[96]. In another, thyroid and medroxyprogesterone were also required[216]. In the third the successful combination was clomiphene plus hCG[184].

Thyroid

Thyroid medication has been available since 1891[274], but for decades no one thought of using it. Gjessing[275], summarizing extensive work on periodic catatonia, prescribed thyroid medication in several male patients with complete recovery, even when the patient had been ill for years or decades. Its effect was demonstrated in a patient who had 33 episodes[135]:

> She received over 90 ECTs, insulin coma treatment, injections of oestrogens, corpus luteum, progesterone and stilboestrol, pituitary and ovarian irradiation, and hysterectomy. All failed to 'disturb the rhythm of the illness'. Finally they drew on Gjessing's experience. Following his regime, they raised the BMR from -18 to +28, causing overactivity and confusion, then allowed it to sink to -10. Initially the episodes continued as before, but eventually the patient recovered while under treatment with thyroid and B vitamins.

Apart from this patient, 14 others have benefited (including two from my series)[95,98,108,115,135,147,215,240]. Almost all had good evidence, including 4 'confirmed cases'[98,108,147]. One patient relapsed when it was withdrawn[115]. But it does not always work[98]. In a review of thyroid treatment in periodic psychosis, 20/38 responded, but it is not known how many had menstrual episodes[215]. The rationale of thyroid medication is unclear – two patients who responded, and relapsed when thyroid was stopped, had no evidence of hypothyroidism[95]. It is interesting that thyroid stimulating hormone is similar in structure to FSH and LH (see page 281).

Summary

At the level of at least five dated episodes, there are, in the literature and my series, 95 'probable' and 24 'confirmed' cases of menstrual psychosis. In the literature, the majority have been reported from Germany, Japan, the United States and France, but most of those in my series were from the United Kingdom.

This disorder is probably distinct from menstrual mood disorder. It may affect about 1/10,000 women, usually with onset in the second decade, often with a brief series of episodes.

In most, the clinical picture is within the bipolar spectrum, but a few have cycloid or catatonic features. A minority have an organic cause, and there may be a variant associated with learning disability.

About one-third have onset in the mid-cycle and two-thirds in the late luteal phase.

There is much evidence of an association with childbearing psychoses. This is from several sources – onset during pregnancy, menstrual relapses after early and late postpartum episodes, 4–13 week onsets, menstrual cure and the occurrence of both psychoses at different epochs of a woman's life.

It is recommended that suspected patients are investigated by prospective diaries, to establish the diagnosis and as a baseline for bespoke therapy. Because of the association with abnormal menstruation, it is important to obtain a gynaecological opinion. In the treatment, there is some evidence for the efficacy of progesterone, clomiphene and thyroid.

Considerable numbers have begun before the menarche, a phenomenon also noticed in diabetes, epilepsy, hypersomnia and migraine psychosis. Others have occurred at the menarche, during phases of amenorrhoea, after the menopause (or oöphorectomy) and in men. These circumstances suggest the direct involvement of hypothalamic nuclei in the triggering of bipolar/cycloid and other psychoses.

References

1   Brockington IF. *Menstrual Psychosis and the Catamenial process.* Bredenbury: Eyry; 2008.

2   Plant TM. Neuroendocrine control of the onset of puberty. *Frontiers in Neuroendocrinology.* 2015;38:73–88.

3   Gore AC. *GnRH: The Master Molecule of Reproduction.* Norwell: Kluwer; 2002.

4   Prevot V, Hanchate NK, Bellefontaine N, Sharif A, Parkash J, Estrella C, et al. Function-related structural plasticity of the GnRH system: a role for neuronal-glial-endothelial interactions. *Frontiers in Neuroendocrinology.* 2010;31:241–258.

5   Sharif A, Baroncini M, Prevot V. Role of glia in the regulation of gonadotropin-releasing hormone neuronal activity and secretion. *Neuroendocrinology.* 2013; 98:1–15.

6   Schally AV, Arimura A, Kastin AJ, Matsuo H, Baba Y, Redding TW, et al. Gonadotropin-releasing hormone: one polypeptide regulates secretion of luteinizing and follicle-stimulating hormones. *Science.* 1971;173:1036–1038.

7   Amoss M, Burgus R, Blackwell R, Vale W, Fellows R, Guillemin R. Purification, amino acid composition and N-terminus of the hypothalamic luteinizing hormone releasing factor (LRF) of ovine origin. *Biochemical and Biophysical Research Communications.* 1971;44:205–210.

8   Popa GT, Fielding U. A portal circulation from the pituitary to the hypothalamic region. *Journal of Anatomy.* 1930;65: 88–91.

9   Scott Struthers R, Nicholls AJ, Grundy J, Chen T, Jimenez R, Yen SSC, et al. Suppression of gonadotropins and estradiol in premenopausal women by oral administration of the nonapeptide gonadotropin-releasing hormone antagonist Elagolix. *Journal of Clinical Endocrinology & Metabolism.* 2008;94:545–551.

10 Cashman FE, Sheppard R. Clomiphene citrate as a possible cause of psychosis. *Canadian Medical Association Journal.* 1982;126:118.

11 Altmark D, Tomer R, Sigal M. Psychotic episode induced by ovulation-initiating treatment. *Israeli Journal of the Medical Sciences.* 1987;23:1156–1157.

12 Kapfhammer HP, Messer T, Hoff P. Psychotische Erkrankung während einer Behandlung mit clomifen. *Deutsche Medizinische Wochenschrift.* 1990;115: 936–939.

13 Oyffe I, Lerner A, Isaacs G, Harel Y, Sigal M. Clomiphene-induced psychosis. *American Journal of Psychiatry.* 1997;154: 1169–1170.

14 Siedentopf F, Horstkamp B, Stief G, Kentenich H. Clomiphene citrate as a possible cause of a psychotic reaction during infertility treatment. *Human Reproduction.* 1997;12:706–707.

15 Parikh AR, Liskow BI. Manic delirium associated with clomiphene-induced ovulation. *Psychosomatics.* 2007;48: 65–66.

16 Grimm O, Hubrich P. Delusional belief induced by clomiphene treatment. *Progress in Neuro-Psychopharmacology & Biological Psychiatry.* 2008;32:1338–1339.

17 Holka-Pokorska J, Piróg-Balcerzak A, Stefanowicz A. "Mid-stimulation psychosis" in the course of *in vitro* fertilization procedure with the use of clomiphene citrate and bromocriptine – case study. *Psychiatria Polska.* 2014;48: 901–916.

18 Haskell CM, Herrmann C, Marsh GG. Clomiphene-induced neurological dysfunction. *Lancet.* 1977;ii:1227.

19 Legro RS, Lin HM, Demers LM, Lloyd T. Rapid maturation of the reproductive axis during perimenarche independent of

body composition. *Journal of Clinical Endocrinology & Metabolism.* 2000;85: 1021–1025.

20 Zhang K, Pollack S, Ghods A, Dicken C, Isaac B, Adel G, et al. Onset of ovulation after menarche in girls: a longitudinal study. *Journal of Clinical Endocrinology & Metabolism.* 2008;93:1086–1094.

21 Rovner P, Santoro N, Chosich J, Allshouse AA, Keltz J, Neal-Perry GS, et al. Unpublished poster at a meeting of the Endocrine Society in San Diego, March 6, 2015.

22 Chao S. The effect of lactation on ovulation and fertility. *Clinics in Perinatology.* 1987;14:39–50.

23 Howie PW, McNeilly AS, Houston MJ, Cook A, Boyle H. Fertility after childbirth: post-partum ovulation and menstruation in bottle and breast-feeding mothers. *Clinical Endocrinology.* 1982;17:323–332.

24 Bonnar J, Franklin M, Nott PN, McNeilly AS. Effect of breast-feeding on pituitary-ovarian function after childbirth. *British Medical Journal* 1975;ii:82–84.

25 Shaaban MM, Sayed GH, Ghaneimah SA. The recovery of ovarian function during breast-feeding. *Journal of Steroid Biochemistry.* 1987;27:1043–1052.

26 Vestermark V, Hogdall CK, Plenov G, Birch M. Postpartum amenorrhoea and breast-feeding in a Danish sample. *Journal of Biosocial Science* 1994;26:1–7.

27 Perez A. First ovulation after childbirth: the effect of breast-feeding. *American Journal of Obstetrics and Gynecology.* 1972;114:1041–1047.

28 Rasgon N, Altshuler LL, Gudeman D, Burt VK, Tanavoli S, Hendrick V, et al. Medication status and polycystic ovary syndrome in women with bipolar disorder: a preliminary report. *Journal of Clinical Psychiatry.* 2000;61:173–177.

29 O'Donovan C, Kusukakar V, Graves GR, Bird DC. Menstrual abnormalities and polycystic ovary syndrome in women taking valproate for bipolar mood disorder. *Journal of Clinical Psychiatry.* 2002;63: 322–330.

30 Rao CK, Moore CG, Bleecker E, Busse WW, Calhoun W, Castro M, et al. Characteristics of perimenstrual asthma and its relation to asthma severity and control. *Chest.* 2013;143:984–992.

31 Murray RD, New JP, Barber PV, Shalet SM. Gonadotropin-releasing hormone analogues: a novel treatment for premenstrual asthma. *European Respiratory Journal.* 1999;14:966–967.

32 Greene R. Phasic insulin resistance associated with the menstrual cycle. *Metabolism.* 1958;7:90–92.

33 Letterie GS, Fredlund PN. Catamenial insulin reactions treated with a GnRH agonist. *Archives of Internal Medicine.* 1994;154:1868–1870.

34 Brown KG, Darby CW, Ng SH. Cyclical disturbance of diabetic control. *Archives of Disease in Childhood.* 1991;66: 1279–1281.

35 Thibodeau LL, Prioleau GR, Manuelidis EE, Merino MJ, Heafner MD. Cerebral endometriosis. *Journal of Neurosurgery.* 1987;66:609–610.

36 Ichida M, Gomi A, Hiranouchi N, Fujimoto K, Suzuki K, Yoshida M, et al. A case of cerebral endometriosis causing catamenial epilepsy. *Neurology.* 1993;43:2708–2709.

37 Vilos GA, Hollet-Caines J, Abu-Rafea B, Ahmad R, Mazurek MF. Resolution of catamenial epilepsy after Goserelin therapy and oöphorectomy: case report of presumed cerebral endometriosis. *Journal of Minimally Invasive Gynecology.* 2011;18:128–130.

38 Marrotte. Recherches sur la menstruation *Revue Médico-Chirurgicale de Paris.* 1851;9:257–267 and 321–329.

39 Icard S. *La Femme pendant la Période Menstruelle.* Paris: Alcan; 1890.

40 Perfect W. *Cases of Insanity, the Epilepsy etc., Successfully Treated.* London: Rochester; 1789. p. 173–179.

41 Logothetis J, Harner R, Morrell F, Torres F. The role of estrogens in catamenial exacerbation of epilepsy. *Neurology.* 1959;9:352–360.

42 Reddy DS. Neuroendocrine aspects of catamenial epilepsy. *Hormones and Behavior*. 2013;63:254–266.

43 Herzog AG, Fowler KM, Sperling MR, Massaro JM. Distribution of seizures across the menstrual cycle in women with epilepsy. *Epilepsia*. 2014. doi 10.1111/epi.12969.

44 Motta E, Golba A, Ostrowska Z, Steposz A, Huc M, Kotas-Rusnak J, et al. Progesterone therapy in women with epilepsy. *Pharmacological Reports*. 2013;65:89–98.

45 Cagnetti C, Lattanzi S, Foschi N, Provinciali L, Silvestrini M. Seizure course during pregnancy in catamenial epilepsy. *Neurology*. 2014;83:339–344.

46 Everke C. Über ovarielle Epilepsie. *Monatsschrift für Geburtshilfe und Gynäkologie*. 1923;61:256–258.

47 Brière de Boismont A. *De la Menstruation considerée dans les Rapports Physiologiques et Psychologiques*. Paris: Baillière; 1842.

48 Muskens LJJ. *Epilepsie, vergleichende Pathogenese, Erscheinungen, Behandlung*. Berlin: Springer; 1926. p. 203–206.

49 Livingstone S. *The Diagnosis and Treatment of Convulsive Disorders in Children*. Springfield: Thomas; 1954. p. 121.

50 Almqvist R. The rhythm of epileptic attacks and its relationship to the menstrual cycle. *Acta Psychiatrica et Neurologica Scandinavica*. 1955; supplement 105: 1–116.

51 Bassetti CL. In: Kryger MH, editor, *Principles and Practice of Sleep Medicine*. 4th ed. Philadelphia: Elsevier; 2005. p. 279.

52 Pomme P. *Traité des Affections Vaporeuses des Deux Sexes*. 2nd ed. Lyon: Benoît Duplain; 1765. p. 130–132.

53 Fischer F. Epileptoide Schlafzustände. *Archiv für Psychiatrie*. 1878;8:200–202.

54 Lhermitte J, Kyriaco N. Hypersomnie périodique régulièrement rythmée par les règles. *Revue Neurologique*. 1929;36: 715–721.

55 Kaplinski MJ, Schulmann ED. Über die periodische Schlafsucht. *Acta Medica Scandinavica*. 1935;85:107–128.

56 Lhermitte J, Dubois E. Crises d'hypersomnie prolongée par les règles chez une jeune fille. *Revue Neurologique*. 1941;73:608–609.

57 Gran D, Begemann H. Neue Beobachtungen bei einem Fall von Kleine-Levin-Syndrom. *Münchener Medizinische Wochenschrift*. 1973;115:1098–1102.

58 Sachs C, Persson HE, Hagenfeldt K. Menstruation-related periodic hypersomnia: a case study with successful treatment. *Neurology*. 1982;32:1376–1379.

59 Bamford CR. Menstrual-associated sleep disorder. *Sleep*. 1993;16:484–486.

60 Ballet G. Du sommeil pathologique. *Revue de Médecine*. 1882;2:945–947.

61 Lecomte R. *Hypersomnie rhythmée par les règles*. Thèse, Paris; 1944.

62 Rocamora R, Gil-Nagel A, Franch O, Vela-Bueno A. Familial recurrent hypersomnia: two siblings with Kleine-Levin syndrome and menstrual-related hypersomnia. *Journal of Child Neurology*. 2010;25:1408–1410.

63 Kahler H. Zur Kenntnis der Narcolepsie. *Jahrbücher für Psychiatrie*. 1921;41:1–17.

64 Villartay. Aménorrhée: sommeil de soixante-douze heures remplaçant les règles. *Revue de Médecine et de Chirurgie Pratiques*. 1850;21:76–78.

65 Aschner B. Neurosen und Psychosen bei Menstruations-störungen (körperliche Behandlung von Geisteskrankheiten). *Wiener Klinische Wochenschrift*. 1931;44:1132–1135.

66 Stadler H. Zur Frage der Beziehung zwischen periodischen und episodischen Dämmerzustände. *Zentralblatt für die Gesamte Neurologie*. 1938;87:695–696.

67 Möller F. Beitrag zur Lehre von dem im Kindesalter entstehenden Irresein. *Archiv für Psychiatrie*. 1883;13:204–215.

68 Papy JJ, Conte-Devolx B. Syndrome d'hypersomnie périodique. *Revue d'EEG et Neurophysiologie*. 1982;12:54–61.

69 Billard M, Guilleminault C, Dement WC. A menstruation-linked periodic hypersomnia: Kleine-Levin syndrome? *Neurology*. 1975;25:436–443.

70　Kleine W. Periodische Schlafsucht. *Monatsschrift für Psychiatrie.* 1925;57: 285–320.

71　Sugimoto T, Ota T. [A case of periodic hypersomnia: the effect of Tokishakuyakusan]. *No To Hattatsu.* 1991;23:303–305.

72　Roth B. *Narcolepsy and Hypersomnia.* Basel: Karger; 1957. p. 53.

73　Sakurai T, and 20 other authors. Orexins and orexin receptors. *Cell.* 1998;92:573–585.

74　De Lecea L, and 14 other authors. The hypocretins. *Proceedings of the National Academy of Sciences.* 1998;95:322–327.

75　Kanbayashi T, Arij J. [Symptomatic hypersomnia due to orexin deficiency in hypothamic lesions]. *No To Hattatsu.* 2006;38:340–345.

76　Petty R. Studies on headache. In: Brush MG, editor, *Functional Disorders of the Menstrual Cycle.* Hoboken, NJ: Wiley; 1988. p. 211–237.

77　Vetvik KG, MacGregor EA, Lundqvist C, Russell MB. Prevalence of menstrual migraine: a population-based study. *Cephalalgia.* 2014;34:280–288.

78　Somerville B. The role of progesterone in menstrual migraine. *Neurology.* 1971; 21:853–859.

79　Somerville B. The role of estradiol withdrawal in the etiology of menstrual migraine. *Neurology.* 1971;22:355–365.

80　Ranzow E. Über Migränedämmerzustände. *Monatsschrift für Psychiatrie und Neurologie.* 1920;47:98–118.

81　Placzek, Dr. Idiopathische passagere Bewusstseinstrübung. *Berliner Klinische Wochenschrift.* 1900;37:705–707.

82　Wenzel U. Periodische Undämmerungen in der Pubertät. *Archiv für Psychiatrie und Zeitschrift für die Gesamte Neurologie.* 1960;201:133–150.

83　Ulrich M. Beiträge zur Ätiologie und zur klinischen Stellung der Migräne. *Monatsschrift für Psychiatrie und Neurologie.* 1912;31:194 and 195.

84　Waldenström J. Studien über Porphyrie. *Acta Medica Scandinavica.* Supplement 82; 1937.

85　Clark EE, Lawrence HE. Acute porphyria: report of a case. *Journal of Nervous & Mental Disease.* 1948;108:502–506.

86　Hopmann P. Akute intermittierende ovulozyklische Porphyrie und ihre Behandlung. *Deutsche Medizinische Wochenschrift.* 1968;93:76–81.

87　Kelényi G, Arató G, Bude V, Orbán S. Urinary excretion of porphobilinogen in acute porphyria. *Lancet.* 1960;i:434.

88　Wojnarowska F, Greaves MW. Progesterone-induced erythema multiforme. *Journal of the Royal Society of Medicine.* 1985;78:407–408.

89　Bauer CS, Kampitak T, Messieh ML, Kelly KJ, Vadas P. Heterogeneity in presentation and treatment of catamenial anaphylaxis. *Annals of Allergy, Asthma and Immunology.* 2013;111:107–111.

90　Hammerbäck S, Ekholm UB, Bäckström T. Spontaneous anovulation causing disappearance of cyclical symptoms in women with the premenstrual syndrome. *Acta Endocrinologica.* 1991;125:132–137.

91　v. Krafft-Ebing R. *Psychosis Menstrualis: eine Klinisch-forensische Studie.* Stuttgart: Enke; 1902.

92　Jolly P. Menstruation und Psychosen. *Archiv für Psychiatrie und Nervenkrankheiten.* 1914; 55:637–686.

93　Lingjaerde P, Bredland R. Hyperestrogenic cyclic psychosis. *Acta Psychiatrica Neurologica.* 1954;29:355–364.

94　Marcé LV. Manie hystérique intermittente à la suite de sevrage: accès revenant à chaque époque menstruelle, traitement infructueux par les toniques, guérison par la diète lactée. *Gazette des Hôpitaux.* 1856;29:526.

95　Hatotani N, Ishida C, Yura R, Maeda M, Kato Y, Nomura J, et al. Psychophysiological study of atypical psychoses – endocrinological apects of periodic psychoses. *Folia Psychiatrica Neurologica Japonica.* 1962;16:248–292.

96　Okuyama T. A case of premenstrual tension syndrome associated with psychotic episodes – on the endocrinological dynamics. *Seishin Shinkeigaku Zasshi.* 1982;84:939–946.

97 Kimura T, Tomonari H, Waseda Y. A case of atypical psychosis responding favourably to bromocriptine. *Japanese Journal of Clinical Psychiatry*. 1988;17:249–256.

98 Cookson BA. Clinical note on the possible use of clomiphene citrate in recurrent psychosis. *Canadian Psychiatric Association Journal*. 1967;11:271–275.

99 Wollenberg R. Drei Fälle von periodisch auftretender Geistesstörung. *Charité-Annalen*. 1891;16:427–476.

100 Schenck CH, Mandell M, Lewis GM. A case of monthly unipolar psychotic depression. *Comprehensive Psychiatry*. 1992;33:353–356.

101 Friedmann M. Über die primordiale menstruelle Psychose (die menstruale Entwicklungspsychose). *Münchener Medizinische Wochenschrift*. 1894;41:4–7, 27–31, 50–53, and 69–71.

102 Thoma E. Über einen Fall von Menstrualpsychose mit periodischer Struma und Exophthalmus. *Allgemeine Zeitschrift für Psychiatrie und Psychisch-gerichtliche Medicin*. 1895;51:590–601.

103 Pötzl O, Hess L. Zur Pathologie der Menstrualpsychosen. *Jahrbücher für Psychiatrie und Neurologie*. 1915;35: 323–387.

104 Ewald G. Bestrahlungsergebnis bei einer menstruell rezidierenden Psychose. *Monatsschrift für Psychiatrie und Neurologie*. 1922;52:6–21.

105 Ewald G. Fraktionerte Kastration mittels Röntgenstrahlen und Operation bei einer menstruell rezidivierenden Psychose. *Münchener Medizinische Wochenschrift*. 1924;71:336–338.

106 Krafft-Ebing R. Untersuchungen über Irresein zur Zeit der Menstruation. *Archiv für Psychiatrie*. 1878;8:65–107.

107 Mendel E. *Die Manie*. Leipzig & Vienna: Urban & Schwarzenberg; 1881. p. 80–83 and 90–93.

108 Kitayama I, Yamaguchi T, Harada M, Okano T, Nomura J, Hatotani N. Periodic psychoses and hypothalamo-pituitary function. *Mie Medical Journal*. 1984;34:127–138.

109 Hergt. Frauenkrankheiten und Seelenstörung. *Allgemeine Zeitschrift für Psychiatrie und Psychisch-gerichtliche Medicin*. 1871;27:657–672.

110 Martini, Zwei Fälle von Menstruationsstörungen und plötzliche Herstellung der Menses durch psychischen Einfluss. *Allgemeine Zeitschrift für Psychiatrie*. 1872;28:657–659.

111 Werner C. *Die Paranoia*. Stuttgart: Ferdinand Enke; 1891. p. 149–151 and 178–179.

112 Hegar A. Zur Frage der sogenannten Menstrualpsychosen. Ein Beitrag zur Lehre der physiologischen Wellenbewegungen beim Weibe. *Allgemeine Zeitschrift für Psychiatrie und psychisch-gerichtliche Medicin*. 1901;58:357–389.

113 Schönthal. Beiträge zur Kenntnis der in frühem Lebensalter auftretenden Psychosen. *Archiv für Psychiatrie und Nervenkrankheiten*. 1892;23:815–833.

114 Horwitz WA, Harris MM. Study of a case of cyclic psychic disturbances associated with menstruation. *American Journal of Psychiatry*. 1935;92:1403–1412.

115 Horwitz WA, Harris MM. Study of a case of cyclic psychic disturbances associated with menstruation. *Archives of Neurology and Psychiatry*. 1936;35:682–685.

116 Takagi R. Periodic psychoses in preadolescence. *Psychiatria Neurologia Japonica*. 1959;61:1194–1208.

117 Abe K, Ohta M. Recurrent brief episodes with psychotic features in adolescence: periodic psychosis of puberty revisited. *British Journal of Psychiatry*. 1995; 167:507–513.

118 Braun-Scharm H. Personal communication; 2000.

119 Rousseau E. *De la folie à l'époque de la puberté*. Thèse, Paris: 1857.

120 Marro A. La pubertà. *Annali di Freniatria*. 1896;5:322 etc.

121 v. Holbeck. See Icard (1890, reference 39), p. 236, case 202; 1869.

122 Wolter R. *Zur Lehre von den menstrualen Psychosen*. Inaugural-Dissertation; Kiel: 1910.

123 Häffner R. Beziehungen zwischen Menstruation und Nerven- und Geisteskrankheiten auf Grund der Literatur und klinischer Studien. *Zeitschrift für die Gesamte Neurologie und Psychiatrie.* 1912;9:154–223.

124 Enachescu SD, Stanescu M. Reflectii asupra unui caz de manie. *Spitalul.* 1936;56: 388–91.

125 Barbier MV. *De l'influence de la menstruation sur les maladies mentales.* Thèse, Paris; 1848.

126 Kowalewski PJ. Der Menstruationszustand und die Menstruations-psychosen. *St. Petersburg Medizinische Wochenschrift.* 1894;19:216–218, 227–229, 238–241, 247–250, 258–260.

127 Sauvet JJ. Réfléxions sur l'emploi des évacuations sanguines dans le traitement des maladies mentales. *Annales Médico-psychologiques.* 1848;12:157–191.

128 Belhomme. Quoted by Icard (1890, reference 39), p. 127, case 47; 1848.

129 Naumoff FA. Eine eigenartige Psychose im Zusammenhang mit einer Funktionsstörung des endokrinen Systems. *Archiv für Psychiatrie.* 1929;88: 226–233.

130 Hauptmann A. Menstruation und Psyche. *Archiv für Psychiatrie und Nervenkrankheiten.* 1924;71:1–54.

131 Delay J, Corteel A, Boitelle G. Hypoluthéinie rélévée par les biopsies cyto-hormonales dans une psychose du post-partum. *Annales Médico-psychologiques.* 1946;104:183–188.

132 Guiraud P, Boitelle G, Rioualt de la Vigne A. État maniaque périodique, remplaçant les règles: action de la progesterone et de la radiothérapie diencephalique. *Annales Médico-psychologiques.* 1946;104:254–256.

133 Knaus H. Menstruelle Zyclus und Psychosen. *Schweizer Archiv für Neurologie und Psychiatrie.* 1949;64:262–280.

134 Maeda M. Endocrinological studies on the female periodic psychoses. *Psychiatria Neurologia Japonica.* 1960;62:35–56.

135 Danziger L, Kindwall JA, Lewis HR. Periodic relapsing catatonia: simplified diagnosis and treatment. *Diseases of the Nervous System.* 1948;9:330–335.

136 Yamashita I. *Periodic Psychosis of Adolescence.* Sapporo: Hokkaido University Press; 1993.

137 Berthier P. *Les Névroses Menstruelles ou la Menstruation dans ses Rapports avec les Maladies Nerveuses et Mentales.* Paris: Delahaye; 1874.

138 Krömer. Beitrag zur Castrationsfrage. *Zeitschrift für Psychiatrie.* 1896;52:1–74.

139 Wilson AE, Christie T. Puerperal insanity; notes of cases treated by injections of ovarian extract (whole gland) from the Dundee Mental Hospital, Westgreen. *British Medical Journal.* 1925;ii:797–798.

140 Gall FJ. *Sur l'Origine des Qualités Morales et des Facultés Intellectuelles de l'Homme et sur les Conditions de leurs Manifestations.* Paris: Bossange; 1822. p. 398–400.

141 Ehrenwald H. Periodisch rezidivierende Katatonie bei einem Knaben, ein Beitrag zur Pathologie der *dementia praecox.* *Archiv für Psychiatrie und Nervenkrankheiten.* 1926;78:264–280.

142 Pipkorn U. Die Bedeutung des Diencephalons bei impulsiv dranghaften Zuständen von Jugendlichen. *Nervenarzt.* 1947;18:505–511.

143 Hitzig E. Über die nosologische Auffassung und über die Therapie der periodischen Geistesstorungen. *Berliner Klinische Wochenschrift.* 1898;35:34–36 and 52–56.

144 Petersen WF, Reese HH. Psychotic and somatic interrelations. *Journal of the American Medical Association.* 1940;115:1587–1591.

145 Grahmann H. Periodische Ausnahmezustände in der Reifezeit als diencephale Regulationsstörung. *Psychiatrie und Neurologie (Basel).* 1958;135:361–377.

146 Schrijver-Hertzberger S. La périodicité mensuelle dans les psychoses. *Encéphale.* 1936;1:185–196.

147 Schrijver-Hertzberger S. Körperliche Erscheinungen in einem Fall von episodischen Verwirrtheitszuständen.

Zeitschrift für die Gesamte Psychiatrie und Neurologie. 1930;125:388–400.

148 Runge W. Die Generationspsychosen des Weibes. *Archiv für Psychiatrie und Nervenkrankheiten.* 1911;48:545–690.

149 Ewald G. Die Generationspsychosen des Weibes. 1. Menstruation. In: Bumke, O, editor, *Handbuch der Geisteskrankheiten, part III.* Berlin: Springer; 1928. p. 118–121; 1928.

150 Dupouy R. La confusion mentale puerpérale. *Consultation.* 1930;34:29–36.

151 Moll A. Waarneming van kraamvrouwelijke krankzinnigheid (*mania puerperalis*). *Tijdschr voor de Geneeskunde (Gorinchem).* 1822;1:217–224.

152 Dubrisay J. Délire extatique éclatant tout à coup dans le cours de la grossesse à la suite d'une émotion morale. *Annales Médico-psychologiques.* 3rd series. 1858;4:428–430.

153 Ribell. Des folie puerpérales. *Revue Médical de Toulouse.* 1877;11:193–205.

154 Ripping LH. *Die Geistersstörungen der Schwangeren, Wöchnerinnen und Säugenden.* Stüttgart, Enke: 1877.

155 Boullé P. Accidents maniaques chez une accouchée; injections intraveineuses d'eau salée; guérison. *Bullétin de la Société d'Obstétrique de Paris.* 1899;2:63–70.

156 Boutet A. *Contribution clinique à l'étude des troubles mentaux d'origine puerpérale.* Thèse, Paris; 1911.

157 Hoch A, Kirby GH. A clinical study of psychoses characterised by distressed perplexity. *Archives of Neurology and Psychiatry.* 1919;1:415–458.

158 Fumarola A. Disturbi mentali e periodi sessuali della donna. *Annali de Ostetricia e Ginecologia.* 1935;57:269–296.

159 Visscher GRA. *Generatie-psychoses en hersenstam: een katamnestisch onderzoek.* Thesis, Groningen; 1949.

160 Bourson Y. *Contribution à l'étude des psychoses puerpérales.* Thèse, Strasbourg; 1958.

161 Schorer CE. Gestational schizophrenia. *Connecticut Psychiatric Association Journal.* 1972;17, supplement 2:SS 259–263.

162 Moisan M. *Psychoses puerpérales: approche psychodynamique.* Thèse, Nantes; 1982.

163 Lehsau HB. *Die menstruationsähnlichen Blutungen in der Schwangerschaft und ihre Häufigkeit.* Inaugural-Dissertation, Münster; 1948.

164 Goecke H. Über die Häufigkeit menstruationsähnlicher Blutungen in der Schwangerschaft nebst einigen Bemerkungen zu ihrer Genese. *Deutsche Medizinische Wochenschrift.* 1951;76: 763–765.

165 Harville EW, Wilcox AJ, Baird DD, Weinberg CR. Vaginal bleeding in very early pregnancy. *Human Reproduction.* 2003;18:1944–1947.

166 Sato H, Yamane K. Menstruation during pregnancy. *Lancet.* 1971;i:79.

167 Esquirol JED. Folies. In: Panckoucke CLF, editor, *Dictionaire des Sciences Médicales.* Paris: Panckoucke; 1816. p. 192–193.

168 Prichard JC. *A Treatise on Diseases of the Nervous System: Part the First, Comprising Convulsive and Maniacal Affections.* London: Underwood; 1822. p. 203–208.

169 Garcia-Rijo M. *De la folie puerpérale.* Thèse, Paris; 1876.

170 Brockington IF, Kelly A, Hall P, Deakin W. Premenstrual relapse of puerperal psychosis. *Journal of Affective Disorders.* 1988;14:287–292.

171 Bailo P, Poloni A. Psicosi puerperali o puerperalità psicotiche. *Quaderni di Clinica Ostetrica e Ginecologica.* 1963;18: 746–759.

172 Blumberg MA, Billig O. Hormonal influence upon 'puerperal psychosis' and neurotic conditions. *Psychiatric Quarterly.* 1942;16:454–462.

173 Dennerstein L, Judd F, Davies B. Psychosis and the menstrual cycle. *Medical Journal of Australia.* 1983;i:524–526.

174 Pagès P, Coll de Carrera J, Lafon R, Billet B. Psychose puerpérale guérie après 16 mois d'évolution par une thérapeutique endocrinienne après échec de thérapeutiques de chocs. *Montpellier Médical.* 1952 ;41–42:869–871.

175 Danziger L, Kindwall JA. Treatment of periodic relapsing catatonia. *Diseases of the Nervous System.* 1954;15:35–43.

176 Franchini C. Contributo allo studio delle psicosi puerperali. *Sistema Nervoso.* 1955;7:81–101.

177 Martin MGL. *Étude sur la folie puerpérale.* Thèse, Lille; 1880.

178 Herzer G. Beitrag zur Klinik der Puerperalpsychosen (Generationpsychosen). *Allgemeine Zeitschrift für Psychiatrie.* 1906;63:244–274.

179 Rees L. The premenstrual tension syndrome in relation to personality, neurosis, certain psychosomatic disorders and psychotic states. In: Reiss M, editor, *Psychoendocrinology.* New York: Grune & Stratton; 1958. p. 82–95.

180 Marcé LV. *Traité Pratique des Maladies Mentales.* Paris: Baillière; 1862. p. 143–147.

181 Staabs G. Einfluss der Menses auf Psyche und Soma bei Geistesgesunden und Kranken. *Psychiatrische-neurologische Wochenschrift.* 1939;39:387–394 and 401–404.

182 Huang MC, Wang YB, Chan CH. Estrogen-progesterone combination for treatment-refractory post-partum mania. *Psychiatry and Clinical Neurosciences.* 2008;62:126.

183 Burger A. *Beiträge zur Kasuistik des sogenannten menstruellen Irreseins.* Inaugural-Dissertation, Bonn; 1909.

184 Koshikawa N. Neuroendocrinological studies on puerperal psychiatric problems: a possible etiology based on the longitudinal examinations of HPG axis in postpartum mental disorders. *Seishin Shinkeigaku Zasshi.* 1991;93:20–58.

185 Hanse A. Beitrag zur Frage der menstruellen Neurosen und Psychosen. *Archiv für Psychiatrie.* 1924;71:643–661.

186 Bartel M. *Ein Beitrag zur Lehre von menstruellen Irresein.* Inaugural-Dissertation, Berlin; 1887.

187 LeGrande du Saulle H. De l'influence de la grossesse, de l'allaitement et du sevrage sur le développement de la folie. *Annales Médico-psychologiques.* third series. 1857;3: 297–303.

188 Jani. Geschichte, Ursachen und Heilart einer Kindbetterinmelancholie. *Archiv für der Geburtshilfe.* 1790;ii:365–377.

189 Ideler KW. Über die *vesania puerperalis. Annalen des Charité Krankenhaus zu Berlin.* 1851;2:121–182.

190 Karel H. Asthenická šilenost opakující se po každém porodu. *Casopis Lékaru Ceských.* 1888;27:579–580.

191 Delay J, Boitelle G, Corteel A. Les psychoses du postpartum: étude cyto-hormonale. *Semaines d'Hôpitaux de Paris.* 1948;24:2891–2901.

192 Durand VJ, Vaneecloo P, Aurières M. À propos de deux cas de psychoses puerpérales. *Annales Médico-psychologiques.* 1978;136:630–638.

193 Atkinson S, Atkinson T. Puerperal psychosis – a personal experience. *Health Visitor.* 1983;56:17–19.

194 Liégey of Rambervilliers. Un cas dans lequel l'exaltation morbide mentale se manifeste dans l'état de grossesse. *Courrier Médicale.* 1868;18:332.

195 Powers EF. *Beitrag zur Kenntniss der menstrualen Psychosen.* Inaugural-Dissertation, Zürich; 1883.

196 Masieri N. Contributo allo studio della patogenesi delle psicosi puerperali. *Rivista Italiana di Ginecologia.* 1925;4: 163–183.

197 Deuchar N, Brockington IF. Puerperal and menstrual psychoses: the proposal of a unitary etiological hypothesis. *Journal of Psychosomatic Obstetrics and Gynecology.* 1998;19:104–110.

198 Easterbrook CC. An attack of epilepsy (*status epilepticus*) followed within 6 weeks by an attack of chorea, occurring in a patient suffering from acute puerperal insanity. *Journal of Mental Science.* 1900;46:114–121.

199 Römer H Jr. Zur Nosologischen und erbbiologischen Beurteilung der Puerperalpsychosen. *Zeitschrift für die Gesamte Neurologie und Psychiatrie.* 1936;155:555–591.

200 Lovestone S. Periodic psychosis associated with the menstrual cycle and increased

blink rate. *British Journal of Psychiatry.* 1992;161:402–404.

201 Lovestone S. Periodic psychosis associated with menstrual cycle and childbirth. *British Journal of Psychiatry.* 1993;162: 424–425.

202 Balduzzi E. La psychose puerpérale: essai d'interprétation pathogénique. *Encéphale.* 1951;40:11–43.

203 Dupouy R. *Les psychoses puerpérales et les processus d'auto-intoxication.* Thèse, Paris; 1904.

204 Ota Y, Mukai T, Gotoda K. Studies on the relationship between psychotic symptoms and the sexual cycle. *Folia Psychiatrica Neurologica Japonica.* 1954;8:207–217.

205 Abély P. Les névroses et les psychoses du post-abortum: leur importance et leur fréquence. *Annales Médico-psychologiques.* 1956;114:399–408.

206 Constantinesco I, Constantinesco D. Résultats à la suite d'un traitment ovarien. *Bullétin de la Société de Psychiatrie (Bucarest).* 1937;2:64–67.

207 Marcé LV. *Traité de la Folie des Femmes Enceintes, des Nouvelles Accouchées et des Nourrices, et Considérations Médico-légales qui se rattachent à ce Sujet.* Paris: Baillière; 1858.

208 Scott DH. Puerperal mania, beneficial effects of belladonna. *Dublin Medical Journal.* 1838;13:442–446.

209 Tuke JB. Cases illustrative of the insanity of pregnancy, puerperal mania, and insanity of lactation. *Edinburgh Medical Journal.* 1867;12:1083–1101.

210 Krasowska J. Les syndromes psychotiques de la tension prémenstruelle à l'age de la puberté. *Annales Médico-psychologiques.* 1960;118:849–876.

211 Algeri G. Le frenopatie in rapporto alla mestruazione. *Archivio Italiano per le Malattie Nervose.* 1884;21:321–345.

212 Matusch. Der Einfluss des Climacterums auf Entstehung und Form der Geistesstörungen. *Zeitschrift für Psychiatrie.* 1890;46:373–437.

213 Näcke. Die Menstruation und ihr Einflusse bei chronischen Psychosen. *Archiv für Psychiatrie und Nervenkrankheiten.* 1896; 28:169–189.

214 Mall G. Zur Diagnostic und Therapie periodisch rezidivierender Psychosen. *Confinia Neurologica.* 1958;18:171–179.

215 Wakoh T. Endocrinological studies on periodic psychosis. *Mie Medical Journal.* 1959;9:351–396.

216 Nomura J, Hatotani N, Yamaguchi T, Inoue K, Kitayama I, Higashimura T. Periodic psychosis as a chronobiological disorder – endocrine studies and treatments. In: Perris C, Struwe G, Jansson B, editors, *Biological Psychiatry.* North Holland: Elsevier; 1981. p. 1235–1238.

217 Abe K, Ohta M. Recurrent brief episodes with psychotic features in adolescence: periodic psychosis of puberty revisited. *Psychiatry & Clinical Neurosciences.* 1998;52, supplement:S313–S316.

218 Burckhart T. Die Beziehungen zwischen Menstruation und Menstruationsstörungen und manischen, melancholischen sowie verwandten Psychosen. *Psychiatrische-neurologische Wochenschrift.* 1941;43: 23–28, 35–38 and 46–49.

219 v. Krafft-Ebing R. Die Bedeutung der Menstruation für das Zustandekommen geistig unfreier Zustände. *Jahrbücher für Psychiatrie.* 1892;10:233–254.

220 Leone BN, Beluffi M. Psicosi premestruali periodiche e farmaci contraccettivi. *Minerva Medica.* 1967;59:3939–3948.

221 Prengowski P. Zur Frage der sogenannten Menstrualpsychosen. *Psychiatrische-neurologische Wochenschrift.* 1927;27: 571–577.

222 Yamashita I, Nakazawa A, Shinohara S, Ito K, Yoshimura Y, Shoji R. Josei seishin byosha no sei shuki ni tomonau henka ni tsuite. *Clinical Psychiatry.* 1962;4:27–32 and 41–47.

223 Kendell RE, Chalmers JC, Platz C. Epidemiology of puerperal psychoses. *British Journal of Psychiatry.* 1987;150: 662–673.

224 Terp IM, Mortensen PB. Postpartum psychoses: clinical diagnoses and relative risk of admission after parturition. *British Journal of Psychiatry.* 1998;172:521–526.

225 Gerada C, Reveley A. Schizophreniform psychosis associated with the menstrual cycle. *British Journal of Psychiatry.* 1988;152:700–702.

226 Altschule MD, Brem J. Periodic psychosis of puberty. *American Journal of Psychiatry.* 1963;119:1176–1178.

227 Trénel. Délires menstruels périodiques. *Annales de Gynécologie et d'Obstétrique.* 1898;49:224–242.

228 Kramer MS. Menstrual epileptoid psychosis in an adolescent girl. *American Journal of Diseases in Childhood.* 1977;131:316–317.

229 Labbate LA, Shearer G, Waldrep DA. A case of recurrent premenstrual psychosis. *American Journal of Psychiatry.* 1991;148:147.

230 Wehr TA, Sack DA, Rosenthal NE, Cowdry RW. Rapid cycling affective disorder: contributing factors and treatment responses in 51 patients. *American Journal of Psychiatry.* 1988;145:179–184.

231 Leibenluft E. Women with bipolar illness: clinical and research issues. *American Journal of Psychiatry.* 1996;153:163–173.

232 Shivakumar G, Bernstein IH, Suppes T. Are bipolar symptoms affected by the phase of the menstrual cycle? *Journal of Women's Mental Health.* 2008;17:473–478.

233 Alaize P. *Le rôle de la fonction interne de l'ovaire et les essais d'opothérapie ovarienne en pathologie nerveuse et mentale.* Thèse, Montpellier; 1906.

234 Berkley HJ. Transitory alienation following distressing pain. *American Journal of Insanity.* 1900;56:515–521.

235 Yamada N, Fukui M, Ishii K, Shibata H, Okabe H, Ohomiya H, et al. [Adult hypercitrullinaemia with consciousness disturbance and marked hypertransaminasemia after delivery]. *Nihon Shokakibyo Gakkai Zasshi.* 1980;77:1655–1660.

236 Wakutani Y, Nakayasu H, Takeshima T, Mori N, Kobayashi K, Endo F, et al. [A case of late-onset carbamoyl phosphate synthetase I deficiency, presenting periodic psychotic episodes coinciding with menstrual periods]. *Rinsho Shinkeigaku.* 2001;41:780–785.

237 Grody WW, Chang RJ, Panagiotis NM, Matz D, Cederbaum SD. Menstrual cycle and gonadal steroid effects on symptomatic hyperammonaemia of urea-cycle-based and idiopathic aetiologies. *Journal of Inherited and Metabolic Disease.* 1994;17:566–574.

238 Mucha H. Ein Fall von Katatonie im Anschluss an die erste Menstruation. *Neurologische Centralblatt.* 1902;21: 937–938.

239 Stein D, Hanokuglu A, Blank S, Elizur A. Cyclic psychosis associated with the menstrual cycle. *British Journal of Psychiatry.* 1993;163:824–828.

240 Okano T Personal communication, 1995.

241 Endo M, Daiguji M, Asano Y, Yamashita I, Takahashi S. Periodic psychosis recurring in association with menstrual cycle. *Journal of Clinical Psychiatry.* 1977;39: 456–466.

242 Grosch H. Periodische Umdämmerung von vierwöchentlichem Rhythmus in der Pubertät. *Deutsche Zeitschrift für Nervenheilkunde.* 1949;160:105–115.

243 Ghadirian AM, Kamaraju LS. Premenstrual mood changes in affective disorders. *Canadian Medical Association Journal.* 1977;136:1027–1032.

244 Martinius J. Periodic psychosis in adolescence. *Zeitschrift für Kinder-und Jugendpsychiatrie.* 1992;20:121–125.

245 Constant M, Abrams CAL, Chasalow FI. Gonadotropin-associated psychosis in perimenstrual behaviour disorder. *Hormone Research.* 1993;40:141–144.

246 Berlin FS, Bergey GK, Money J. Periodic psychosis of puberty: a case report. *American Journal of Psychiatry.* 1982;139:119–120.

247 Otsuka K, Sakai A, Okudera T, Shibata E, Matoh K, Kawamura S. Oral contraceptive administration prevents relapse of periodic psychosis with hyperprolactinaemia. *Psychiatry & Clinical Neurosciences.* 2007;61:127–128.

248 Andreou C, Syngelakis M, Karavatos A. Metformine for psychosis associated with the menstrual cycle in a patient with polycystic ovary syndrome. *Archives of Women's Mental Health.* 2008;11: 387–388.

249 Morinobu S, Ikiji S, Morioko Y, Totsuka S, Negishi K. Three cases of atypical psychosis appearing in puberty. *Clinical Psychiatry.* 1985;27:1013–1022.

250 Fauré-Amiel P. *Les états psychotiques et névrotiques de la puerpéralité.* Thèse, Toulouse; 1962.

251 Yui K, Ishiguro T. The psychosomatic investigation and treatment of periodic psychosis of puberty. Paper read at the 4th Congress of the International College of Psychosomatic Medicine, Kyoto; 1977.

252 Dazzi P. Le psicosi puerperali. *Rivista di Neuropsichiatria e Scienze Affini.* 1957;3: 1–162.

253 Dauby E. *Quelques considérations sur la menstruation dans ses rapports avec la folie.* Thèse, Paris; 1866.

254 Machado Rodrigues JD, Santos Lapa MG, Brockington IF. Psychotic episode secondary to gonadotropins. *General Hospital Psychiatry.* 2014;36:549e7–549e8.

255 Riecher-Rössler A, Kulkarni J. Estrogens and gonadal function in schizophrenia and related psychoses. In: Neill JC, Kulkarni J, editors, *Biological Basis of Sex Differences in Psychopharmacology.* Berlin & Heidelberg: Springer; 2011.

256 Daly RJ, Kane FJ, Ewing JA. Psychosis associated with the use of a sequential oral contraceptive. *Lancet.* 1967;ii:444–445.

257 Moos RH. The development of the Menstrual Distress Questionnaire. *Psychosomatic Medicine.* 1968;30:853–867.

258 Brockington IF, Meltzer HY. Documenting an episode of psychotic illness: the need for multiple information sources, multiple raters and narrative. *Schizophrenia Bulletin.* 1982;8:485–492.

259 Hu LY, Chen PM. Olanzepine treatment of premenstrual onset psychosis: a case report. *General Hospital Psychiatry.* 2013;35: 452e1–452e3.

260 Santos Cubiña J, Castaing-Lespier PA, Sabaté N, Torres-Martin A, Quiñones-Fernandini VM. Menstrual psychosis: presenting symptom of bipolar disorder not otherwise specified in a 13-years-old Hispanic female. *Bulletino de l'Associatión de Puerto Rico.* 2013;105:53–65.

261 Teja JS. Periodic psychosis of puberty. *Journal of Nervous & Mental Disease.* 1976;162:52–57.

262 Kymissis P, Padrusch B. The use of lithium in cyclical behavioural disorders of adolescence: case report. *Mount Sinai Journal of Medicine.* 1979;46:700–702.

263 Felthous AR, Robinson DB, Conway RW. Prevention of recurrent menstrual psychosis by oral contraceptive. *American Journal of Psychiatry.* 1977;137: 245–246.

264 Von Hagen KO. Mental illness following pregnancy. *California and Western Medicine.* 1943;58:324–327.

265 Schmidt HJ. The use of progesterone in the treatment of post-partum psychosis. *Journal of the American Medical Association.* 1943;121:190–192.

266 Gayral L, Fénier Y. Confusion mentale onirique grave prémenstruelle par hyperfollicullinie. *Toulouse Médical.* July 1951; 618–619.

267 Leetz KL, Rodenhauser P, Wheelock J. Medroxyprogesterone in the treatment of periodic menstrual psychosis. *Journal of Clinical Psychiatry.* 1988;49:372–373.

268 Ambelas A. Cyclic psychosis, menstrual cycle and adolescence. *British Journal of Psychiatry.* 1994;163:709.

269 Abély P. *Introduction à l'Étude de l'Endocrino-Psychiatrie.* Paris: Sedes; 1949. p. 154–158.

270 Fernando MD, Grizzaffi J, Crapanzano KA, Jones GN. Catamenial psychosis in an adolescent girl. *BMJ Case Reports.* 2014. doi 10.1136/bcr-2014-206589.

271 Sadurni MC, Rodie JU, de Montagut LM, Autet MS. The use of oral contraceptives as a prevention of recurrent premenstrual psychosis. *Psychiatry Research.* 2009;170:290–291.

272 Hatotani N, Nishikubo M, Kitayama I. Periodic psychoses in the female and the reproductive process. In Zichella L and Pancheri, P editors, *Psychoneuroendocrinology in Reproduction.* North-Holland: Elsevier; 1979. p. 55–67.

273 Matsunaga H, Sarai M, Taniguchi N, Kagomoto T, Inui M, Kameda H. Gonadal function in young female affective illness associated with the menstrual cycle – in relation to the polycystic ovary syndrome. *Seishin Shinkeigaku Zasshi.* 1992;94:738–758.

274 Murray GR. Note on the treatment of myxoedema by hypodermic injections of an extract of the thyroid gland of a sheep. *British Medical Journal.* 1891;ii: 796–797.

275 Gjessing R. A review of periodic catatonia. *Biological Psychiatry.* 1974;8:23–45.

The Challenge and the Opportunity

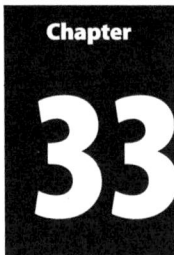

What Is Known

Introduction

What is known is what has been established by the concomitance of evidence from many sources. This knowledge is held at three levels of confidence:

- Provisional: in the literature here reviewed, there are many claims and theories that await replication by other researchers with a different data set.
- Probable: some findings are based on substantial evidence, but with reservations; this is knowledge held 'on the balance of probability'.
- Confirmed: when there is much solid evidence without reservations, one can use the term 'beyond reasonable doubt'.

This brief review of what is known will distinguish between 'provisional', 'probable' and 'confirmed' findings. For probable and confirmed findings, it will consider their present status and acceptance.

What is Known about the Psychoses of Childbearing

Postpartum Psychoses are Heterogeneous

Before the turn of the eighteenth century, this was already obvious: three neuropsychiatric disorders (infective delirium, eclamptic psychoses and parturient delirium) were described before Osiander's[1] *mania lactea* (puerperal mania). The existence of many organic brain diseases, presenting with psychosis in pregnancy, parturition or the puerperium, is beyond doubt – indeed they make up a substantial proportion of the literature. Now that they have almost disappeared from high income nations, this diversity has to some extent been forgotten.

Some may believe that what remains – the non-organic psychoses that complicate about 1/1,000 births throughout the world – are a homogeneous group of 'affective' or bipolar disorders. The present study has found that they are also complex; this is a provisional finding that requires confirmation by other large series followed long term and subjected to a formal, multi-rater diagnostic analysis.

There are Several Distinct Reproductive Triggers

Only early postpartum episodes are frequent enough to be detected by state-of-the-art epidemiological surveys, and some may consider that they are the sum total of 'puerperal psychoses'. The present study has accumulated evidence that these early onset episodes start, beyond reasonable doubt, on day 1 (as known to Esquirol[2]), and, on the balance of probability, during labour (as known to Macdonald[3]); they may even start shortly before the onset of labour.

In addition to the early puerperium group, there is evidence of four other onset groups – post-abortion, prepartum, late postpartum (4th–13th week) and weaning. This evidence was presented in Section 4, Chapters 20 and 21. The conclusion, with the reservations, will be presented here.

Abortion Trigger

- Several surveys and Roldan's cohort study[4] have claimed that post-abortion episodes are more common than postpartum episodes.
- In my series, 14 per cent of abortions were followed by a psychotic episode.
- There is overwhelming evidence of a link between post-abortion episodes and prepartum and postpartum episodes.
- Steinmann's case[5], and three in my series, followed long term, showed a statistical association between episodes and abortions.

The reservation is that few single bipolar/cycloid episodes have been reported in the literature, when compared with the huge number of postpartum episodes. A possible explanation is that abortion, especially miscarriage, is a much less prominent event than the full term birth of a child.

> In line with this explanation, one mother, interviewed 18 years after her 1st episode, described three episodes, which she claimed had followed major stress; one of these occurred when she was forced to make redundant a number of loyal employees; she failed to mention a termination, which I discovered in her medical records.

The high proportion of recurrent to single episodes is consistent with this explanation – post-abortion psychoses are not reported in their own right, but only if they come to light through association with other reproductive episodes.

In conclusion, abortion is on the balance of probability a trigger of bipolar/cycloid episodes. It is possible that this factor operates only in women subject to postpartum episodes. If so, it does not apply to all of them, because three mothers in my series had many abortions without this complication.

Prepartum Trigger

- Authors have described up to 12 prepartum episodes, without details.
- A total of 41 mothers in the literature and 9 in my series had serial prepartum psychosis without any other childbearing episodes, the highest proportion for any time frame.
- In my series, 20 per cent of recurrences of bipolar/cycloid psychoses were prepartum.
- In five cases, studied long term, sporadic episodes were statistically unlikely.
- There are 117 cases of recurrent psychosis with prepartum and other reproductive episodes.

The reservation is that there are already a number of possible reasons for the development of a psychosis during the nine months of pregnancy – sporadic episodes, chronic psychoses relapsing when prophylaxis is stopped, first trimester presentations that started before conception, Runge psychoses and perhaps precocious early postpartum psychoses; in addition, the prepartum episode may be due to stress, for example, the fear that the baby would be removed, as in one mother in my series, who killed her first infant.

The conclusion is that, on the balance of probability, there is, in addition to all these, a trigger of bipolar/cycloid episodes, acting in mid-term and late pregnancy.

4–13 Week Onset Trigger

- In the literature, almost 400 episodes have been reported, a higher rate/trimester than prepartum and post-abortion cases.
- Surveys have found a raised admission rate in the second and third months after childbirth.
- Eight mothers in the literature and four in my series had two 4–13 week onsets.
- Although the distribution of onsets failed to show a bimodal distribution in the bipolar/cycloid group, it did show a steep fall in onset numbers, beginning 14–15 days after the birth.

There are two reservations: first, the onset of a psychosis can seldom be precisely identified, and delayed presentation is an alternative explanation for late onset postpartum psychoses. Secondly, my series had fewer cases than would be expected from a study of the literature, and a low ratio of bipolar/cycloids.

With these *caveats*, the conclusion is that, on the balance of probability, Marcé was right to identify a second form of postpartum bipolar disorder distinct from that beginning shortly after childbirth.

Weaning Trigger

In the literature 32 cases have been described in detail, of which 8 are relatively convincing, and 4 had two or more episodes. With the reservations that most of them were published many years ago, and that I have never seen a case in more than 30 years of practice in this field, weaning is, on the balance of probability, a trigger of bipolar/cycloid episodes.

These four additional triggers are seldom mentioned. They profoundly affect the search for the causes of this group of psychoses.

Many Non-Organic Postpartum Psychoses are Bipolar or Cycloid

The link with manic depression has been established beyond doubt, and includes the prophylactic effect of lithium. The present study has also found evidence that bipolar and cycloid episodes belong to the same rubric: this is provisional, and requires confirmation by state-of-the-art diagnostic studies. If it is confirmed, it will lead to a revision in the nosology of the psychoses, similar to that which occurred when schizo-affective mania was annexed to bipolar disorder.

Non-Organic Postpartum Psychoses Relapse and Recur

Recurrences were first noted in the sixteenth century and are universally recognized; but the complexity of these recurrences, involving a variety of reproductive triggers (indicating links among them), has not been grasped. The risk may be higher in mothers with both reproductive and unrelated episodes.

In addition, a substantial minority (especially of bipolar/cycloid disorders) relapse, sometimes repeatedly; this was noticed by Esquirol[6], is a prominent feature and beyond reasonable doubt, but is seldom mentioned.

Investigations

It is beyond doubt that early onset non-organic postpartum psychoses are more common in first time mothers, and have a genetic component. The genetics may be distinct from that of bipolar disorder – a finding supported by long-term studies. A particular chromosome has provisionally been identified.

The Role of Menstruation

On the balance of probability, there is an association of puerperal and menstrual psychoses, based on 21 well-studied cases.

Table 33.1 summarizes the harvest of 200 years of research (on the next page).

Table 33.1 What is known about the psychoses of childbearing

Area	Confirmed	Probable	Provisional
Nosology	There are many organic psychoses (forgotten)		Non-organic cases are also heterogeneous
	A large minority of non-organic psychoses are bipolar (accepted)		A large minority are cycloid; the bipolar and cycloid cases belong to the same group
Triggers of bipolar episodes	Most begin during the first three weeks after the birth (accepted) This includes day 1 (forgotten)	They may start intrapartum (rarely mentioned) They may occur after abortion (rarely mentioned)	They may begin shortly before parturition The limit is 15 days not three weeks
		They may occur in the second and third trimesters of pregnancy (rarely mentioned)	They may occur periodically in pregnancy, starting in the first month (Runge psychoses)
		They may begin 4–13 weeks after the birth (rarely mentioned)	Childbearing and other triggers of bipolar psychoses are distinct
		They may occur after weaning (forgotten)	
Course	Non-organic psychoses often recur in subsequent pregnancies (accepted)		The risk may be higher in mothers with both reproductive and unrelated episodes
	These recurrences may have all the preceding onsets not just early postpartum onset (rarely mentioned)		
	They often relapse or run a phasic course (rarely mentioned)		These relapses are menstrual
Associations	Early postpartum onset is more common in *primiparae* (accepted)	There is an association with menstrual psychosis (rarely mentioned)	
	There is a genetic component (accepted)		There is a link to chromosome 16p13
Treatment		Lithium is prophylactic (accepted)	

What is Known about Menstrual Psychosis

An Association between Psychosis and the Menstrual Cycle is beyond Doubt

This association is based on more than 100 probable and confirmed cases, and a few surveys. Many psychiatrists seem unaware of this, but how many have studied the evidence?

It is also beyond doubt that the majority are bipolar/cycloid disorders. There may be organic variants.

There are provisionally two triggers within the menstrual cycle – ovulation and the collapse of luteal support before menstrual bleeding.

On the balance of probability, episodes can occur before and at the menarche, during amenorrhoea and after childbirth. The reservation here is that the evidence is from an accumulation of single cases, without the support of surveys or neuro-scientific studies. There is weaker evidence for their occurrence during the early months of pregnancy, after the menopause and in males.

Associations

In addition to its association with childbearing bipolar/cycloid psychoses, menstrual psychosis is provisionally associated with abnormal menstruation and learning disability.

Treatment

On the basis of uncontrolled data from single cases, progesterone, clomiphene and thyroid may be efficacious.

Cause

At the level of hypothesis, the *locus* of interaction between the menstrual process and the bipolar/cycloid diathesis is in the hypothalamus.

Table 33.2 lists the result of 175 years of research.

Table 33.2 What is known about menstrual psychosis

Area	Confirmed	Probable	Provisional
Nosology	Psychoses are associated with the menstrual cycle (widely disbelieved) Most are bipolar (not known)		A few are organic
Triggers			Within the cycle, there are mid-cycle and paramenstrual triggers
		Before and at the menarche (not known)	In early pregnancy
		During amenorrhoea (not known)	After the menopause
		In the postpartum period (rarely mentioned)	In men
Treatment			Progesterone, clomiphene and thyroid are best
Associations		With bipolar/cycloid childbearing psychoses	With abnormal menstruation With learning disability
Cause			Involves the gonadorelin neuronal complex or arcuate nucleus

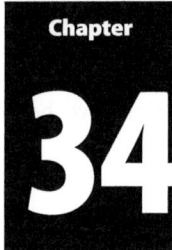

Chapter

34

Obstacles to the Growth of Knowledge

Introduction

During the twentieth century, in which almost every area of medicine made astonishing and revolutionary progress, one can count few advances in the knowledge and treatment of the psychoses of childbearing and menstruation.

On the Psychoses of Childbearing:

- Before the end of the nineteenth century it was known that a substantial proportion of cases were due to infection, eclampsia, chorea, pernicious vomiting or cerebral venous thrombosis. By their control through antibiotics and improved antenatal care, these disorders have almost been eliminated from high income nations.
- Several new but rare organic psychoses have been identified.
- As the organic psychoses diminished, it became clearer that the non-organic psychoses were more common in first-time mothers, although this is a small effect and applies only to those of early postpartum onset.
- The discovery of ECT and neuroleptic medication has reduced the duration of non-organic postpartum psychosis from 6–8 months to as many weeks.
- The development of mother & baby units has improved the treatment milieu for mothers in some countries.
- With a shift in nosological boundaries, the link between non-organic postpartum psychosis and bipolar disorders was perceived, leading to treatment and prevention by lithium.
- There is evidence from genetic studies and the long-term studies reported here that puerperal and other triggers of bipolar/cycloid disorder are distinct.

On the Menstrual Psychoses:

Before 1850, the flair of some French pioneers had spotted the link, and, by 1902, the exemplary thoroughness of some German clinicians established an association between psychosis and the menses; cases had already been observed during amenorrhoea, after childbirth, before and at the menarche and in males. This was a solid base for further studies. Surveys were the next stage, and building up registers for genetic and epidemiological studies. After 1960, treatment trials and neuroendocrinological studies became possible. This has not happened. In 2016, we were still at baseline, approaching the problem anew. As in the early nineteenth century, in the twenty-first century isolated authors are publishing sporadic cases, without having gained anything from the lessons learned about clinical methodology 100 years ago.

Despite widespread neglect, single case studies have contributed some new (provisional) knowledge – the Runge psychoses, several organic causes and treatment with progesterone, clomiphene and thyroid. The anatomical and neurochemical basis of menstruation has been clarified, and hypothalamic cells that may be involved have been located.

The Obstacles

On the Psychoses of Childbearing

The small number of scientific teams worldwide, and of publications, shows that this is an unfavoured area of psychiatric research. For a group of 20 or more distinct disorders, known for many years, it is a sparse literature; in Fürstner's words[7], these psychoses have been *etwas stiefmütterlich behandelt* [treated in a somewhat stepmotherly fashion]. It is not clear why psychiatrists should focus so little attention on psychoses causally linked to events whose physical and psychological effects are complex but well understood and that can be precisely located in time. It is a research opportunity that has been widely neglected.

The kraepelinian classification in use throughout the twentieth century has not helped the identification of cases, and has made it difficult to focus research on the group; this impediment has been consolidated by *DSM-V*.

Nosology (classification) is of primary importance, an essential first stage. All investigations lose their power and cutting edge if the patients studied are heterogeneous, and include more than one distinct entity. 'Puerperal psychosis' is a paradigm for other heterogeneous group of disorders, treated as unitary and distinct. The heterogeneity is two-fold:

- Diagnostic analysis of my series indicated that, in spite of the elimination of many organic cases, the non-organic group is not homogeneous: only about two-thirds are bipolar/cycloid.
- Focusing on the bipolar/cycloid group, there are (on the balance of probability) several reproductive triggers, which may be related, but cannot be assumed to be the same; in addition there is a smaller number of non-reproductive triggers such as steroids, surgery, thyrotoxicosis and bromocriptine.

In my series, eliminating those not bipolar/cycloid, and without early postpartum episodes, would remove 46 per cent of the whole group of childbearing psychoses, leaving just more than half suitable for epidemiological, neuroscientific and genetic investigation.

There is a lack of longitudinal studies. It reflects no credit on psychiatry that, in 200 years of research, the majority of mothers studied in detail and followed for more than 20 years have been collected by one clinician.

The clinical methods employed by some scientists do not match the precision of the investigations. Genetics, epidemiology and neuroendocrinology require expert knowledge and training. But there is also a discipline of clinical observation:

- Because of the error in all psychiatric observations (especially errors of omission), multiple information sources are required[8]. Each modality contributes to the totality of the data.

- Because clinical phenomena rely mainly on ratings, not measurement, multiple raters are necessary; consensus ratings are substantially more reliable than ratings made by single observers[9].

- 'Lifetime' or longitudinal diagnoses, based on several episodes, are preferable to episode diagnoses: they confirm episode diagnoses and provide the background for their interpretation. They also require multiple information sources, especially the study of case records[10]: the psychiatric records provide information on psychopathology and course, and the general practice records contain summaries of most psychiatric admissions and consultations, as well as information on medical, surgical, gynaecological and obstetric events.

- Because psychiatric terminology is in a state of flux, narrative description is preferred to professional jargon[11]. It allows the interpretation of clinical descriptions written years ago, and will be useful as new concepts are introduced.

- Because of the imperfection of the nosology of the psychoses, it is best to employ Kendell's polydiagnostic technique[12], using different definitions of each clinical concept.

It is obvious that the use of structured interviews, rated by inexperienced research workers working alone, whose 'reliability' is borrowed from studies conducted by co-trained experts under special conditions, falls well below these standards. Until epidemiological, neuroscientific and genetic studies are allied to rigorous clinical methods, the postpartum psychoses (and other psychoses) will remain 'a picture puzzle'[13].

On Menstrual Psychoses

The main obstacle is the widespread and obstinate denial of its existence, and ignorance of the substantial knowledge already obtained. Before any systematic studies can be initiated, there is a need to alert psychiatrists to its occurrence, with its unusual therapeutic and research opportunities. Adult and child/adolescent psychiatrists will occasionally encounter periodic psychoses, and those working with learning disability have a particular opportunity. But the best sources will be clinics dealing with bipolar disorder, and mother–infant services receiving referrals of puerperal psychosis.

Many clinicians have failed to achieve the minimal standards of clinical observation required to substantiate the diagnosis, which requires the dating of onsets.

The Neglect of Published Work

A potent reason for the stagnation in the growth of knowledge, common to both groups of disorders, is the neglect of the literature. Even the few publications that have appeared have not been studied. Citation analyses expose the depth and degree of this universal neglect, which has clinical as well as scientific consequences: there are striking examples of poor care because what was long ago discovered is no longer known. This may be part of the culture of academic medicine, which rewards research activity not scholarship. Given the choice between obtaining fresh data, and studying published work, there can be no contest; but this is a false dichotomy – the two activities are complementary, serving the shared aim of increasing knowledge. It is pointless to plan, fund or conduct research without locating the growing point. It is disproportionate to spend years on a field study, and not to spare a few days or weeks comparing the findings with all other relevant studies. It is futile to pour out publications, with the expectation that they will be integrated into the body of knowledge, and not to reciprocate by respecting and studying the work of other clinicians and scientists.

Research Suggestions

The purpose of a review, such as this monograph, is to establish a basis for future research. This chapter will consider these opportunities under the headings of epidemiology, patient panels, the study of acute episodes, long-term studies, genetic and neuroscientific studies, clinical observation and the review of all published cases.

Epidemiology

There are impressive Scandinavian epidemiological surveys, based on hospital diagnoses. In addition, a community survey should be undertaken. With disorders that affect only 1/1,000 births, it would be necessary to screen 100,000 mothers, yielding about 100 puerperal and 10 menstrual psychoses. This would occupy a small team for several years. The second stage, requiring a similar resource, would involve interviewing those identified, studying their records and their lifetime course.

Patient Panels

Other nations should follow the example set by Jackie Benjamin, and forge links between mothers who have suffered from 'puerperal psychoses'. Panels like 'Action on Puerperal Psychosis' (set up in the 1990s) and 'Action on Menstrual Psychosis' (established in 2011) support mothers, and provide a platform for research.

The Study of Acute Episodes

In the postpartum psychoses, there are opportunities for the study of acute episodes, using measurements of sex steroid hormones, and other methods, in collaboration with gynaecologists, to chart the menstrual process. It can be anticipated that a substantial minority of bipolar/cycloid cases will follow a relapsing or phasic course, which can be investigated. The relapse phenomenon (whether menstrual or not) could be used as a research strategy to study the pathogenesis of psychosis. This is similar to the strategy already employed[14,15] using pregnant mothers with a history of puerperal psychosis, who are studied by hormone challenge tests in the early puerperium. A similar opportunity arises when (rarely) women present with frequent menstrual episodes; both these strategies require difficult and expensive case finding. It would be easier to focus on mothers hospitalized with acute postpartum psychoses, knowing that a substantial minority will relapse after a few weeks, and a few will relapse repeatedly.

As for psychoses that start 4–13 weeks (or more) after the birth, it is of interest to know whether their frequency and timing are affected by lactation, and to refute or confirm Marcé's hypothesis about their menstrual status. If mother–infant psychiatrists would date onsets with care, and study the menstrual process by hormonal and other measurements, 10 years of research would show whether or not the menstrual hypothesis survived close scrutiny, and end years of speculation and uncertainty.

Long-Term Studies

In both childbearing and menstrual psychoses there is a need for longitudinal studies. Here there are opportunities for all clinicians who care for mothers referred to specialist services. There are many consultants in Britain, Australia and other countries, appointed early in their careers to work on mother & baby units, who can look forward to 20 years of prospective data collection, and accumulate at least 200 mothers with puerperal psychosis. With forethought they can form an alliance with their patients for long-term follow-up, which will clarify the effect of reproductive events, the menopause, intercurrent medical disorders, surgical intervention and stress. This is work that requires no funding, just a good standard of clinical practice.

Clinical academics, following a large series of mothers long term, with full verbatim descriptions of episodes, and using two-rater consensus diagnoses, could conduct a more detailed exploration of the Matrix of Associations reported on pages 209 and 222.

Menstrual psychosis usually presents in the second decade. There is a need to enrol these young women in a longitudinal study of the effect of pregnancy, childbirth and other events.

Genetic and Neuroscientific Studies

Using registers, sufficient sufferers will in time be collected to conduct molecular genetic studies. Occasional patients with serial relapses or frequent menstrual episodes are suitable for neuroendocrinological studies. In menstrual psychosis, because of the probable involvement of a small area in the hypothalamus, it may be feasible to employ positron emission tomography to study particular ligands.

These investigations require a high standard of clinical assessment. Best would be to recruit mothers followed long term, with multiple episodes and lifetime diagnoses. Because of the error in identifying symptoms, and the subjectivity of judgements about personality and social context, experienced clinicians should be involved in the processing of clinical data. If senior researchers, absorbed in the scramble for funding, cannot afford the time for this, homogeneity can be improved by these exclusions:

- Focus on acute episodes with manic or cycloid features, eliminating depressive or paranoid psychoses, as well as those with evidence of chronic disorders, pre-eclamptic toxaemia or any alternative diagnosis. Cohort studies of bipolar women are essentially the same strategy
- Focus on mothers with early postpartum onsets, eliminating episodes with other reproductive or non-reproductive triggers. Later studies can focus on late postpartum, prepartum, post-abortion and weaning onsets.

Clinical Observation

This is the *incunabula* [cradle] of medicine. It is important for various reasons:

- Clinical classification (which is all we have, at present, in psychiatry) is the essential preliminary to all other studies. It is based on case lore – one's own and that in the literature. Classificatory concepts may be endorsed by expert committees, but are created by the intuition of those working at the clinical coalface.

- The non-organic childbearing psychoses are brain diseases, whose causation should yield to molecular genetics and neuroscientific investigation, but what we know now was established by clinical observation before the end of the nineteenth century.
- There are a number of disorders, which may be important in developing nations, on which the only source is the early nineteenth century literature; millions of Medical Research Council monies spent in high-income nations, would probably not discover a single case.
- As for menstrual psychoses, almost every case is informative. Unaided clinical observation has already (provisionally) found a needle in the haystack – the gonadorelin neuronal network – as the site of interaction between the menstrual process and the bipolar/cycloid diathesis.

The role of the clinician is not just to pigeonhole patients into an official contemporary classification. This may help with management; but medicine also has the responsibility to discover the causes of diseases so that they can be prevented, a task that involves finding aetiological clues. Clinicians should approach those under their care with an enquiring mind, asking, 'What can be learned from this case?' This approach has fallen into neglect, but, in the twenty-first century, still offers opportunities for progress. My 14 years of experience on mother & baby units must be modest compared with that of many consultants, but I have encountered *inter alia* mole pregnancies, menstrual and other associations and some (now rare) parturient psychoses; 97 sufferers from my own series have served as examples in this monograph. A renewed recognition of the value of clinical enquiry in the search for causal clues will give all clinicians an opportunity to contribute.

The Review of All Published Cases

This monograph is largely based on the review of all published cases, irrespective of language or epoch. This is a strategy comparable to the Cochrane reviews, focused on case description rather than treatment trials. The classification of the psychoses is unsatisfactory, and attention to detail may improve it. There is a role here for seasoned practitioners, who have the experience to interpret what they read.

Literature review has its own methodology. The first step is to obtain the original publication, and study the text, especially the methods and results, and any case descriptions; major works often require repeated study and comparison with other reports. Is this enough? Selecting important elements from a mass of detail involves judgement. Judgement is difficult[16], and should benefit from collaboration. The activity is similar to the rating of symptomatology, where studies of co-rating have established the advantage of consensus ratings. A rigorous standard of literature and case review may also require more than one mind. In mother–infant psychiatry, the material exists: I have collected it from all over the world over several decades, and now hold it all in one place, available to study. I hope that other scholars – and there are many with the language skills – will improve on the analysis reported in this monograph.

The study of *all* published cases could be a way forward for psychiatry, applicable to other areas, especially psychoses, with a literature (ancient and modern) in many languages, but limited to a few thousand works. It leads to sharper definitions, improved classification, a radical revision of the problem to be solved, and fresh lines of enquiry.

References

1   Osiander F B (1797) *Neue Denkwürdigkeiten für Ärzte und Geburtshelfer*, Göttingen, Rosenbusch, volume 1, p. 52–89, 90–128.

2   Esquirol J E D (1818) Observations sur l'aliénation mentale à la suite de couches. *Journal Général de Médecine, de Chirurgie et de Pharmacie Françaises et Étrangères* 62: 629–648.

3   Macdonald J (1847) Puerperal insanity. *American Journal of Insanity* 4: 113–163.

4   Roldan F (1994) *Bipolar Disorder of Early Onset: Effect of Pregnancy and Abortion on the Illness*. Masters thesis, Birmingham.

5   Steinmann I (1935) Die Verursachung der Wochenbettpsychosen. *Archiv für Psychiatrie und Nervenkrankheiten* 103: 552–579.

6   Esquirol J E D (1816) Folies. In C L F Panckoucke (editor), *Dictionaire des Sciences Médicales*, Paris, Panckoucke, pages 192–193.

7   Fürstner C (1875) Über Schwangerschafts- und Puerperalpsychosen. *Archiv für Psychiatrie und Nervenkrankheiten* 5: 505–543.

8   Downing A R, Francis A T, Brockington I F (1980) A comparison of information sources in the study of psychotic illness. *British Journal of Psychiatry* 137: 38–44.

9   Brockington I F, Roper A, Meltzer H Y, Altman E, Perry R (1992) Multiple Raters. *International Journal of Methods in Psychiatric Research* 2: 187–190.

10 Brockington I F, Roper A, Edmunds E, Kaufman C, Meltzer H Y (1992) A longitudinal psychopathological schedule. *Psychological Medicine* 22: 1035–1043.

11 Brockington I F, Meltzer H Y (1982) Documenting an episode of psychotic illness: the need for multiple information sources, multiple raters and narrative. *Schizophrenia Bulletin* 8: 485–492.

12 Brockington I F, Kendell R E, Leff J P (1978) Definitions of schizophrenia: concordance and prediction of outcome. *Psychological Medicine* 8: 387–398.

13 Paffenbarger R S (1961) The picture puzzle of the postpartum psychoses. *Journal of Chronic Diseases* 13: 161–173.

14 Wieck A, Kumar R, Hirst A D, Marks M N, Campbell I C, Checkley S A (1991) Increased sensitivity of dopamine receptors and recurrence of puerperal psychosis. *British Medical Journal* 303: 613–616.

15 Meakin C J, Brockington I F, Lynch S E, Jones S R (1995) Dopamine supersensitivity and hormonal status in puerperal psychosis. *British Journal of Psychiatry* 166: 73–79.

16 Hippocrates (5th century BC) Aphorism 1 includes 'η δε κρισις χαλεπη [judgment is difficult]. Aphorisms, book 1. Translated by W H S Jones, 1931. London, Heinemann. p. 98 and 99.

Appendix: The Anne Roper Interview

General Description

This is a medical interview covering family history, relationships with the family of origin, childhood, employment record, marital and sexual relationships, relationships with children, social life and interests, personality, general medical and surgical history, menstrual history, fertility, miscarriages, childbirth, psychiatric history and lifetime psychopathology.

It usually takes 4–5 hours to administer (range 2 hours 30 minutes to 9 hours, mean 5 hours 10 minutes, median 4 hours 40 minutes).

It can be self-administered.

No ratings are made. Interviewers are instructed to record in narrative the answer to probes, and clarifying questions, so that they can be studied by them and others on a later occasion.

Section A Family History of Mental Illness

1a. What was your maiden name?

1b. Please give the following details for each member of your family:

- First name
- Dates of birth (and death)
- Any mental illness

List family members in the following order:

- Mother
- Father
- Any sisters and their children
- Any brothers and their children
- Your own children
- Mother's parents
- Mother's brothers and sisters
- Father's parents
- Father's brothers and sisters

Section B Personal History

2 Relationships with Family of Origin

Give a brief description of the personality ('What sort of a person') of each of the following. Say how close your relationship was with each of them in childhood, and how close it is now. Where do they live now, and how often do you see them?

- Mother
- Father
- Any brothers
- Any sisters

2a. How well did your parents get on together?

2b. How did your parents treat you as a child?

2c. What was the atmosphere of your childhood home?

(If your parents were divorced or widowed, please give details of any step-parents and any associated family members).

(If you were looked after by someone else, apart from your natural parents, please give details of your relationship with them.)

2d. Did your family have any special problems, for example poverty, migration, illness, one parent being away, or dependent relatives?

3 Childhood

3a. Where were you born, and where did you spend your childhood?

3b. What do you remember as particularly good about your childhood?

3c. What were the main problems you faced as a child?

3d. Please give details of any illnesses you had.

3e. Did you suffer from any nervous problems? Give details.

3f. Did you have any learning problems? Give details.

3g. What were your highest educational achievements?

3h. How good were your relationships with your teachers?

3i. How good were your relationships with children of your own age? (How many close friends did you have?)

3j. What were your main recreational interests (games, hobbies)?

3k. Did you get into any difficulties as a child (truancy, trouble with the law, referral to a child guidance clinic)?

4 Employment Record

List all the jobs you have done, giving the approximate dates, and a general comment about each.

Give the reason for any change in occupation.

5 Marital and Sexual Relationships

Give a brief account of your main long-standing relationships, with approximate dates, and any comment you wish to make.

As to your present relationship, describe the personality of your husband (partner), and the quality of your relationship.

5a. What are the main strengths in your relationship?

5b. What are the main sources of friction?

5c. What happens when you disagree?

5d. Has either of you threatened to terminate the relationship?

5e. Are there any sexual problems or difficulties?

6 Relationships with Children

List your children, and give details of:

- Year of birth
- Boy or girl
- First name

- Personality
- Quality of relationship
- Any problems

7 General Comment on Your Home Life

7a. What do you feel most happy or satisfied with, in your home and family life?

7b. What would you most like to change?

7c. What are your main sources of emotional support?

7d. Has there ever been a time when you suffered from a lack of material or emotional support?

8 Social Life and Interests

8a. Friends: list by first name any close friends, giving the duration of the relationship, frequency of meeting and shared interests.

8b. Do you have anyone to whom you can confide private matters?

8c. How much free time do you have each week?

8d. How do you spend it?

8e. Do you feel satisfied with your social life at present? If not, how would you like to develop it?

9 Personality

9a. How would you describe your own personality? What sort of a person are you?

9b. What are your strong points?

9c. What are your main failings (things you would change if you could)?

9d. What do other people think of you?

9e. What sort of a person would you like to be?

Section C The Main Events in Your Life

List them, with dates.

Section D Medical History

If the answer to any of these questions is 'yes', give brief details of the dates, duration of treatment and hospital concerned.

10 General Medical and Surgical History

10a. Was your own birth complicated, for example, by forceps delivery, Caesarean section or foetal distress?

10b. Have you ever had a serious medical illness (for which you required admission to hospital or other medical treatment)?

10c. Have you ever had a surgical operation?

10d. Have you ever had an accident or head injury?

10e. Have you ever had epilepsy or any other disorder of the nervous system?

10f. Have you suffered from any gynaecological illness?

10g. What drugs have you received as treatment for any illness?

11 Menstrual History

11a. What was the date of your menarche (beginning of menstruation)?

11b. Have you suffered from any menstrual abnormalities?

11c. Have you suffered from premenstrual tension? If so, describe the symptoms, timing and duration, any investigations or treatment you received, and any change after the birth of your children.

12 Fertility, Miscarriages and Terminations

12a. Have you ever suffered a spontaneous abortion (miscarriage)? Please give the date and details, especially the duration of the pregnancy.

12b. Have you ever had a termination of pregnancy? Please give the details as for 12a, and the reasons for termination.

12c. Have you ever had difficulty in conceiving, or received treatment for infertility?

12d. Have you ever taken 'the pill' as a contraceptive method? Please give details of the hormone combination, and dates.

13. Childbirth

For each child born, record:

(a) the date of delivery

(b) whether the pregnancy was planned, welcomed or a source of conflict

(c) whether there were any complications during the pregnancy

(d) whether any drugs were prescribed during the pregnancy

(e) the duration of the pregnancy (to the nearest week)

(f) the hospital where delivery took place and (if possible) the name of the obstetrician

(g) the duration of labour, method of delivery and whether there were any complications

(h) whether any drugs were given at or after delivery

(i) the birth weight of your baby (or babies)

(j) any health problems of your baby

(k) details of breast feeding including duration and any drugs taken to suppress lactation

(l) any social problems during or after this pregnancy, for example lack of support, marital friction or other major events

(m) any difficulties in your relationship with your baby, for example, delayed 'bonding'.

Section E Psychiatric History

Please deal with each episode of illness in turn, labelling them 'episode 1', 'episode 2' and so on. Under each episode, give the following details:

14a. The dates of the onset of the illness, recovery, admission to hospital and discharge; the name of the hospital and the consultant in charge.

14b. The context of the illness, i.e. what was happening at the time the illness began, and in the weeks before it. Were you under stress at the time (for example from lack of support, marital friction, problems with other relationships, upsetting events or other burdens, worries or difficulties?

14c. A <u>description</u> of the illness, in the order in which things happened, from the beginning to the end.

Did you have any strange experiences? How often did they occur? How long did they last?

Did you hold any unusual ideas or preoccupations?

What was your emotional state (for example depression, elation, fear)?

If you were depressed, were you also despondent and suicidal?

Did the illness affect your sleep, appetite or energy?

Did you suffer from confusion or memory difficulties?

Did others notice that you were ill? How did they react?

14d. What <u>treatment</u> was given, and what helped you to recover? Did you recover completely? What residual symptoms or disabilites were you left with?

14e. Did you have a pattern of recovery and relapse soon afterwards? Were the relapses related to menstruation? If so give dates.

14f. What do you feel about the way this episode was handled?

15 Effect of Psychiatric Illness on Your Life

15a. Has your experience of postpartum psychiatric illness affected your wish to have further children? Has it led to taking measures to prevent further childbirth?

15b. Has it affected your marriage?

15c. Has it affected other relationships, for example with your family of origin, or children?

15d. Has it had any other effects, for example on your career, or the attitude of friends and others?

List of Symptoms and Behaviours

When you have finished giving an account of each episode, consider this list of symptoms and behaviours sometimes found in psychiatric illness. Use it to remind you of what happened during your illness(es), and add to the account which you have given of each episode, describing the symptom and its onset, frequency and duration.

If you have experienced any of these symptoms at other times (not as part of your illness), give the details.

Self-depreciation and guilt (feeling excessively guilty or unworthy)

Hypochondriasis (feeling excessively concerned about your health, perhaps believing you were ill when you were not)

Grandiosity (believing you or yours were more famous, talented, powerful or special than you are)

Misinterpretation (believing that things were going on which referred to you, for example, newspaper articles, television or radio programmes about you, people talking about you, or setting things up to test you)

Persecution (people trying to harm or injure you) – who, how and why?

Auditory hallucinations ('voices' heard when no one is speaking). What did they say? What explanation did you have at the time?

Visual hallucinations (seeing things which were not there)

Other hallucinations (peculiar or unusual smells or tastes, feeling you were being touched or interfered with, without actual basis)

Experiences of thought-interference (thoughts, impulses or emotions put into your mind, or removed from it, by an outside force, thoughts spoken out loud, echoed, or broadcast to others)

Ideas of influence, possession or control (beliefs that your mind was being controlled or possessed by something outside you)

Incoherent speech (talking in such a way that other people could not understand you)

Depersonalization (feeling completely different from usual, perhaps unreal, dreamy or detached; the world seeming strange, perhaps flat and colourless like a stage set, perhaps more colourful and detailed; feeling that your body or mind was changing in some way)

Self-injury (inflicting damage on yourself in any way)

Suicidal ideas, plans or acts; please describe the build-up, what you intended to do, and what happened; did you take any precautions to prevent people saving you?

Bizarre actions (any strange things you would not normally do)

Depression (feelings of intense sadness, emptiness or misery)

Euphoria (feelings of exceptional happiness)

Anxiety (great fear, panic or agitation)

Phobias (avoiding things because of anxiety, putting restrictions on your life)

Anger (unusual feelings of rage, resentment or vengefulness)

Perplexity (feeling confused, bewildered or puzzled by what was going on around you or inside you)

Cyclothymia (moods going up and down without apparent cause) – something you might experience when you were not ill

Manic behaviour (feeling more active and energetic than usual; overtalkativeness; distractibility so that you don't finish tasks, or what you are saying before going on to something else; requiring less sleep than usual without fatigue; ideas racing through your mind; increase in sexual drive)

Loss of appetite and weight. How much?

Insomnia (including difficulty in falling asleep, frequent awakening and early waking). How many hours sleep did you get, compared with normal? What kept you awake?

Retardation (feeling slowed up, lifeless, moving slowly as if it were an effort to move)

Self-neglect (losing interest in your appearance, losing your standards in home care)

Hysterical conversion symptoms. (This means suffering from paralysis, loss of sensation, blindness, deafness, or loss of memory for which there is no physical cause)

Index